Environmental Health and Nursing Practice

Barbara Sattler, RN, DrPH

Dr. Barbara Sattler is the Director of the Environmental Health Education Center at the University of Maryland School of Nursing where she is an Associate Professor. The Environmental Health Education Center, a multi-disciplinary center in Baltimore, is engaged in training, education, and research related to environmental health. Dr. Sattler is the principle investigator and co-investigator on several projects including a new "Healthy Homes Initiative" funded by the U.S. Department of Housing and Urban Development and an EPA-funded, continuing education initiative with the American Nurses Association. Dr. Sattler is the PI for "Community Outreach" for the EPA Hazardous Substance Research Center at the Johns Hopkins University Department of Geography and Environmental Engineering in which the University of Maryland is a collaborator and she and staff are working with communities concerned about hazardous waste sites. And, Dr. Sattler is the PI on a grant from Health Services Resource Administration within DHHS to create a graduate degree program in environmental health for nurses at the University of Maryland, the first in the country. This program is nested within the Master's Degree in Community/Public Health Nursing.

Dr. Sattler is on the Education Committee of the Children's Environmental Health Network where she has helped to develop a train-the-trainer program for medical and nursing faculty on children's environmental health. During the summer, she organizes a summer institute for school-based nurses on environmental health. She is the manager of a Kellogg-funded project for nursing faculty development on environmental health, a project that spans the 16-state southern region and is also currently funded by the Bauman Foundation to improve knowledge and increase advocacy among health care professionals in the area of safe drinking water. Dr. Sattler's particular areas of interest are community-based environmental health assessments/ interventions, "right to know" issues, and risk communication.

Dr. Sattler's past positions have included Director of the National Center for Hazard Communication, Health and Safety Staff to the United Steelworkers of America, and Director of the Maryland Committee on Occupational Safety and Health (COSH). She is a Registered Nurse with both a Masters and Doctorate in Public Health from the John Hopkins University School of Hygiene and Public Health. She holds joint appointments in the Department of Epidemiology at the University of Maryland School of Medicine and an Adjunct Appointment in the Department of Health Policy and Management at the Johns Hopkins University School of Public Health.

Jane Lipscomb, RN, PhD, FAAN

Dr. Jane Lipscomb is an Associate Professor at the University of Maryland at Baltimore (UMAB) School of Nursing. She has conducted research into the occupational hazards facing health care workers for the past twenty years. She was faculty for a Kellogg funded grant to conduct nursing faculty development in environmental health. She is active within the American Public Health Association leadership. Prior to joining the faculty at UMD, Dr. Lipscomb spent three years as a senior scientist in the Office of the Director of the National Institute for Occupational Safety and Health (NIOSH). At NIOSH, Dr. Lipscomb assisted in the development and implementation of the National Occupational Research Agenda (NORA). Prior to NIOSH, Dr. Lipscomb was an Assistant Professor at the University of California, at San Francisco (UCSF) School of Nursing and Director of their graduate Occupational Health Nursing program. While at UCSF, Dr. Lipscomb received federal research support to develop and implement a model for integrating occupational and environmental content into baccalaureate nursing curricula. Dr. Lipscomb earned a MS in Occupational Health Nursing from the Boston University/Harvard School of Public Health and PhD in Epidemiology from the University of California at Berkeley. Her dissertation examined the Epidemiology of Symptoms Reported by Persons Living Near Hazardous Waste Sites.

Environmental Health and Nursing Practice

Barbara Sattler, RN, DrPH
Jane Lipscomb, RN, PhD, FAAN
Editors

 Springer Publishing Company

Springer Publishing Company, Inc.
536 Broadway
New York, NY 10012-3955

Acquisitions Editor: Ruth Chasek
Production Editor: Janice Stangel
Cover design by Joanne Honigman

03   04   05   /   5   4   3   2

Library of Congress Cataloging-in-Publication Data

Environmental health and nursing / Barbara Sattler, Jane Lipscomb, editors.
    p. ; cm.
    Includes bibliographical references and index.
    ISBN 0-8261-4282-6
      1. Environmental health.   2. Nursing.   3. Industrial nursing.
  I. Sattler, Barbara, DrPH.   II. Lipscomb, Jane.
    [DNLM: 1. Environmental Health.   2. Environmental Exposure.
  3. Nursing Care. WA 30 E638706 2002]
    RA566 .E575 2002
 615.9—dc21   2002017022

Printed in the United States of America by Maple-Vail Book Manufacturing Group

CONTENTS

**Part III Environmental Health Risks in
Specific Populations and Settings**

Part IV Integrating Environmental Health into Nursing Practice

Contributors

Brenda Afzal, RN, MS
Staff
Behavioral/Community Health
   Nursing
University of Maryland

Maria Alvarez Amaya, PhD,
   WHNP-C
Associate Professor of Nursing
School of Nursing, University of
   Texas at El Paso

Sophie Balk, MD
Associate Professor of Pediatrics
Children's Hospital at Montefiore
Albert Einstein College of
   Medicine

Erin Belka
Vista Volunteer, Environmental
   Health Education Center at
   University of Maryland

Pat Bertsche, MPH, RN, COHN-S
Manager, Corporate Occupational
   Health Services
Abbot Laboratories

Charlotte Brody, RN
Executive Director
Health Care Without Harm

Patricia Butterfield, PhD, RN
Associate Professor
Montana State University

Phillip Butterfield, PhD, PE
Assistant Research Professor,
   Center for Biofilm Engineering
   and Department of Civil
   Engineering
Montana State University-
   Bozeman

Jackie Hunt Christensen
Administrative Director
Food and Health Program
Institute for Agricultural and Trade
   Policy

Marian Condon, RN, MS, BA
Research Assistant,
  Environmental Health Education
   Center at University of
   Maryland

Tonya McKee
Vista Volunteer,
Environmental Health
Education Center at University
of Maryland

Kathleen McPhaul, RN, MPH
Doctoral Student, University of
Maryland

Lillian Mood, RN, MPH, FAAN
Director of Risk Communication
and Community Liaison
(retired)
South Carolina Department of
Health and Environmental
Control

Ralph O'Connor, PhD
Assistant Director for Science
Division of Health Education and
Promotion
Agency for Toxic Substances and
Disease Registry

Gary Orr, PE, CPE
Alexandria, VA

**Dorothy Powell, Ed.D., RN,
FAAN**
Associate Dean and Associate
Professor
Allied Health Sciences Pharmacy
and Nursing
Howard University
Washington, D.C.

**Cherryll Ranger, RN, BSN,
GCPH**
Health Education Specialist/Nurse
Health Educator for the Health
Education
Division for Health Education and
Promotion Agency for Toxic
Substances and Disease
Registry

Diann Slade, MSN, RN
Instructor
Allied Health Sciences Pharmacy
and Nursing
Howard University
Washington, D.C.

Karen Sova RN. MS
Silver Spring, MD

Susan Wilburn, RN, MPH
Senior Specialist of Occupational
Safety and Health
American Nurses Associates

Foreword

In the report produced by the Institute of Medicine Committee on Nursing, Health and Environment in 1995, nurses are identified as key resource people on environmental issues affecting human health. The compelling arguments for nurses' involvement in environmental health include the facts that (1) nurses are the largest group of health professionals, (2) nurses are present in every health care setting in every community, and (3) environment is an integral part of nursing's heritage.

Historic nursing figures like Florence Nightingale and Lillian Wald paved the way and set a high standard for nurses to follow as they compiled data, presented persuasive public policy initiatives, and involved themselves fully in affecting all the determinants of health for individuals and communities. It was clear to them, as it is today, that people cannot be healthy unless they have healthy places to live, work, and play.

The publication of *Nursing, Health & Environment* in 1995 sparked the interest of nurses in a dimension of practice that had been undervalued and overlooked. It has been heartening for longtime practitioners and advocates, like the authors of this book, to see the energy and feel the support of a broader range of nurses in addressing environmental factors that affect health. Significant work in preparing faculty in environmental health has been led by the University of Maryland. Practicing nurses and students involved in environmental projects across the country are coming to the forefront. Meaningful work with communities, like the Mississippi Delta project and its environmental curriculum, is getting deserved attention. Nurses are leading the way in making the health care industry more environmentally responsible.

When we are interested and involved, nurses want to be informed practitioners. A number of public surveys indicate that nurses and doctors are the most trusted sources of information on environmental health risks. That is a positive finding in terms of public trust, but it only remains positive if nurses have an accurate understanding and information to share with inquiring patients and the public. Nurses have a long history as advocates for patients and communities, and our advocacy, to be effective, must be based on sound data and current science.

Environmental health is a multidisciplinary enterprise. Engineers, geologists, chemists, toxicologists, and epidemiologists are just some of the willing partners and valuable resources for nurses as we explore environmental health issues. There is a world of scientific environmental literature and experts to draw from for nursing practice. The social scientists have added to the literature their research and guidance on risk communication, community organization, and advocacy. What has been missing is an integration of these rich resources with the science and art of nursing to provide guidance for nurses, especially those just beginning to incorporate environmental concerns into their practice, whatever their setting.

We have been relying on papers, articles, presentations, and a few book chapters from nurses to illustrate the synergy between nursing practice and environmental health. To my knowledge, this book will be the first full book devoted to environmental health in nursing practice. What a welcome addition it is! I can think of no one more highly qualified to bring the information together and make it come alive for nurses than Barbara Sattler and Jane Lipscomb. Barbara has been a true pioneer in bringing environmental content to health professionals and Jane has had a stellar career in occupational health nursing. Both were instrumental in the Institute of Medicine study and have been key players in faculty preparation initiatives. Both have amazing networks of interdisciplinary colleagues and the respect of a host of environmental professionals. Most of all, both have a heart for communities, families, and individuals whose lives are disrupted and forever changed by environmental exposures and a commitment to preventing problems before they occur.

I know that I voice the gratitude of thousands of nurses to the contributors to this book. Thank you for putting meat on the bones of our desire to help, for making new and somewhat intimidating content readable and understandable, and for your living examples of what it can mean to a society to have strong, informed nurses addressing environmental health issues.

Lillian Mood, RN, MPN, FAAN

Introduction

Environmental health comprises those aspects of human health, including quality of life, that are determined by physical, chemical, biological, and social and psychological problems in the environment. It also refers to the theory and practice of assessing, correcting, controlling, and preventing those factors in the environment that can potentially affect adversely the health of present and future generations.

World Health Organization , 1993

As we enter the new millennium, we are aware of the radically different environment in which we live compared to a mere century ago. Tens of thousands of man-made chemicals have been introduced to our environment, which did not exist before the 1940s. These synthetic chemicals can be found in our food, air, soil, and water, and in our workplaces, schools, homes, and communities. Many can be found in our bodies (including breast milk) in measurable amounts. Unfortunately, we have virtually no information regarding the human health effects associated with much of this steady and unnatural stream of chemicals in our lives. Of the 3,000 chemicals that are the high-production industrial chemicals, publicly accessible toxicity data are not available for 71% of them. There is however cause for concern based on existing, although limited, information about the contaminants in our daily environments.

Exposure to chemicals in our environment is one factor which combined with our genetic make-up, diet and smoking habits, exposure to sunlight, radiation, viruses, and other factors, determines our health and illness profile. The relative contribution of environmental and genetic factors to disease expression is the subject of much study and debate. In a recent epidemiologic study of twins, wherein researchers set out to identify the "genes versus environment" determinants of cancer, the environment was found to have the principal role in causing cancer (Lichtenstein et al., 2000).

Environmental health is not new to nursing. Florence Nightingale was a pioneer in the field of environmental health and eloquently promoted the need and value of assessing and controlling environmental causes of disease. Professional nursing is just now rediscovering its strong environmental health roots. In 1997, the American Nurses Association House of Delegates passed a resolution to reduce the production of toxic pollution within the health care sector, thereby contributing to the reduction of the carcinogen load in our environment, as well as other non–cancer-causing toxins (ANA, 1997). In this resolution, nurses committed to educate other nurses about medical waste issues, explore alternatives to polyvinyl chloride (PVC) plastics (which when incinerated cause carcinogenic air pollutants), create mercury-free health care delivery settings, reduce dioxin emissions from hospital waste incinerators, and develop standards for by-products from the use of laser and electrosurgery units. Nurses are gradually becoming environmental health pioneers within the modern health care industry. When provided with the background knowledge that to date has not been part of their traditional training, nurses will be prepared to expand their practice into the critical area of environmental health. The primary goal of this book is to alert nurses to the importance of environmental health to nursing practice. Until now, nurses have had to depend on consumer information and the popular press to educate themselves about environmental health issues. This book was written to complement this knowledge by providing an overview of environmental health principles, specific information on common environmental health hazards, and resources essential to the successful integration of environmental health into practice. To date, little nursing literature on environmental health and nursing practice. Nursing in the 21 century must regain its focus on the control of environmental causes of disease and begin to build this body of knowledge. This will make a critical contribution to prevention strategies that will reduce the chemical load in our food, water, and air and thereby improve human health. Nurses need to develop and ultimately share their expertise in this area of health. They must understand the mechanisms and pathways of exposure to environmental health hazards; basic prevention and control strategies; the interdisciplinary nature of effective interventions; and the role of research, advocacy, and policy. This knowledge must include pollution prevention, product design, engineering controls, purchasing choices, and education.

There are a few nurses who have been active in environmental health issues. Hollie Shaner is an environmental health pioneer and a proud member of the nursing profession. For years, Hollie would painstakingly sort the waste produced by her family into piles of paper, plastic, aluminum, and so on and make sure that it was appropriately recycled or reused. She would leave her environmentally friendly home and go to work as a floor nurse in her Vermont hospital only to throw everything into a red bag— paper, plastic, food waste, Styrofoam cups, batteries, medical equipment, everything. The red bags would then be incinerated. The dissonance between her home and work practices wore on Hollie until she decided that she needed to amend the hospital's ways. A woman of great conviction and friendly persuasion, Hollie was soon able to create a culture of recycle and reuse at her hospital, thus reducing the ecological footprint of her hospital. Paper and plastic are now recycled, food waste is taken off-site where it is composted, and Hollie has written four books for the American Hospital Association waste management. (She is also a founding member of the Nightingale Institute for the Health and Environment, website: www. nihe.org.) Over the years, Hollie has worked with the Health Care Without Harm Campaign and has provided inspiration to many nurses who are trying to reconcile their nursing and environmentalist philosophies and practices.

Another modern day hero is Charlotte Brody, who wrote chapter 5 on advocacy for this book and has been a major creative and leadership force in the Health Care Without Harm Campaign. In her chapter, Charlotte chronicles the efforts and activities of a unique coalition of organizations and individuals who are looking at the environmental health impacts of the health care industry. The coalition is composed of the American Nurses Association and a number of nursing subspecialty organizations including the national organization representing operating room nurses. What is it about contemporary health care delivery that threatens patients, the environmental health of the health care workers, and community members? Health Care Without Harm has helped to answer these questions and has set an agenda to raise awareness and change practices in the health care sector. The mission of Health Care Without Harm is to transform the health care industry so it is no longer a source of environmental harm by eliminating pollution in health care practices without compromising safety or care by: (1) promoting comprehensive pollution prevention practices; (2) supporting the development and use of environmentally safe materials, technology, and products; and (3) educating and informing health care institutions, providers, workers, consumers, and all affected constituencies about the environmental and public health impacts of the health care industry and solutions to its problems. (see website: www.noharm.org)

This book is divided into four parts and concludes with a section on resources. The first part, "The Environment and the Health Care Workplace," discusses environmental and occupational hazards associated with health care. All nurses, regardless of practice and setting, must be informed about the impact the health care industry has on our environment and what nurses can do to minimize harmful effects. Even more critical is the need for nurses to understand the risks they face on the job and to advocate for safe health care workplaces. Part II, "Environmental Health Basics," provides a framework for understanding and describing nursing activities within the context of environmental health. Contained within this framework of risk assessment and risk management are all the elements of environmental health and nursing practice. Within the context of risk assessment, the basic principles of the disciplines of toxicology and epidemiology are presented, as well as a discussion of risk communication. Additionally, common environmental exposures found in water, air, soil, and food are discussed. Part III, "Environmental Health Risks in Specific Populations and Settings," focuses on risks to children, workers, and in schools, along with cross-cultural issues in environmental health. Part IV, "Integrating Environmental Health into Nursing Practice," describes nursing processes such as history taking, education, and advocacy around environmental issues. A description of the environmental and occupational health infrastructure in the US and related health policy is included here to assist nurses in all roles, particularly in the role of community advocate. This book is written as a primer for nurses on environmental health—the first acquisition in a library of books to eventually collect on the subject. In anticipation of this, we have provided a list of resources in the appendix to assist in the pursuit of this area of inquiry and practice.

PART I

The Environment and the Health Care Workplace

CHAPTER 1

Pollutants Produced by the Health Care Industry

Barbara Sattler

As mentioned in the Introduction, the health care industry itself is a source of environmental health hazards. This chapter outlines the major hazardous substances produced as by-products of health care. Much of this chapter was framed by a conference sponsored by Health Care Without Harm held in the fall of 2000, entitled "Setting Healthcare's Environmental Agenda," during which time concept papers were commissioned. The sections below follow closely several of these paper topic areas.

MERCURY POLLUTION AND THE HEALTH CARE INDUSTRY

Mercury is a highly toxic element that is widely used in the health care industry. It is neurotoxic, especially during fetal and early child development, creating a wide array of symptoms including tremors, impaired vision and hearing, insomnia, emotional instability, and attention deficit. Mercury's use in health care settings includes sphygmomanometers, thermometers, and some gastrointestinal device in which the mercury is used to add weight to the tubing so that it will be easily swallowed and dropped into the esophagus and stomach. It is also found ubiquitously in our homes, offices, and health care environments in the ballasts of fluorescent lights, the switches on thermostats, and other products.

When mercury pollution is released into the environment it has a negative impact on wildlife and it accumulates in our lakes and streams. In the lakes and streams, it interacts with microorganisms and organic materials and is transformed to methyl mercury, which is particularly toxic to fish and then to the people who eat the mercury-laden fish. In 2000, the Environmental Protection Agency (EPA) warned pregnant women to limit their fish consumption because of the critical mercury poisoning of our fresh and ocean waters. Forty states have issued advisories for dangerous levels of mercury in fish. Through medical waste incineration, the health care industry is now the fourth largest source of mercury pollution in the environment. Approximately 4–5% of the mercury in waste water is produced by the health care industry. In response, the EPA and the American Hospital Association have signed a Memorandum of Understanding to virtually eliminate mercury from hospitals by 2005.

Recommendations for reducing mercury exposure (Harvey, 2000) include

- Eliminate the purchase of any new mercury-containing equipment
- Hold a mercury roundup
- Provide yearly training on mercury pollution prevention, including spill training and information about labeling mercury-containing products
- Replace all mercury-containing equipment (sphygmomanometers, laboratory and patient thermometers, gastrointestinal equipment)
- Eliminate the use of mercury-containing fixatives and reagents
- Introduce a purchasing procedure that preferentially selects lowest mercury content
- Replace all mercury-containing pressure gauges on mechanical equipment
- Eliminate distribution of mercury thermometers to new parents
- Initiate florescent bulb and battery collection programs
- Support legislation that prohibits the sale of mercury-containing equipment

POLYVINYL CHLORIDE PLASTIC

Polyvinyl chloride (PVC) is a chlorinated plastic polymer used in a wide variety of plastic medical products, accounting for 27% of the hospital-use plastics in the U.S. (Ross, & Schettler, 2000). In 1996, approximately 445 million pounds of PVC plastic were consumed in IV tubing, blood bags, gloves, medical trays, catheters, and testing and diagnostic equipment. There are two key public health issues involving PVC. When it is used in IV tubing and IV bags, the plasticizer added to the PVC to make it flexible can leach into the IV fluids. Once in the IV fluids, this toxic plasticizer (di-2-ethylhexyl phthalate—DEHP) causes direct patient exposure. The greatest exposures can occur during dialysis, extracorporeal membrane oxygenation, exchange transfusion, or repeated blood transfusions in newborns and preterm babies. The National Toxicology Program of the National Institute of Environmental Health Science (2000) has expressed serious concern for the possibility of adverse effects on the developing reproductive tract of male infants exposed to high levels of DEHP from medical procedures such as those used in neonatal intensive care units.

A second point of public health concern is that when PVC is manufactured, and when it is incinerated as a method of final disposal, dioxin and furans are released into the environment. There are limited opportunities for PVC recycling and if it is added to non-PVC plastic for recycling, it can contaminate the process. The EPA has identified municipal and medical waste incineration as the leading source of dioxins and furans in our air pollution. PVC is usually the largest chlorine source in these incinerators.

Dioxins and furans are extremely toxic environmental contaminants. They affect many growth and developmental processes in animals and humans. In animals, dioxin causes cancer in multiple organ systems. Prenatal exposure in rodents causes breast cancer later in life. Human epidemiological studies indicate that it is also carcinogenic in humans. Additionally, it affects reproduction and development. Minute exposures in utero have caused permanent disruption of male sexual development in rodents, including delayed testicular descent, decreased sperm count, and feminized sexual behavior. Small dietary exposures in primates have shown increased risk and severity of endometriosis. In humans, women with endometriosis have higher body levels of dioxin.

Dioxin is toxic to the immune system as well, creating increased susceptibility to infection. Low levels of exposure during pregnancy also alter thyroid hormone levels in mothers and offspring. Through ordinary dietary consumption, the general population carries a current body burden of dioxin that is near or above the levels that cause adverse effects in animal studies. Human breast milk concentrates dioxin and passes it on to the nursing infant at a rate 60 to 100 times greater than average adult exposure. Dioxins are man-made, persistent toxic chemicals that can be found in the body of every human on earth. Health professionals can play a critical role in reducing the earth's load of this unnecessary toxic pollutant. The authors of the PVC white paper, Rossi and Schettler (2000) suggest the following steps to reduce PVC-related environmental health risks:

- Cease all non-essential incineration
- Eliminate the use of IV tubing with DEHP
- Conduct a PVC audit/develop a PVC reduction plan / phase out the use of PVC

- Require vendors to disclose PVC and DEHP content in their products /establish a PVC-free purchasing policy
- Eliminate large sources of chlorine from incinerator waste feed
- Separate out PVC waste and send it to a landfill
- If incineration is used, ensure optimum working conditions to reduce dioxin and furan creation
- Educate staff on the life cycle of hazards of PVC and the toxicity of DEHP

(Adapted from Rossi, M. and Schettler, T. Healthcare's Environmental Agenda, White Paper on PVC, 2000)

There are a few model health care institution programs that are evolving regarding PVC and DEHP elimination. Catholic Healthcare West requires its group purchasing organization to identify products that contain PVC. Kaiser Permanente is phasing out the use of PVC (and latex examination gloves). DEHP-free products are being requested by neonatal intensive care units. Internationally, the Persistent Organic Pollutants (POPS) Treaty negotiations arose over demands to eliminate global releases of persistent and bioaccumulative chemicals. For example, in 1996, the International Experts Meeting on POPS recommended the "virtual elimination from the environment of POPS that meet scientifically-based persistence, bioaccumulative, and toxicity criteria." Dioxins and furans are two of the twelve priority POPS.

WASTE MANAGEMENT

American hospitals generate over 2 million tons of waste each year. In 1998, the EPA and the American Hospital Association signed a Memorandum of Understanding to reduce health care waste by 33% by 2005 and by 10% more by 2010. This is a voluntary initiative that is going to require a concerted effort by the health care industry. Kathy Herwig, the author of the white paper on waste management (2000), has several recommendations for improving hospital waste management.

First, everyone in the institution from the top down must be involved and must share the sponsorship of an environmentally sound and sustainable waste management program in order for it to be successful (Gerwig, 2000). Training and education are critical. Systems must be in place to support the new waste management practices. Suppliers should be alerted to the need for less packaging, recycled materials, and reusable products. Gerwig suggests that we understand our organizational waste stream, for handling and disposal may be dictated by regulations and policies. There is solid waste (trash), but there is also hazardous waste (chemicals, mercury, etc.), and regulated medical waste (biohazardous waste, although this is a very small component). There are recyclables such as paper and cardboard, construction debris, and industrial waste water.

Knowledge of where the waste goes will be important to the development of waste management improvements. Is everything being incinerated or is it being separated and more environmentally soundly disposed of, recycled, composted and so on? Gerwig suggests that goals be set for waste minimization and expectations for everyone's behavior. This would include the expectation that double-sided written materials be used. Construction and demolition waste should be salvaged and reused or recycled, whenever possible. In the reference section of this chapter you will find many helpful websites and guidebooks for environmentally healthy and safe waste management. Nurses at all levels of the hospital hierarchy can play a role in creating a culture of awareness about the environmental impacts of the health care settings and promote the adoption of sound policies and practices.

Participating in the Health Care Without Harm Campaign, which you will learn more about in chapter 5, can provide structure, support, and camaraderie for nurses who are interested in making the health care industry as healthy as possible for everyone. The broad and important campaign goals are as follows:

1. To work with a wide range of constituencies for an ecologically sustainable health care system
2. To eliminate the nonessential incineration of medical waste and promote safe materials use and treatment practices
3. To phase out use of polyvinyl chloride (PVC) and persistent toxic chemicals, and to build momentum for a broader PVC phase-out campaign
4. To phase out the use of mercury in the health care industry
5. To develop health-based standards for medical waste management to recognize and implement the public's right to know about chemical usage in the health care industry
6. To develop just siting and transport guidelines that conform to the principles of environmental justice: "no communities should be poisoned by medical waste treatment and disposal."
7. To develop an effective collaboration and communication structure among campaign allies

Specific web site and other resources are in the Resource Section in the Appendix of this book.

REFERENCES

Eliminating Mercury Use in Hospital Laboratories: A Step toward Zero Discharge: Public Health Reports, July/August 1999 Volume 114 p. 353–358.

Healing the Harm: Eliminating the Pollution from Health Care Practices. Mercury Thermometers and Your Family's Health.

How to Plan and Hold a Mercury Fever Thermometer Exchange Making Medicine Mercury Free.

20 minute video and guidebook Mercury Use in Hospitals and Clinics. Minnesota Office of Environmental Assistance, 520 Lafayette Road N., 2nd Floor, St. Paul, MN 55155; (612) 296-3417; (800) 657-3843.

The case against mercury: Rx for pollution prevention. U.S. Environmental Protection Agency, Region 5, Chicago, IL. 1995.

Medical waste pollution prevention. Keep mercury out of the wastewater stream. U.S. Environmental Protection Agency, Region 5. Chicago, IL.

Mercury. Western Lake Superior Sanitary District. Duluth, MN.

Western Lake Superior Sanitary District Blueprint for Mercury Elimination; 2626 Courtland St. Reduction Project Guidance for Wastewater Duluth, MN 55806-1894 Treatment Plants (38-page book of interest 218-722-3336, beyond wastewater treatment plants, free).

Monroe County, New York, Department of Health (also available in hardcover)

Mercury Work Group Site,

(Massachusetts) Medical, Academic and Scientific Community Organization (MASCO) www.masco.org/mercury.

Massachusetts Water Resources Authority www.mwra.state.ma.us.

The Wisconsin Mercury Sourcebook contains chapters on Hospitals and Clinics, http//www.p2pays.org/ref/04/03851.

A Memorandum of Understanding between USEPA and the American Hospital Association (http://www.epa.gov/glnpo/toxteam/ahamou.htm) commits to seeking virtual elimination of mercury from the hospital waste stream.

European Commission. 2000. Green Paper on Environmental Issues of PVc. Webpage: http://www.europa.eu.int/comm/environment/pvc/index.htm

European Commission. 2000, Five PVC studies:

1. The Influence of PVC on the Quantity and Hazardousness of Flue Gas Residues from Incineration
2. Economic Evaluation of PVC Waste Management
3. The Behavior of PVCs in Landfills
4. Chemical Recycling of Plastics Waste (PVC and Other Resins)
5. Mechanical Recycling of PVC Wastes Webpage: http://www.europa.eu.int/comm/environment/waste/factsen.htm

National Toxicology Program, Center for the Evaluation of Risks to Human Reproduction (CERHR). 2000. CERHR Evaluation of Di (2-ethylhexyl) Phthalate, Intermediate Draft. Webpage: http://ntp-server.niehs.nih.gov/htdocs/liason/ CERHRPhthalatesAnnct.html.

Rossi, M. (2000). Neonatal Exposure to DEHP and Opportunities for Prevention. Falls Church, VA: Health Care Without Harm. Webpage: http://www.noharm.org

Schether, T. 1999. "Do We Have a Right to Higher Standards? C. Everett Koop, MD and an ACSH panel review the toxicity and metabolism of DEHP." Webpage: http://www.noharm.org.

Tickner, Joel, et al. 1999. The Use of Di-2-Ethylhexyl Phthalate in PVC Medical Devices: Exposure, Toxicity, and Alternatives. Lowell: Lowell Center for Sustainable Production, University of Massachusetts Lowell. Webpage: http://www.noharm.org.

University of Massachusetts Lowell, Sustainable Hospitals Project. (2000). "Alternative Products." Webpage: http://www.sustainablehospital.org

US EPA. 2000. Draft Exposure and Human Health Reassessment of 2,3, 7,8-Tetrachlorodibenzo-p-Dioxin (TCDD) and Related Compounds. Webpage: http://www.epa.gov/ncea/pdfs/dioxin/partland2.htm.

American Hospital Association, An Ounce of Prevention: Waste Reduction Strategies for Health Care Facilities [Order number 057-007. To order: call 1(800) AHA-2626].

Kaiser Permanente, Waste Minimization Starter Kit, [To order kit, call Kathy Gerwig (510-267-2624)].

EPA's WasteWise site offers links and information to help reduce solid waste. They have an online fact sheet to hospital waste reduction. http://www.epa.gov/ epaoswer/nonhw/reduce/wstewise/main.htm.

CHAPTER 2

Occupational Health Risks in the Health Care Industry

Jane Lipscomb

Ironically, health care workers, dedicated to promoting health through treatment and care for the sick and injured, all too often face serious risks to their own health in the course of this work. Health care workers now report a rate of work-related injuries greater than that of construction workers, farmers, miners, and manufacturing workers—all highly hazardous occupations (Bureau of Labor Statistics, 1998). Exposure to airborne and bloodborne infectious agents, workplace assault, ergonomic hazards, toxic drugs and other chemicals, radiation, and work stress often due to or exacerbated by inadequate staffing have resulted in increasing rates of injuries over the past two decades. Thus health care workers often struggle to provide quality and compassionate care in an inherently dangerous work environment.

According to Bureau of Labor Statistics (BLS) data, the number of injury and illness cases recorded among health services workers increased 130% between 1983 and 1993, while total employment in the category grew only 46% (BLS, 1995). The number of injuries has remained relatively stable since 1993. By 1988, nursing and personal care workers reported a worker injury and illness rate that eclipsed the rate for workers employed in construction (Fig. 2.1). In 1996, when private sector injury and illness rates decreased 5% to a rate of 7.4 per 100 employees, hospital employers reported an injury and illness rate increase of nearly 10%. The nursing home segment of the health care industry deserves special note in that it has consistently reported injury and illness rates significantly higher than those for the most hazardous industries, as high as 14.2 per 100 as recently as 1998. This rate is more than double the incident rate of 6.7 for the industry as a whole, (BLS, 1998). In 2000, 593,400 Occupational Safety and Health Administration (OSHA) recordable injuries and illnesses were reported among workers employed in health services; 283,400 of these occurred in the hospital setting (www.bls.gov). It should also be noted that *actual* number and rates of injuries and illnesses experienced by health care workers are considerably higher than those reported due in part to significant underreporting of needlestick injuries. It is estimated that 64% to 96% of the 600,000 to 800,000 needlesticks occurring each year in the U.S. go unreported (Henry & Campbell, 1995; Ippolito et al., 1997).

Furthermore, in the health care work environment, workers are not the only ones who suffer when occupational safety and health threats are not adequately identified and addressed. Patient care also deteriorates. A recent National Academy of Sciences, Institute of Medicine study (IOM, 1999)

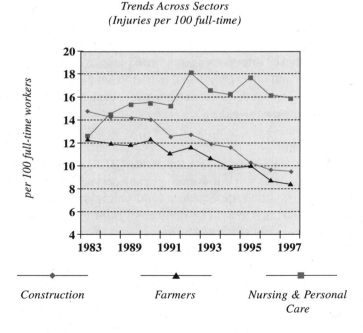

FIGURE 2.1 Work injuries and illnesses per 100 full-time workers in nursing and personal care compared with construction workers and farmers (U.S. Department of Labor, Bureau of Labor Statistics, 1983–1997, Annual Survey of Occupational Injuries and Illness. National Institute for Occupational Safety and Health, 2000).

examined the problem of medical errors and identified work conditions, specifically inadequate staffing, as a risk factor for medical errors. In response to this report, the National Institute for Occupational Safety and Health (NIOSH) and the Agency for Healthcare Research and Quality (AHRQ) have undertaken an initiative to examine the intersection between working conditions for health care workers and quality patient care.

This chapter provides an overview of the leading hazards faced by health care workers and discusses these hazards within the historical, social, and cultural contexts in which health care is performed.

A HISTORICAL CONTEXT

The practice of occupational health and safety in the U.S. dates from the late 19th century, with the first occupational health nurse employed by industry in 1895 (Rogers, 1994). Despite decades of knowledge regarding infection disease risks facing health care workers, concerns about occupational health and safety in the health care industry were totally overshadowed by concerns about patient care and in most cases largely ignored or denied. As recently as the 1950s there was still no consensus regarding the occupational risk of tuberculosis (TB) exposure, in part due to fears that young women would avoid nursing if they knew the risks involved and that liability issues might surface. It was not until TB declined significantly in the general population, while remaining elevated among medical workers, that TB was fully recognized as an occupational hazard (Sepkowitz, 1994).

It was not until the 1980s and the documentation of occupationally transmitted HIV infections that the risks facing health care workers were finally acknowledged by the industry, the government, and the public at large. This was despite the fact that up until this time approximately 200 health care workers were dying from hepatitis B infections each year— many more deaths than have ever officially been associated with occupationally transmitted HIV (Shapiro, 1995). So why has it taken so long for health care workers to attract the concern afforded other workers? Possible explanations include the following (Lipscomb & Borwegen, 2000; Lipscomb & Rosenstock, 1996):

• *A false perception that the industry is self-regulated.* Nurses and other health care professionals are all too familiar with the Joint Commission on the Accreditation of Health Care Organizations (JCAHO) that conducts preannounced inspections of most hospitals every three years.

JCAHO accreditation is primarily directed at assessing the quality of patient services and therefore little attention is directed at workplace exposures and hazards during inspections.

- *An industry that employs mainly females must be a safe industry.* Seventy-six percent of all hospital workers, 83% of nursing home workers, and 93% of home care workers are female. Among the nursing work force, close to 95% of registered nurses are female.

- *A focus on curative rather than preventive medicine.* Health care expenditures are primarily dedicated to curative medicine rather than to preventive medicine and public health, which includes occupational health and safety. We need only examine the data on the cost of end of life care to vividly demonstrate this point.

- *A low unionization rate within the health care sector.* Today, only 13.5% of hospital workers, the most unionized segment of the health care industry, are covered by a collective bargaining agreement. As a consequence, compared with workers in more heavily unionized industries, health care workers have little voice and power to effectively negotiate for and improve workplace health and safety conditions.

- *The lack of attention by governmental agencies responsible for health and safety.* Little research has been conducted and few governmental standards have been issued for the hazards causing most injuries to health care workers. It was not until 1991 and the passage of OSHA's blood-borne pathogen standard that health care workers finally received protection from exposure to hepatitis B via mandatory, employer provided, hepatitis B vaccine. Even more appalling is the fact that it has taken health care workers an additional decade to win enhanced protection against other deadly infections, namely hepatitis C, by passage of the Needlestick Safety and Prevention Act signed into law early in 2001.

CHARACTERISTICS OF THE WORK FORCE AND WORK SETTING

The health care sector employs over 12 million health care workers, having grown by three million workers between 1980 and 1997. Nurses and aides comprise almost 38% of this work force (4,390,000 individuals; NIOSH, 2002). BLS projections for the 10 fastest growing occupations from 1996 to 2006 include six health-related occupations: personal and home care aides, physical and corrective therapy aides, home health aides, medical assistants, physical therapists and occupational therapists, all projected to increase by 70% to 85% during this period (BLS, 1997). As is reflected in these projections, health care workers are increasingly being employed outside the acute care or hospital setting. The majority of RNs still work in hospitals (60%), but an increasing proportion work in community/public health settings (17%), in ambulatory care settings (9%), and in nursing homes (8%). For the purpose of this discussion, the term *health care workers* includes both health care professionals and support staff members working in hospitals, outpatient clinics, nursing homes, home health care settings, medical laboratories, dental offices, and veterinary settings.

Patient care, although the primary source of injuries and illnesses to nursing staff, is not the only activity that impacts health care workers' health and safety. All patient care and treatment areas, sterilization areas, pharmacies, support laboratories, housekeeping, maintenance, and waste disposal areas include exposures and activities that may pose health and safety hazards to workers. In addition, the generation and disposal of biologic, chemical, and radiological wastes pose risks to the communities surrounding health care facilities and beyond, in particular if these facilities incinerate their waste on-site. The widespread use and resulting incineration of plastics containing chlorine compounds, such as polyvinyl chlorine (PVC)-containing products, have the potential to create and release into the atmosphere dioxins, among the most toxic substances known.

HAZARDS OF HEALTH CARE WORK

Health care organizations consist of many separate industries all housed within the walls of the facility. Hazards range from the biologically associated, with airborne and bloodborne exposures to infectious agents, to industrial strength disinfectants and cleaning compounds in use throughout the facility. Hazards associated with food preparation and waste disposal are also present in health care. In addition, chemical hazards include waste anesthetic and sterilant gases, antineoplastic drugs, and other therapeutic agents. Physical hazards include exposure to ionizing and non-ionizing radiation, safety and ergonomic hazards, violent assaults, and psychosocial and organizational factors, including psychological stress and shiftwork (Table 2.1).

MUSCULOSKELETAL INJURIES

Musculoskeletal injuries rank second among all work-related injuries, with the greatest number occurring among health care workers. Exposures include the requirement to lift, pull, slide, turn, and transfer patients; move

TABLE 2.1 Selected Hazards, Health Effects and Control Strategies in Health Care

Biological Hazards	Health Effects	Control Strategies
• Viral (hepatitis B virus, hepatitis C virus)	Acute febrile illness, liver disease, death	Safer needle devices, hepatitis B vaccine
• Bacteria (mycobacterium tuberculosis)	Tuberculosis (TB) infection, TB illness, multiple drug resistance, death	Isolation of suspect patients, respirators, ulttraviolat (UV) light, negative pressure rooms
• Natural rubber latex proteins (and rubber chemical additives)	Range from Type IV delayed hypersensitivity to rubber additives to Type 1 immunologic response, anaphylactic shock, death	Substitution with low latex protein powderless gloves or nonlatex gloves and supplies
Chemical Hazards		
• Ethylene oxide	Peripheral neuropathy, cancer, reproductive effects	Substitution, enclosed systems, aeration rooms
• Formaldehyde	Allergy, nasal cancer	Substitution, local ventilation
• Glutaraidehyde	Mucous membrane irritation, sensitization, reproductive effects	Substitution, local ventilation
• Antineoplastic drugs	Cancer, mutagenicity, reproductive effects	Class 1 ventilation hoods, isolation of patient excreta
• Waste anesthetic gases	Hepatic toxicity, neurologic effects, reproductive effects	Scavenging systems, isolation of off-gassing patients
• Mercury	Neurologic effects, birth defects	Substitution with electronic thermometers
Physical Hazards		
• Patient handling	Back pain, injury	Patient handling devices, lifting teams, training
• Static postures	Musculoskeletal pain and injury	Rest breaks, exercise, support hose and shoes
• Ionizing radiation	Cancer, reproductive effects	Isolation of patients, shielding and maintenance of equipment

TABLE 2.1 (continued)

• Lasers	Eye and skin burns, inhalation of toxic chemicals and pathogens, fires	Local exhaust ventilation, equipment maintenance, respirators and face shields
• Physical assault	Traumatic injuries, death	Alarm systems, security personnel, training
Psychosocial/Organizational		
• Violence threat and physical assault	Traumatic injury, death, posttraumatic stress disorder	Training, postassault debriefing
• Restructuring	Mental health disorders, exacerbation of musculoskeletal injuries, traumatic injuries, burnout	Acuity-based staffing, employee involvement in restructuring activities
• Work stress (other than above)	Mental health disorders, burnout	Stress prevention and management programs
• Shiftwork	Gastrointestinal disorders, sleep disorders	Forward, stable and predictable shift rotation

equipment; and stand for long hours. Among all occupations, hospital and nursing home workers experience the highest number of occupational injuries and illnesses involving lost workdays due to back injuries. Nurses' aides report a greater percentage of their injuries as back injuries than any other occupations. A three-year review of BLS annual survey data indicates that "nursing personal care facilities" have an occupational musculoskeletal injury and illness rate of 4.62 per 100 workers per year—the highest among all three-digit Standardized Industrial Classification (SIC) codes (BLS, 1997).

Back injuries continue to take a huge economic and personal toll within the health care sector. The nursing home industry alone spends over $1 billion each year in workers' compensation premiums, even though the implementation of engineering and administrative controls such as safe staffing levels, lifting teams, and use of newer mechanical patient handling devices have been shown to reduce dramatically both injury rates and workers' compensation premiums in nursing homes.

One study of a large nursing home found that nursing assistants working in a nursing home experienced four episodes of low back pain on average in a three-year period, but that assistive devices (a mechanical lift and transfer belt) were used for less than 2% of all transfers. Patient safety and comfort, lack of accessibility, physical stresses associated with the devices, lack of skill, increased transfer time, and lack of staffing were some of the reasons cited for not using these devices. Ironically, when patients and residents were surveyed, it was found that they actually preferred mechanical lifts and stated that mechanical lifts made them feel more secure (Garg & Owen, 1992).

The use of lifting teams in hospitals or other health care settings has also been shown to be a cost effective control strategy. In one large acute care public hospital in Northern California, annual lost-time injuries decreased from 16 to 1 following one-year deployment of a lifting team with a savings of $144,000 (Charney, 1994).

In November 2000, OSHA promulgated a final Ergonomics Program Standard. Ten years in the making, this standard was considered to be the most important worker safety action developed in the agency's history. Most provisions of the standard were to have been in place by October 2001. At a minimum, the standard required employers to provide basic information to their employees about musculoskeletal disorders (MSDs). In the event that an MSD incident is reported in the workplace, the standard required the employer to do a job hazard analysis to determine whether MSD hazards are present in a job. If a hazard is present on the job, the employer would be required to reduce the MSD hazard to the extent feasible. In the case of health care workers this may include the use of assistant lifting devices or lifting teams. Tragically for U.S. workers, within months of his inauguation President Bush (and the Republican-controlled Congress) passed legislation overturning the ergonomics standard. Workers have suffered over two million ergonomic injuries since this action (aflcio.org 2002).

WORKPLACE VIOLENCE

The health care sector also has the dubious distinction of leading all other industry sectors in incidence of nonfatal workplace assaults. In 1999, 43% of all nonfatal assaults against workers resulting in lost workdays in the U.S. occurred in the health care sector. Among all nonfatal workplace assaults resulting in lost workdays occurring in health services occupations, nursing aides and orderlies suffer the highest proportion—61% compared to 3% for police and guards. In 1999, BLS reported a rate of 14 per 100 full time equivalents (FTEs) and 9 per 100 FTEs for social services and health services, respectively. By comparison the national average was 1.8 nonfatal assaults per 100 workers. (BLS, 1999). Among these assault victims, 30% were government employees, even though they comprise only 18% of the work force. Across all industries, in 45% of reported cases of nonfatal workplace assault, the perpetrator of the assault is a health care patient. In contrast, only 8% of these injuries are perpetrated by a coworker; yet media and employer attention is disproportionately directed to coworker violence (BLS, 1996).

In mental health the risk is particularly high. In a Washington psychiatric facility, 73% of staff surveyed had reported at least a minor injury related to an assault by a patient during the past year. Only 43% of those reporting moderate, severe, or disabling injuries related to such assaults had filed for workers' compensation. When workers were directly surveyed regarding their assault experiences in the past year, they reported 437 per 100 employees, while the hospital incident reports and workers' compensation claims indicated a rate of only 35 per 100 and 13.8 per 100 employees respectively (Bensley et al., 1997). These data provide a dramatic example of the magnitude of the problem of underreporting of occupational injuries and illnesses. They also demonstrate that in this industry, workers' compensation is an underutilized remedy for work-related injuries.

Emergency department personnel face a significant risk of fatal injuries from assaults by patients or their families. Weapon carrying in emergency departments, reported to be as high as 25% in major urban hospitals, creates the opportunity for severe or fatal injuries when they occur (Wassenberger, Ordog, Kolodny, & Allen, 1989). Although mental health and emergency departments have been the focus of attention and research on the subject, no department within a health care setting is immune to workplace violence. Consequently, all departments should have violence prevention programs.

A number of environmental risk factors have been associated with assaults by patients regardless of health care setting, including poor security, inadequate staffing patterns, time of high activity, and containment activities. Inadequate training and a lack of clear policies and procedures have also been identified as contributing to the incidence of assaults (Lipscomb & Love, 1992).

In 1996, OSHA issued *Guidelines for Preventing Workplace Violence for Health Care and Social Service Workers*. These guidelines provide direction on how to establish a comprehensive safety and health program directed at violence prevention and include the following five elements: visible, high level *management commitment* to violence prevention; meaningful *employee involvement* in policy development, joint management and worker violence prevention committees, and overall program implementation; *work site analysis* that includes regular walkthrough surveys of all patient care areas and the collection and review of all reports of worker assault; *hazard prevention and control* that includes alarm systems and other security measures; and *training and education.*

NEEDLESTICK INJURIES

Exposure to conventional unsafe needles that transmit bloodborne infections to health care workers continues to be the most life-threatening risk facing health care workers in a wide variety of settings (Lipscomb & Borwegen, 2000). Fortunately, data exist demonstrating that the elimination of unnecessary sharps and the use of safer needles can dramatically reduce needlestick injuries (Centers for Disease Control, 1997a). The recent passage of the federal Needlestick Safety and Prevention Act, effective April 2001, should afford all health care workers protection from this unnecessary and deadly hazard. Not only does the Act require that safer needles be made available, but that employees, namely nurses, be involved in identifying and choosing the device. Therefore, it is critical that nurses understand some basic distinctions among available devices.

Safer needle devices have integrated safety features built into the product that prevent needlestick injuries. The term "safer needle device" is broad and includes many different devices, from those that have a protective shield over the needle to those that do not use needles at all. Needles with integrated safety features are categorized as "passive" or "active." Passive devices offer the greatest protection as the safety feature is automatically triggered following use, without the need for the health care worker to take any additional steps. An example of a "passive" device is a spring-loaded retractable syringe or self-blunting blood collection device (Figure 2.2). An example of an "active" safety mechanism is an employee-activated self-sheathing needle.

As of 1998, the FDA had approved over 250 safer needle-bearing products. In 1997, the CDC reported on an eight-hospital study that demonstrated that during such high risk procedures as drawing blood, needlesticks could be reduced up to 76% with the use of safer needles (CDC, 1997a). Yet in 1998, fewer than 10% of the needles purchased by health care

Examples of "Active" and "Passive" Safety Devices

cample of an "active" safety mechanism, requiring the healthcare worker to pull the sheath over the needle after use.

Before use

After use

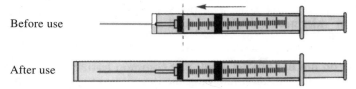

Thi is an example of a "passive" safety mechanism, where the needle retracts automatically into the barrel when the plunger is depressed after use..

Before use

After use

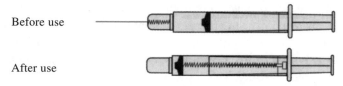

FIGURE 2.2 Examples of "Active" and "Passive" Safety Devices. From SEIU's *Guide to Preventing Needlestick Injuries*, Service Employees International Union, 1998

employers had these integrated safety features. The health care industry's reluctance to embrace safer devices to date has resulted in the needless injury, illness, and death of additional health care workers. It is for this reason that health care workers have fought hard for the passage of the Needlestick Safety and Prevention Act. It is hoped that the force of this law will dramatically advance the use of safer devices. Unfortunately, any government regulation is only as effective as the enforcement capability of the agency responsible for its implementation. Federal OSHA and OSHA approved state programs conducted approximately 90,000 annual inspections in both 1997 and 1998, focusing inspection on the most hazardous industries (Ashford, 2000). At its current enforcement capacity, it could take inspectors more than 50 years to inspect all five million workplaces covered by the OSH Act. Recognizing that at the present time needlestick injuries continue to sicken and disable health care workers, a review of the risk of acquiring various infections follows.

After a needlestick injury, the risk of developing occupationally acquired hepatitis B in the nonimmune health care worker ranges from 2% to 40% depending on the hepatitis B e-antigen status of the source patient (Gerberding, 1995). The risk of transmission from a positive source for hepatitis C is between 3% and 10% (Gerberding) and the average risk of transmission of HIV is 0.3% (CDC, 1991). However, the risk of transmission increases if the injury is caused by a device visibly contaminated with blood, if the device is used to puncture the vascular system, or if the stick causes a deep injury. All of these diseases are associated with significant morbidity and mortality and only the hepatitis B virus can be prevented by vaccine. Tragically, all health care workers, laundry workers, and housekeeping workers are all too often engaged in duties that create an environment for these high-risk needlestick injuries.

The above data figures translate into the estimate that each year more than 1,000 health care workers will contract a serious infection, such as hepatitis B or C virus or HIV, from an occupational needlestick injury. The majority will become infected due to the growing spread of hepatitis C, which infects 560 to 1,120 health care workers in the U.S. each year (Gibas, Blewett, Schoenfeld, & Dienstag, 1992), with 85% becoming chronic carriers. One health care worker per week will eventually die from occupational exposures to HIV occurring today (Ippolito et al., 1997). Some groups of workers, such as phlebotomists, experience a particularly high risk of needlesticks and subsequent infections. According to a 1994 survey of this group of workers, 24% of health care workers who drew blood were stuck by a needle in the previous year.

LATEX ALLERGY

Despite the success of the 1991 Bloodborne Pathogen Standard in preventing occupationally acquired hepatitis B infections, the increased use of exam and surgical gloves required by this standard is in part responsible for the epidemic of latex allergy now affecting health care workers. In 1997, NIOSH issued guidelines for preventing allergic reactions to natural rubber latex in the workplace, including recommending the use of powderless, low-protein latex gloves for protection from bloodborne pathogens in health care and other settings (www.cdc.gov/niosh). The publication of this guidance along with health care professional advocacy for latex-free environments appears to be having an impact. NIOSH is currently evaluating the effectiveness of these recommendations in a series of clinical intervention trials (see chapter 3).

CHEMICAL HAZARDS

Health care workers are exposed to a wide range of chemical disinfectants, anesthetic waste gases, and chemotherapeutic drugs that are known to affect human health, and others for which no or inadequate testing has been conducted. NIOSH estimates that the average hospital contains 300 chemicals—twice the number of the average manufacturing facility. Among disinfectants, formaldehyde is a carcinogen and has been linked to occupational asthma in the hospital setting. Glutaraldehyde is used as a cold sterilizer and disinfectant to clean and disinfect heat-sensitive equipment. It is also used as a tissue fixative in the history and pathology labs and as a hardening agent in the development of x-rays. Mucous membrane irritation, headaches, allergic contact dermatitis, asthma and asthma-like symptoms, hives, and nausea have been reported among hospital workers exposed to glutaraldehyde. Ethylene oxide (ETO), a gas sterilant, is a neurotoxin, a carcinogen, and a reproductive health hazard. Thousands of health care workers were exposed to harmful levels of ETO prior to the 1984 OSHA standard for ETO. This chemical continues to be of concern to central supply hospital workers due to leaks from distribution lines, especially when changing gas cylinders.

Anesthetic agents, used in large amounts in hospitals, pose a threat to health care workers when operating room scavenging systems are poorly maintained. Health care workers are also exposed when patients are transferred to the recovery room and exhale anesthesia gases. Specially designed nonrecirculating general ventilation systems with adequate room air exchanges are necessary in these areas.

Antineoplastic agents, frequently administered in both inpatient and outpatient services, manifest their cytotoxic effects among workers who handle and administer them. Health effects associated with handling antineoplastics include the acute effects of the drugs themselves, such as nausea, fatigue, reproductive effects, and cancer. Safe handling guidelines were published in the mid-1980s by the National Institutes of Health, and later by OSHA, to control dermal and inhalation exposure associated with the mixing and administration of these drugs. The use of gloves composed of the proper material is critical, as most of these substances easily penetrate regular latex gloves. Aerosolized medications pose unique threats because of how they are administered. Included among them is ribavirin, a potential human teratogen.

ORGANIZATION OF WORK

Organization of work refers to management and supervisory practices as well as production processes and their influence on the way work is performed (National Occupational Research Agenda NORA, 2002). The way work is organized and scheduled and how staffing decisions are made are thought to have a significant impact on worker injury and illness rates. The U.S. health care industry has been in a constant state of change over the past decade, including organizational mergers; downsizing; changes in employment arrangements such as contract work, job restructuring, and redesign; and worker–management relations. Undoubtedly the emergence of managed care and its cost containment priority has prompted or contributed to many of these changes.

The widespread concern about the adequacy of nursing staffing levels across a variety of health care organizations is directly related to the issue of organization of work. Between 1981 and 1993, total hospital employment grew steadily, but nursing personnel declined by 7%, while adjusting for the severity of the illness of the patients under their care. The decline in nursing personnel was 20% to 27% in Massachusetts, New York and California, all of which had high managed care penetration rates (Arellano, 1996).

Inadequate staffing has a direct impact on the quality of patient care. In 1996, two-thirds of 5,000 registered nurses polled reported an increase in the number of patients assigned to them, three-fourths reported increased severity of the illness of patients under their care as well. Staffing reductions, combined with replacement of registered nurses with unlicensed personnel, have led to work speed-up for many nurses. Two-fifths of responding nurses said they would not want a family member to receive care at the institutions where they worked (Shindu-Rothchild, Berry, & Long-Middleton, 1976). The Minnesota Nurses Association examined 200 OSHA worker injury and illness logs at 86 Minnesota hospitals over a four-year period; it found a 65% increase in injuries and illness reported by nurses while nursing staff was reduced by 9%. Needlestick and back injuries contributed most to the increase of reportable incidents (Shogren, 1996).

Finally, a nursing shortage is currently gaining much attention from the media, the health care industry, and the nursing profession. The explanations most frequently given for the current shortage are an aging nursing work force and the phenomenon of women having other career choices. The profession and industry would be wise to turn their attention to the quality of the work life of nursing, including health and safety on the job, if they are serious about attracting qualified candidates into professional nursing.

SUMMARY

Health care workers, including nurses, face a wide range of workplace hazards, many of which are associated with significant morbidity and mortality. They often sacrifice their own health in the course of providing health care to others in need. The industry, the public, and the government have been slow to acknowledge the hazards and to provide adequate protection. In the absence of this protection, they must advocate for their own health and safety and educate the public and their health care organizations about their right to a healthy and safe workplace and the improvement in patient care that will result.

BIBLIOGRAPHY

Aiken, L. H., Sochalski, J., & Anderson, G. F. (1996). Downsizing the hospital nursing workforce. *Health Affairs, 15*, 82–92.

Alter, M. J. (1993). The detection, transmission and outcome of hepatitis C virus infection. *Infectious Agents and Disease, 2*, 155–166.

Ashford, N. (2000). Government regulations in occupational health and safety. In B. S. Levy, & D. H. Wegman (Eds.), *Occupational health: Recognizing and preventing work-related disease and injury* (pp. 211–236). Philadelphia: Lippincott, Williams & Wilkins.

Bensley, L., Nelson, N., Kaufman, J., Silverstein, B., Kalat, J., & Wlaker, J. (1997). Injuries due to assaults on psychiatric hospital employees in Washington State. *American Journal Ind Medicine, 31*, 92–99.

Bureau of Labor Statistics. (1995). *U.S. Department of Labor, Survey of Occupational Injuries and Illnesses.*

Bureau of Labor Statistics. (1997). *U.S. Department of Labor, Survey of Occupational Injuries and Illnesses.*

Bureau of Labor Statistics. (1998). *U.S. Department of Labor, Survey of Occupational Injuries and Illnesses.*

Bureau of Labor Statistics. (1997). *U.S. Department of Labor, Survey of Occupational Injuries and Illnesses.* 1996–2006 Employment Projections 1997. USDL 97-429.

Centers for Disease Control and Prevention. (1991). Recommendations for preventing transmission of human immunodeficiency virus and hepatitis B virus to patients during exposure prove invasive procedures. *MMWR Recommendations and Reports, 40(RR-8)*, 1–9.

Centers for Disease Control and Prevention. (1997a). Evaluation of blunt suture needles in preventing percutaneous injuries among health-care workers during gynecologic surgical procedures—New York City, March 1993–June 1994. *MMWR, 46*, 25–29.

Centers for Disease Control and Prevention. (1996). Evaluation of safety devices for preventing percutaneous injuries among health-care workers during phlebotomy procedures—Minneapolis-St. Paul, New York City, and San Francisco, 1993–1995. *MMWR, 46,* 21–25.

Charney, W. (1994). The lift team method for reducing back injuries: A 10 hospital study. *AAOHN J, 45,* 300–304.

Garg, A., & Owen B. D. (1992). Reducing back stress to nursing personnel: an ergonomic intervention in a nursing home. *Ergonomics, 35,* 1353–1375.

Gerberding, J. L. (1995). Prophylaxis for occupational exposures to bloodborne viruses. *New England Journal of Medicine, 332,* 444–455.

Gibas, A., Blewett, D. R., Schoenfeld, D. A., & Dienstag, J. L. (1992). Prevalence and incidence of viral hepatitis in health workers in the prehepatitis B vaccination era. *American Journal of Epidemiology, 136,* 603–610.

Henry, K., & Campbell, S. (1995). Needlestick/sharp injuries and HIV exposure among health care workers: National estimate based on U.S. hospitals. *Minn Med, 78,* 1765–1768.

Institute of Medicine. (1999). *To err is human: Building a safer health system.* Washington, DC: National Academy Press.

Ippolito, G., Pura, V., Petrosillo, N., Pugliese, G., Wispelwey, B., Tereskerz, et al. (1997). *Prevention, management and chemoprophylaxis of occupational exposure to HIV.* Charlottesville, VA: International Health Care Workers Safety Center, University of Virginia.

Lipscomb, J. A., & Love, C. C. (1992). Violence toward health care workers: An emerging occupational hazard. AAOHN Journal, 40, 219–228.

Rogers, B. (1994). *Occupational Health Nursing.*

Sepkowitz, K. A. (1994). Tuberculosis and health care workers: An historical perspective. *Annals of Internal Medicine, 120,* 71–79.

Shapiro, C. N. (1995). Occupational risk of infection with hepatitis B and hepatitis C virus. *Surgical Clinics of North America, 75*(6), 1047–1056.

Shindu-Rothchild, J., Berry, J., & Long-Middleton, E. (1996). Where have all the nurses gone? Final results of our patient care survey. *American Journal of Nursing, 96,* 25–39.

Shogren, E. (1996). Restructuring may be hazardous to your health. *American Journal of Nursing, 96,* 64–66.

Wassenberger, J., Ordog, G. H., Kolodny, M., & Allen, K. (1989). Violence in a community emergency room. *Archives of Emergency Medicine, 6,* 266–269.

CHAPTER 3

_____

Latex Allergy in Health Care

Susan Wilburn

_____

Allergy to natural rubber latex products emerged as a significant occupational hazard for health care workers in the 1990s as the use of latex medical gloves increased. This followed the publication of the Centers for Disease Control and Prevention (CDC) recommendations for universal precautions in 1987 and the 1991 Occupational Safety and Health Administration's (OSHA) Bloodborne Pathogens Standard requiring the use of universal precautions.

It is important for nurses to know about this potentially life-threatening and disabling allergy in order to protect themselves from unnecessary exposure to the allergen, to ensure early identification of symptoms of the allergy and to care for latex-allergic patients safely.

In 1997, the National Institute for Occupational Safety and Health (NIOSH) issued the following warning:

WARNING!

Workers exposed to latex gloves and other products containing natural rubber latex may develop allergic reactions such as skin rashes; hives; nasal, eye, or sinus symptoms; asthma; and (rarely) shock.

There is no safe contact with products containing natural rubber latex for an individual with a latex allergy. Continued exposure can result in the progression of illness from dermatitis to anaphylaxis.

BACKGROUND

Latex products are manufactured from a milky sap-like fluid derived from the rubber tree, *Hevea brasiliensis* (Subramanian, 1995). The term *latex* has been applied to natural and synthetic materials sharing characteristics

27

of flexibility and strength. "Natural rubber latex" (NRl) describes products derived from natural rubber. These are different from synthetic latexes that are used in water-based paints, which generally do not contain natural substances. Latex, as used in this chapter, refers to natural rubber latex products.

Most of the natural rubber latex medical gloves in use in the United States are produced in Southeast Asia and Malaysia. The latex is obtained by tapping the rubber tree in a process similar to tapping a maple tree for maple syrup. Several chemicals, which are known to cause allergic reactions in and of themselves, are added to the latex fluid during the manufacturing process. These chemicals, including thiurams and mercaptobenzothiazole, cause a chemical contact dermatitis that can be confused with latex allergy and delay appropriate treatment until the correct differential diagnosis is made (Kelly, 1999).

This delayed-hypersensitivity contact dermatitis from chemicals in rubber has been recognized since the 1930s (ANA, 1997; Truscott and Roley, 1995). But except for rare early reports, clinicians did not recognize systemic allergic reaction to latex proteins until 1979, when case reports began to appear in Europe (Granady and Slater, 1995). Latex allergy erupted in the United States shortly after the CDC introduced universal precautions in 1987. By late 1992, the Food and Drug Administration (FDA) received 1133 reports of serious allergic reactions and anaphylaxis occurring in patients and health care staff associated with 30 classes of medical devices. There were 15 patient deaths associated with latex barium enema catheters, which were subsequently removed from the market (Granady, 1995; Levy 1993). The FDA estimated that these reports represented only 1% of actual occurrences (Levy, 1993). By 1999, the FDA received five reports of health care worker deaths associated with latex glove use (Jacobson, 1999). Researchers hypothesize that the latex allergy outbreak is the result of multiple factors including deficiencies in manufacturing processes, increased latex exposure, hand care practices, immunological cross-reactivity, and changes in latex agricultural practices (Hamann, 1993; Truscott, 1995b).

Latex exposure occurs through contact with the skin or mucous membrane and by inhalation, ingestion, parenteral injection, or wound inoculation. Respiratory exposure occurs when glove powder, which acts as a carrier for NRl protein, becomes airborne when the gloves are donned or removed (Kinnaird et al., 1995; Korniewicz and Kelly, 1995). Scientific data regarding the natural progression of latex allergy are incomplete. The exact dose and duration of exposure required to produce sensitization are not known; however exposures at very low levels can trigger allergic reactions in some sensitized individuals (Charous, 1994; Kelly, 1995).

Risk factors include occupational exposure to latex (including during the manufacture of latex products and use of latex gloves), multiple surgical procedures or mucosal instrumentation involving latex, and a personal or family history of allergies (Sussman and Beezhold, 1995).

Symptoms of latex sensitization range from mild to severe and life threatening. Mild reactions involve skin redness, hives, or itching. More severe reactions may involve respiratory symptoms such as runny nose, sneezing, swollen and itchy eyes, asthma (difficulty breathing and wheezing), and, rarely, anaphylactic shock. Symptoms may present gradually and progress, although some individuals skip this progression and experience an abrupt onset of anaphylaxis or asthma (Kelly, 1995).

Table 3.1 describes the types of glove-associated reaction including latex allergy, time of onset, symptoms, and treatment.

The prevalence of latex allergy is 1–6% in the general population and 8–17% of the exposed health care work force. Individuals with spina bifida have shown to be at highest risk for latex sensitivity with a prevalence of 18–68% (Kelly, 1999; Kinnaird et al., 1995; Slater, 1992).

A wide variety of products contain latex: medical supplies, personal protective equipment, and numerous household objects (e.g., catheters, gloves, tubings, drains, IV ports, anesthesia equipment, nipples, pacifiers, teething rings, toys, elastic, condoms, diaphragms, sports equipment, and many more). All medical products must be labeled if they contain natural rubber latex or dry natural rubber. Lists of latex medical and consumer products and their non-latex alternatives are available from the Spina Bifida Association of America (800 621-3141) and other latex allergy support networks (www.netcom.com/~nam1latex_allergy.html).

Latex allergy is also associated with allergies to certain foods, especially avocado, potato, banana, tomato, chestnuts, kiwi fruit, and papaya (Beezhold et al., 1996; Charous, 1994).

DIFFERENTIAL DIAGNOSIS

Early diagnosis and avoidance of all latex products are essential for individuals with a Type I hypersensitivity. Because irritant dermatitis and chemical contact dermatitis (Type IV delayed hypersensitivity) are often confused with an IgE-mediated response (latex allergy), it is important to see an allergy and/or immunology specialist to establish a differential diagnosis.

TABLE 3.1 Types of latex and other glove-associated reactions (ANA, 1997; Burton, 1997; OSHA, 1999)

Type of Reaction and Time of Onset	Symptoms/Signs	Cause	Prevention/ Management
Irritant contact dermatitis (nonallergic), gradual onset over days	Scaling, drying, cracking of skin	Direct skin irritation by gloves, powder, soaps/ detergents, scrubs, incomplete hand drying	Identify reaction, avoid irritant product, and dry hands completely after washing and prior to donning gloves; use cotton glove liner
Allergic contact dermatitis (Type IV delayed hypersensitivity) 6–48 hours after contact	Blistering, itching, crusting (similar to poison ivy reaction)	Accelerators (e.g., thiurams, carbamates, benzothiazoles), processing chemical (e.g., biocides, antioxidants)	Identify reaction chemical; select alternative glove materials without chemical
Natural rubber latex allergy— IgE/histamine mediated (Type I immediate hypersensitivity), occurs within minutes of contact		Natrual Rubber Latex (NRL) proteins: direct contact with or breathing NRL proteins including glove powder containing proteins, from powdered gloves or the environment	Identify reaction, allergy consultation; substitute nonlatex gloves for affected worker and other nonlatex products
A) Localized contact urticaria that may be associated with or progress to B) Generalized reaction	Hives in area of contact with latex Includes generalized urticaria (beyond area of contact), rhinitis, wheezing, swelling of mouth, shortness of breath; can progress to hypotension and anaphylactic shock		Eliminate exposure to glove powder; substitute nonlatex examination gloves for all workers as a primary prevention measure and to accommodate latex-allergic patients and workers safely Clean NRL-containing powder from environment

The most sensitive and specific test for latex allergy is a skin test. Currently in the U.S., however, there is no FDA-approved skin test reagent on the market. In Canada, Bencard is available for skin testing (Kelly, 1999). Blood tests available to measure latex antibodies have more false positive and false negative results than the skin test. A strong history of symptoms improves the predictive value of these tests. General screening of the health care population is not recommended without a history of exposure to latex products and symptoms related to latex use.

GLOVE STANDARDS AND SELECTION

Latex gloves were originally developed in 1889 by William Halstead to protect the badly chapped hands of his scrub nurse from harsh disinfectants and germs of diseased patients (Truscott, 1995b). The purpose of medical glove use today is similar to that of 1889: to prevent health care worker and patient exposure to infectious materials such as HIV and hepatitis B and C viruses, and to protect from exposure to cleaning agents, hazardous drugs, and other chemicals.

OSHA's 1991 Bloodborne Pathogens Standard mandates that "gloves shall be worn when it can be reasonably anticipated that the employee may have hand contact with blood, other potentially infectious materials, mucous membranes and non-intact skin, when performing vascular access procedures . . . and when handling or touching contaminated surfaces" (29 CFR 1910.1030).

OSHA's 1994 Personal Protective Equipment Standard discusses the fact that no gloves provide protection against all potential hazards and "commonly available glove materials provide only limited protection against many chemicals" (29 CFR 1910.132 and 1910.138). Further, no glove can protect against a needlestick injury. Safer needle devices as required by the Federal Needlestick Safety and Prevention Act are necessary to prevent needlestick injuries. Personal protective equipment such as medical gloves are at the low end of the industrial hygiene hierarchy of controls and are less effective than hazard elimination and engineering controls for preventing bloodborne exposures (Olishifski, 1988).

Understanding the purpose of protective gloves and the physical properties of gloves is necessary to ensure that the right gloves are used for specific tasks. The FDA regulates medical gloves as "Class I" medical devices, requiring that they meet the general controls established by the FDA for most medical devices. In 1999, the FDA published a proposed regulation to reclassify medical gloves as Class 2, indicating that the agency believes general controls are insufficient to provide reasonable assurances of safety and effectiveness especially in the following areas: barrier integrity, degradation of quality during storage, contamination, exposure to natural rubber latex allergens, and the role of glove powder as a carrier of airborne NRL allergens (FDA, 1999).

FDA specifies defect levels for adulteration of patient examination and surgical gloves (21 CFR 800.20). This rule defines defects as leaks, tears, mold, embedded foreign objects, and so forth, and requires that for surgical gloves, the leak rate should not exceed an Acceptable Quality Level (AQL) of 2.5% and for patient examination gloves 4%.

Ironically, the FDA does not require viral or chemical barrier testing, exposure to such hazards being the primary reason for wearing medical gloves.

The FDA relies on manufacturers' voluntary conformance with consensus standards in order to provide a reasonable assurance of safety for many other aspects of medical gloves. The consensus standards are issued by the American Society for Testing and Materials (ASTM).

ASTM voluntary consensus standard specifications for medical gloves include tensile strength, minimum percentage elongation, and thickness. In addition, ASTM has standards for viral barrier penetration (ASTM F1671-97a), chemical permeability (ASTM G 739-96), and standard measurement tests for powder and protein levels (no specific amount required). The FDA allows a low protein-labeling claim when the extractable protein is 50 micrograms per gram of glove.

Because FDA regulations do not cover the essential tests for gloves for viral and chemical barrier penetration, it is necessary for consumers and purchasers of glove products to ensure that the appropriate testing has been carried out to meet the requirements for glove use in their settings. Product evaluation committees should ask manufacturers to provide the results of independent testing for the above referenced FDA and ASTM standards to assist with product selection. As with all products used in patient care and for protecting workers, frontline health care workers, especially those affected by latex allergy, should be involved in the evaluation, selection, and testing of new products.

It is also important to know what chemical additives are present in each type of glove evaluated. The same accelerator chemicals that cause a chemical contact dermatitis are present in both latex gloves and in some of the synthetic alternatives. The FDA glove-labeling rule in 1997 prohibited the use of the term "hypoallergenic" in relation to medical gloves (FDA, 1997).

This term had been used to describe gloves that are low in chemical additives but not low in latex protein allergens which is confusing to those people trying to avoid latex. The current FDA guidance for labeling as reduced potential for chemical sensitization requires a modified Draize-95 test (FDA, 1997). The manufacturer's verification of this testing should be required by the purchasing authority for health care organizations.

The following is a synthesis of recommendations for medical glove use by leading regulatory, scientific, and professional organizations.

- Gloves shall be worn when it can be reasonably anticipated that the employee may have hand contact with blood, other potentially infectious materials, mucous membranes, and nonintact skin.
- Employers shall ensure that appropriate gloves in appropriate sizes are accessible to employees, including alternatives for those employees who are allergic to the gloves normally provided.
- The most appropriate glove for a particular application should be selected and it should be determined how long it can be worn. The performance characteristics of gloves relative to the specific hazard anticipated should be known.
- Unnecessary exposure to natural rubber latex proteins should be reduced for all workers and patients. Latex gloves should be used only in those situations requiring protection from infectious agents.
- Patients and employees with a latex allergy should avoid all contact with latex gloves and other latex-containing products. Non-latex glove choices that have comparable barrier effectiveness to latex should be provided.
- All medical facilities should provide synthetic non-latex gloves for general physical examinations, especially for all mucosal examinations (e.g., oral, vaginal, rectal).
- Non-latex gloves should be used for activities that are not likely to involve contact with infectious materials (food preparation, routine housekeeping, maintenance, etc.). Because most serious reactions result from mucosal exposure to latex antigens, all food preparation services should use only non-latex gloves to prepare food. (American Academy of Dermatology, 1998; American College of Allergy, Asthma and Immunology and American Academy of Allergy, Asthma and Immunology, 1997; ANA, 1997; CDC, 1998; NIOSH, 1997; OSHA, 1991, 1994, 1999)

Substitution of synthetic gloves for nrl gloves reduces the exposure of patients and glove wearers to latex allergens. Synthetic materials are sometimes superior to latex in resisting permeation by certain chemical agents. Some synthetic gloves, however demonstrate inferior flexibility, durability, and viral barrier penetration properties compared with latex (Korniewicz and Kelly, 1995; Rego and Roley, 1999).

Other concerns include synthetics' own potential chemical allergenicity (see chemical sensitivity labeling claims above) because some synthetic gloves contain chemical additives known as accelerators. The production and disposal of polyvinyl chloride gloves creates another environmental hazard, dioxin, a known carcinogen and endocrine disrupter.

Synthetic alternatives to latex include vinyl, polyethylene, polyurethane, nitrile, neoprene, and tactylon. Table 3.2 presents synthetics with their advantages and disadvantages.

TABLE 3.2 Glove Materials

Material	Composition	Advantages	Disadvantages
Vinyl	Polyvinyl chloride	No protein allergens; resists acids, alkalies, fat, alcohols; resists aging Increased barrier breakdown	Moderate flexibility, limited fit & feel, fatigues quickly, contains irritating chemicals Not durable Environmentally toxic
Nitrile	Acrylonitrile and butadiene	No protein allergens; resists cuts, abrasions, and punctures; resists solvents better than latex or neoprene Comparable viral barrier to latex	Contains sensitizing chemicals Limited feel and flexibility, slow memory, aging compromises barrier protection
Neoprene	Chloroprene	Resists chlorinated solvents, alcohol, alkalies, oil, & petroleum	Reduced elasticity, limited fit, feel & flexibility; contains sensitizing chemicals
Tactylon	Styrene-ethylene, Butylene-styrene	Tactility, elasticity, resists oxidation, no protein or sensitizing chemicals	Soluble to some solvents
Plastic	Polyethylene	Lightweight	Limited fit, feel, & flexibility; limited strength

(Hamann, 1993; Korniewicz and Kelly, 1989, 1995; Rego and Roley, 1999; Sustainable Hospitals Project, 2000).

SUMMARY

Latex allergy is a disabling, career- and life-threatening occupational illness affecting hundreds of thousands of health care workers in the United States. Because the only effective treatment is complete avoidance of latex exposure, it is necessary to reconsider the use of latex medical products, especially gloves, for all purposes and to implement institutional and legislative changes to make the environment safe for exposed workers, allergic workers, and patients.

Latex allergy results from the use of products designed to protect the very health care workers who are sickened. It is important to remember the principle of "first do no harm" in relation to health care worker health and safety and implement a policy of testing any new chemical, medicine, or personal protective equipment prior to its implementation to ensure that the therapeutic measure does not cause additional problems.

BIBLIOGRAPHY

American Nurses Association. (1997). Position Statement on Latex Allergy.

American Academy of Allergy, Asthma, and Immunology and American College of Allergy, Asthma, and Immunology. (1997). Joint Statement Concerning the Use of Powdered and Non-powdered natural rubber latex gloves.

American Academy of Dermatology. (1998). Position paper on latex allergy.

American College of Allergy, Asthma, and Immunology position Statement. Latex allergy—an emerging health care problem. (1995). *Ann Allergy Asthma Immunology, 75*(1):19–21.

American College of Allergy, Asthma, and Immunology. Latex Allergy home page includes Guidelines for the Management of Latex Allergy and Safe Latex Use in Health Care Facilities.

Beezhold, D. H., Sussman, G. L., Liss, G. M., and Chang, N. S. (1996). Latex allergy can include clinical reactions to specific foods. *Clinical and Experimental Allergy, 26*(5):416–422.

Burton, A. D. (1997). Latex allergy in health care workers. McDiarmid MA & Kessler ER, eds. The Health Care Workers. *Occupational Medicine: State of the Art Reviews 12*(4), 609–634.

Bolyard, E. A., Tablan, O. C., Williams, W. W., Pearson, M. L., Shapiro, C. N., and Deitchman, S. D. The Hospital Infection Control Practices Advisory Committee. (1998). *Guideline for Infection Control in Health Care Personnel. Centers for Disease Control and Prevention. American Journal of Infection Control, 26:*289–354.

Centers for Disease Control and Prevention (CDC) (1989). Guidelines for prevention of transmission of human immunodeficiency virus and hepatitis B virus to health-care and public-safety workers. *MMWR 38(S-6):*1–37.

Charous, B. L. (1994). The puzzle of latex allergy: Some answers, still more questions. *Annals of Allergy, 73*(4), 277–281.

Department of Labor. Occupational Safety and Health Administration. (1999). Technical Information Bulletin: Potential for Allergy to Natural Rubber Latex Gloves and Other Natural Rubber Products.

Department of Health and Human Services, Centers for Disease Control and Prevention, National Institute for Occupational Safety and Health (NIOSH) (1997). NIOSH Alert: Preventing Allergic Reactions to Natural Rubber Latex in the Workplace.

Grandy, L. C., & Slater, J. E. (1995). The history and diagnosis of latex allergy. *Immunology and Allergy Clinics of North American, 15*(1), 21–29.

Hamann, C. P. (1993). Natural rubber latex protein sensitivity in review. *American Journal of Contact Dermatitis, 4*(1), 4–21.

Hamann, C., & Nelson, J. (1993). Permeability of latex and thermoplastic elastomer gloves to the bacteriophage X174. *Am. J. Infect Control, 21*:289–96.

Jacobson, E. (1999). Testimony of the Center for Devices and Radiological Health, Food and Drug Administration, Department of Health and Human Services before the Subcommittee on Oversight and Investigations Committee on Education and the Workforce, U.S. House of Representatives.

Kelly, K., Sussman, G., & Fink, J. (1996). Stop the sensitization. *J Allergy Clinical Immunology, 98*(5):857–858.

Kelly, K. (1995). Management of the Latex-allergic patient. *Immunology and Allergy clinics of North American, 15*(1), 139–157.

Kelly, K. (1999). Latex Allergy. CD-Rom. Medical College of Wisconsin.

Kinnaird, S. W., McClure, N., & William, S. (1995). Latex allergy: an emerging problem in health care. *Nursing Clinics of North American, Sept 30*(3):475–93.

Korniewicz, D. M., & Kelly, K. F. (1995). Barrier protection and latex allergy associated with surgical gloves. *AORN J. June; 61*(6), 1037–44.

Laughon, B., Butz, A., & Larson. (1989). Integrity of Vinyl and Latex Procedure Gloves. *Nursing Research, 38*(3):144–146.

Levy, D. A. (1993). Report on the International Latex Conference: Sensitivity to Latex in Medical Devices. Baltimore, MD, USA 5–7 Novemeber, 1992. *Allergy, 49 (4, suppl.) I-9.*

Olishifski, J. B. (1988). Methods of Control. In Plog BA. Fundamentals of Industrial Hygiene. Chicago: National Safety Council, pp. 457–474.

Occupational Safety and Health Administration (OSHA) (1994). Personal Protective Equipment Standard. 29 CFR 1910.132; 29 CFR 1910.138. OSHA Bloodborne Pathogens Standard. (1991). 29 CFR 1910.1030.

Rego, R., & Roley, L. (1999). In-use barrier integrity of gloves: Latex and nitrile superior to vinyl. *American Journal of Infection Control, 27*:405–10.

Slater, J. E. (1992). Allergic reaction to natural rubber. *Annals of Allergy, 68*(3), 203–209.

Slater, J. E. (1994). Latex allergy. *Journal of Allergy and Clinical Immunology, 94 (2, Pt 1),* 139–150.

Subramaniam, A. The chemistry of natural rubber latex. *Immunology and Allergy Clinics of North American, 15*(1), 1–19.

Sussman, G., & Beezhold, D. (1995). Allergy to latex rubber. *Annals of Internal Medicine, 122*:43–36.

Sustainable Hospitals Project (2000). Web site on gloves selection. University of Massachusetts—Lowell. www.uml.edu/centers/LCSP/hospitals/.

Truscott, W., & Roley, L. (1995). Glove-associate reactions: Addressing an increasing concern. *Dematology Nursing, 7*(5), 283–292.

Truscott, W. (1995b). The industry perspective on latex. *Immunology and Allergy Clinics of North America, 15*(1), 89–121.

Tarlo, S. M., Sussman, G. L., Contala, A., & Swanson, M. D. (1994). Control of airborne latex by use of powder-free latex gloves. *Journal of Allergy and Clinical Immunology, 93*(6), 985–989.

Swanson, M. C., Bubak, M. E., Hunt, L. W., et al. (1994). Quantification of occupational latex aeroallergens in a medical center. *Journal of Allergy and Clinical Immunology, 94(3, Pt. 1)*, 445–451.

U.S. Food and Drug Administration. (1997). Final Rule: Natural Rubber-Containing Medical Devices; User Labeling. Federal Register. September 30; 62(189); 51020–51030.

CHAPTER 4

Ergonomics

Pat Bertsche and Gary Orr

rgonomics is the science of designing jobs, selecting tools, and modifying work methods to better fit workers' capabilities and to prevent work-related musculoskeletal disorders (MSDs), such as back strain, tendinitis, and carpal tunnel syndrome. An MSD hazard is a physical risk factor that by itself or in combination with other physical risk factors has a sufficient level of intensity, duration, and/or frequency to cause a substantial risk of MSDs. This is particularly true with repeated exposure. Jobs in which the employee's typical work activities include specific physical risk factors such as awkward posture; high hand force; contact stress; highly repetitive motion; or heavy, frequent, or awkward lifting require hazard analysis. Once a hazard analysis is complete and the root cause(s) of the risk factors identified, a control strategy needs to be developed and implemented to prevent or minimize the occurrence of MSDs.

Table 4.1 shows selected data on work-related injuries and illnesses among various health care providers reported to the Bureau of Labor Statistics in 1998. Overexertion injuries due to lifting clearly represent the greatest number of injuries among patient handlers. On May 8, 2000, Mary Foley, President of the American Nurses Association (ANA), testified in Washington, DC in a public hearing on the Occupational Safety and Health Administration's (OSHA) proposed Ergonomics Program Standard. She stated: "Recent changes in the health care environment have lowered staffing levels (downsizing) requiring individual nurses to care for more patients and with fewer people to assist" (ANA, 2000). Ms. Foley also stated that between 1994 and 1997 there was an 8.8% increase in the average number of patients for whom a registered nurse (RN) cared and a 7.2% decrease in the number of RNs employed.

TABLE 4.1 Bureau of Labor Statistics: Nonfatal Injuries and Illnesses Among Health Care Providers in 1998

Occupation	Total cases	Selected exposures or events leading to an injury or illness			
		Overexertion lifting	Repetitive motion	Exposure to harmful substances	Assaults and violent acts
Registered nurses	24,979	5,586	513	1,150	1,522
Licensed practical nurses	10,847	3,233	173	635	645
Nursing aides, orderlies	84,128	26,139	647	2,260	5,607
Total	119,954	34,958	1,333	4,045	7,774

It is essential for nurses and other health care providers to understand ergonomics in order to facilitate the prevention of their own MSDs and MSDs among the people for whom they have responsibility. This understanding will also facilitate a more comprehensive assessment of the needs of their clients and the development of client care plans, including patient education in the prevention of MSDs. The purpose of this chapter is to acquaint the reader with MSD risk factors and control strategies. It is important to realize that control strategies vary, depending on the job and type of industry; however, the risk factors are essentially the same.

MUSCULOSKELETAL DISORDER RISK FACTORS

A combination rather than any single risk factor may be responsible for the occurrence of MSDs. Therefore, it is important to identify all the work-related risk factors that may be present in an existing job or a job that is being designed. The risk factors associated with the occurrence of MSDs include

1. *Awkward Postures.* Postures determine which muscles are used in an activity and how forces are translated from the muscles to the object being handled. It is important to allow flexible joints like the wrist, shoulder, neck, hips, and ankles to move. Usually awkward postures become a concern when there is little opportunity to move (static pos-

tures) or if awkward posture is combined with other risk factors, such as repetition and forceful exertions. Factors to consider include the following.

- Greater muscular force is required when awkward postures are used because muscles cannot perform efficiently.
- Fixed awkward postures (e.g., holding the arm out straight for five minutes) contribute to rapid muscle and tendon fatigue and joint soreness.
- Forces on the spine increase as the center of gravity of the torso extends beyond the feet. Therefore bending forward or backward will increase the muscle contraction in the back in relation to the degree of awkward posture.
- Forces on the spine also increase when lifting, lowering, or handling objects with the back bent or twisted. This occurs because the muscles must handle the body weight in addition to the load in the hands.

2. *Forceful Exertions.* Tasks that require forceful exertions place higher loads on the muscles, tendons, and joints. As the force increases the muscles fatigue more quickly. A thorough study by Marras, Davis, Kirking, and Bertsche (1999) on patient handling activities showed that many of the lifts and transfers performed by health care workers place very high forces on the spine. In addition to transfers, repositioning a patient in bed (where the patient has little ability to assist), even with two people, places very high forces on the L5/S1 disc. The amount of force exerted depends upon

- Weight and distribution of the load handled or lifted (bulky loads are more difficult to lift than compact loads);
- Speed of movement (for higher speed of movement, force capacity is reduced);
- The friction characteristics of objects handled (the more slippery the object, the more force required to hold it).
- Vibration through contact with a tool or work surface (localized vibration from hand tools can increase the grip force requirements);
- The type of grip used: pinch or power. Pinch grips usually place three to four times more force on the tendons than power grips.

3. *Repetition or frequency.* Repetition refers to the tasks or series of motions that may be performed over and over again with little variation. If tasks or motions are repeated frequently (e.g., every few seconds), fatigue and muscle tendon strain can accumulate, and can result in permanent tissue damage. Tendons and muscles can often recover from the effects

of stretching or forceful exertions if sufficient time is allotted between exertions. Frequent repetition of the same work activities can also exacerbate the effects of awkward postures and forceful exertions.

4. *Duration.* Duration refers to the amount of time a worker is exposed to risk factors. The duration of job tasks can have a substantial effect on the likelihood of both localized and general fatigue. In general, the longer the period of continuous work (muscle contraction), the longer the recovery or rest time required.

5. *Contact stresses.* High contact forces (due to hard or sharp objects such as desk edges or small diameter tool handles) may create pressure over one area of the body (such as the forearm, palm of the hand, or sides of the fingers) that can inhibit nerve function and blood flow.

6. *Vibration.* Vibration is usually divided into two areas: localized (sometimes called segmental) and whole body. Exposure to localized vibration occurs when a part of the body comes in contact with a vibrating object, such as a powered hand tool. Localized vibration from handheld power tools can increase grip force, reduce blood flow, and produce symptoms of carpal tunnel syndrome. Exposure to whole body vibration can occur while standing or seated in vibrating environments or objects, such as trucks or heavy machinery. Prolonged exposure to whole body vibration has been associated with back and neck MSDs.

7. *Cold temperatures.* Cold temperatures can reduce the dexterity and sensitivity of the hand, causing a person to apply more grip force to hold tool handles and objects. There is also evidence that cold tends to exacerbate the effects of localized vibration.

8. *Workplace conditions.* Workplace conditions that can cause or influence the presence and magnitude of MSD risk factors include but are not limited to the following.
   - *Poorly fitting gloves.* Poorly fitting gloves or tight gloves can reduce sensory feedback from the fingers and thus result in an increased grip force being used.
   - *Obstructions.* Obstructions such as bed rails, furniture, and IV stands that hamper smooth, free lifting and reaching motions, can increase awkward postures and reaches that result in higher forces required to accomplish the task. Tight spaces such as small bathrooms and showers can require employees to bend, twist, or make long or awkward reaches while handling a patient.
   - *Standing surfaces.* Prolonged standing on hard surfaces increases back and leg fatigue. Standing on slopes, uneven surfaces, or differ-

ent levels places stress on the spine and hip. Standing on wet surfaces can increase the risk of sudden forces acting against the spine while trying to prevent slips and falls.

- *Prolonged high visual demands.* Processing information quickly, making decisions rapidly, and visually scanning complicated vital sign monitors for slight evidence of abnormality can increase fatigue and increase muscle tension.
- *Glare/poor light.* Glare (direct and indirect) or inadequate levels of light can contribute to the occurrence of static (fixed) awkward postures so that fatigue may set in rapidly. Tasks where adequate light levels are important include those requiring reading, computer operations, and inserting catheters or other invasive procedures.

9. *Work organization.* MSD risk factors can be intensified by work organization characteristics, such as

- *Inadequate work–recovery cycles.* Inadequate work–recovery cycles may not allow enough time between exertions, and may contribute to fatigue and overexertion.
- *Excessive work pace and duration.* Excessive work paces may not allow enough recovery time between exertions and may contribute to fatigue and overexertion. Excessive duration, such as overtime (voluntary and involuntary) and long work shifts, may increase the exposure to risk factors present in the job, as well as reduce the available recovery time. Work activities that can be handled in a regular work shift may not be acceptable for longer periods because of increased exposure to risk factors and decreased availability of recovery time. Even when adequate work–recovery cycles are implemented, overtime or long work shifts may increase the risk of MSDs.
- *Unaccustomed work.* Unaccustomed work may require employees to use muscles for a longer duration or use different muscles, creating soreness. The soreness can be in the muscles, tendons, or joints. Usually, it subsides as the employee adapts to the activity. Unaccustomed work can occur for employees who are new, have transferred from another job, or are returning from extended absences (e.g., return from injuries, vacations, or layoffs). Unaccustomed work can also occur when there is an increase in activity (e.g., increased production standards or increased hours of work) that may add to the repetitiveness of the job. This includes dealing with new patients or patients with different needs, new equipment, malfunctioning equipment and tools, increasing force requirements, repetition due to start-

ing a procedure over again, or an increase in exposure to vibration from poorly maintained tools. When the job has risk factors that contribute to MSDs, then the soreness attributable to conditioning may linger or intensify over time. During conditioning the affected body parts are gaining strength, flexibility, and endurance needed to perform a task. However, the adaptation process has limits. MSDs are likely to occur when the job requirements exceed the capabilities of employees, or there is inadequate recovery time.

- *Lack of task variability.* High levels of routine or similar work load may increase mechanical load due to lack of changes in posture. Time pressures can cause hurried movements, resulting in high accelerations. Time pressures can also produce an increase in the number of cycles of repetitive movements and contribute to static or awkward trunk postures.

- *No control over work pace.* When the employee has no control over work pace, it is reasonable to assume that pace has an amplifying rather than a mitigating role in the development of unwanted physical and mental effects (Salvendy & Smith, 1981). Sources of pacing pressure include coworkers, supervisors, or the need to earn the maximum pay allowance in an incentive job (Rodgers, 1986). Reward systems that pay employees extra money for increased time on the job or number of patients handled may result in fewer recovery breaks and increase exposure to risk factors, or may influence or cause other risk factors, such as using long reaches instead of moving to the other side of the bed, or manual handling instead of using the appropriate equipment.

CONTROL STRATEGIES

Risk factors can be controlled either in the design of a job or after the work has started. There are opportunities to provide very effective controls for a small proactive investment in design. Once the work has begun, reactive or retrofit changes can still be implemented, but usually require modifications to the equipment that has been installed. Reactive changes also require employees to change work patterns. Implementing a change after habits have been formed requires communication with the employee(s) in order to be successful. The individual whose job will be changed needs to know why the change is needed, what will be changed, and the time frame and consequences of the change. One way to ensure that information is properly communicated is through employee involvement in the design and change process.

When risk factors for MSDs are identified, it is essential to identify control measures that reduce or if possible eliminate the risk. Traditional classification of control measures distinguishes between engineering controls and administrative controls. The opportunities to implement engineering and administrative controls differ, depending on if the risk factor is associated with a new job/process or a existing job/process.

Engineering controls are the preferred method to reduce or eliminate exposure to MSD risk factors. They involve physical changes to the workstations, equipment, and facility, such as the installation of ceiling-mounted lifts or any other relevant aspect of the work environment to reduce or eliminate risk factors. Engineering controls are typically permanent controls.

Administrative controls are procedures that significantly limit daily exposure by control or manipulation of the work schedule or manner in which work is performed. Administrative controls require the employer to periodically audit the job to ensure that the controls are used. These examples in the health care setting include lifting teams for all patient transfers, adequate staffing levels, and employee training in lifting techniques and proper body mechanics.

Table 4.2 lists controls that have been used in health care settings to eliminate or reduce MSD risk factors.

SUMMARY

Musculoskeletal disorders such as back strain, tendinitis, and carpal tunnel syndrome are significant problems in the workplace today. Risk factors that can cause or contribute to these disorders were described in this chapter, in addition to the types of ergonomics controls currently available to reduce or minimize such disorders. Health care professionals must have an understanding of these risk factors and control strategies to prevent MSDs among themselves and to assist their clients in the prevention of these potentially disabling conditions. Jobs need to be designed and modified to match the capabilities of the employees who perform them.

BIBLIOGRAPHY

Alexander, D. C., Orr, G. B. (1992). The Evaluation of Occupational Ergonomics Programs, Proceeding of the Human Factors Society 36th Annual Meeting, pages 697–701, Human Factors Society, Santa Monica, California.

Alexander, D. C., Pulat, B. M. eds, (1985). *Industrial ergonomics: a practitioner's guide*, Industrial Engineering and Management Press, Norcross GA.

TABLE 4.2 Controls for musculoskeletal disorder risk factors that have been applied in the health care industry

I. Controls for lateral transfers—transferring a patient from one horizontal position to another—(e.g., bed to gurney)

Lift sheet	This may be a strong draw sheet preferably with handles. A trained person is on each side of the patient. The sheet is lifted or pulled up in a bed or pulled over to a gurney. These should be used in conjunction with a friction reducing device.
Roller board/ roller mat	The board is approximately 6 feet by 2 feet, some have rollers with a vinyl covering. The bed and gurney are pushed together and the board is placed between them. The patient is positioned on the board and rolled onto the gurney. The employees use a push/pull technique rather than a lift.
Slide board or beasy board	The patient is positioned onto the board (approximately 6 feet × 2 feet), then the board is pushed/pulled onto the new location. The board can be used in combination with a lift sheet. Air assisted sliding boards are also an option.
Flat gurneys with transfer aids	Height-adjustable gurneys are available with mechanical means of transferring a patient on and off a stretcher. Some are motorized, while others use a hand crank.
Transfer mats	Two low friction mats are used. One mat is slid under the shoulders and the other mat under the hips. Straps secure the mat to the patient. The mats are pulled to the new position.
Jordan frame	A metal frame is assembled around the patient. Plastic slides are moved under the patient and attached to the frame.
Convertible wheelchairs	Some wheelchairs can be converted into gurneys.
Inflatable mats	Air mats are placed under the patient, then inflated. The mat uses air to reduce friction so that the transfer force is greatly reduced.
Mechanical transfers	A small motorized device is used to pull the patient and draw sheet onto the bed or gurney.

II. Controls to move between sitting and standing—patient is cooperative and can bear weight

Chairs that lift	The chair is equipped with a lift. When the lift is activated the chair slowly raises upward and tilts forward. The chair is stationary.
Lift cushions	A spring action lift cushion can be placed on any chair that has a hard seat. A lever activates the spring lift to assist the patient out of the chair.

TABLE 4.2 *(continued)*

Gait belt	A belt (about 2 inches wide) is fastened securely around the patient's waist so that it does not slide up when the employee pulls the belt. The belt does not have handles, so the employee grips the belt to pull or lift the patient
Posey belt or lower walking belt with handles	The belt (about 4 inches wide) is fastened snugly around the abdomen (hip area). The employee grips the handles to pull the patient to a standing position. The handles should allow the employee to obtain a comfortable secure grasp. Employees should be taught to rock and pull, and not lift, while using the belt.
Wheelchairs with removable armrest	Patient does not have to be lifted over the armrest. The wheelchair should also have a swing out footrest.
Patient transfer sling	The sling (about 8 inches wide, 20 inches long) has cutouts in the material for hand holds. Some slings have rings attached for the employee to grip. One side of the sling is textured to increase the grip on the patient. The sling is tucked securely around the patient with the bottom of the sling at the hip, but the sling is not fastened to the person.
Pivot disc	For the patient who can assist in moving, the pivot disc is used to rotate the person 90 degrees. The disc is placed on the floor so the patient can stand on the disc and turn to be seated in a chair or bed.
Sit/stand lift assist	This hoist can be used to assist the employee in transfers to/from a seated position.

III. Controls to reposition—patient with upper body strength

Slide boards	The board enables the patient who has upper body strength to slide from one location to another. The board is rectangular with a smooth slippery surface for ease of transfer.
Hand blocks	The patient uses hand blocks to lift high enough off the mattress to reposition on the bed or chair.
Push-up bar	Through the use of this bar the patient can lift up for repositioning or move to a standing position. The bar can be positioned behind the patient to push up in bed or ease into a seated position
Trapeze bar	The trapeze bar is suspended from an overhead frame. The patient can grasp the bar to reposition in bed.

(continued)

TABLE 4.2 *(continued)*

IV. Controls for toileting and bathing

Hip lifter	An inflatable lift is positioned under the hips of the patient and can be inflated with a pump. The hips are elevated so a specially designed bedpan can be positioned.
Bath boards	The board is level with the bath and allows the patient to move between a wheelchair and the tub or hand held shower.
Toileting/shower chair	A heavy chair with a padded removable seat. The seat is adjustable and the arms are removable to improve access during lifting. The chair rolls and has brakes, and comes with a safety belt. The chair must be able to fit over the toilet.
Shower cart	The shower cart can be wheeled next to the bed and the patient transferred with a lift sheet or sliding board. The patient can be showered, dried, and dressed at a level conducive to good posture and then returned to bed.
Height adjustable bath	At the lowest setting, the bath can be utilized by independent patients. The height can be adjusted so the employee can stand while bathing the patient.
Sit/stand lift assist	The sit/stand lift assist allows patients with some upper body strength to be moved from a sitting position to a standing position with mechanical assistance. The lift assist supports the patient while the employee prepares the patient for toileting or the shower.

American Conference of Government Industrial Hygienists, (2000), TLV for physical agents in the work environment, *ACGIH*, Cincinnati, OH.

American Nurses Association. (2000). Testimony of Mary Foley, President, at public hearing on OSHA's proposed ergonomics standard. Available at (http://www.nursingworld.org/gova/federal/legis/testimon/2000/ergomf.htm). Also available at U.S. Department of Labor—OSHA Docket Office, Washington, DC (Docket Number S777, p. 15877).

Benson, J. D. (1987). Control of low back pain using ergonomic task redesign techniques. *Professional Safety, 32(9)*, 21–25.

Bureau of Labor Statistics (1998). Lost-worktime injuries and illnesses: Characteristics and resulting time away from work [*USDOL 00-115, Table R12*]. Washington, DC: U.S. Government Printing Office. Retrieved April 20, 2000, from www.bls.gov.

Chaffin, D. B., Anderson, G. B. J. (1991). *Occupational Biomechanics* New York: John Wiley & Sons.

Corlett, E. N., Bishop, R. P. (1976). A technique for assessing postural discomfort. *Ergonomics, 25*, 315–322.

Eastman Kodak Co. (1983). *Ergonomic design for people at work, Volume 1*. New York: Van Nostrand Reinhold.

Fragala, G. (1996). *Ergonomics: How to Contain On-the-Job Injuries in Health Care*, Joint Commission on Accreditation of Healthcare Organizations, Illinois: Oakbrook Terrace.

Greenberg, L., & Chaffin, D.B. (1977). *Workers and Their Tools*. Midland, MI: Pendell.

Holmer, I. (1994). Cold stress: Part I—Guidelines for the practitioner. *International Journal of Industrial Ergonomics, 14*, 139–149.

Human Factors Society (1988). American National Standard for Human Factors Engineering of Video Display Terminal Workstations. *ANSI/HFS Standard 100-1988*, Santa Monica, CA.

International Standards (ISO 1986). Guidelines for the Measurement and Assessment of Human Exposure to Hand Transmitted Vibration, *ISO/DIS 5349.2* (Geneva: International Standards Organization).

Jurgens, H. W., Aune, I. A., & Pieper, U. (1990). International Data on Anthropometry. *International Labor Office, Occupational Safety and Health Series No. 65*, Geneva, p. 21–41.

Karasek, R., Theorell, T. (1990). *Healthy work: stress, productivity, and the reconstruction of working life*, (pp. 31–82). New York: Basic Books, Inc.

Keyserling, W. M., Armstrong, T. J., Punnett, L. (1991). Ergonomic Job Analysis: A Structured Approach for Identifying Risk Factors Associated with Overexertion Injuries and Disorders. *Applied Occupational Environmental Hygiene, 6(5)*, 353–363.

Kilbom, A. (1994). Repetitive work of the upper extremity: Part I—Guidelines for the Practitioner. *International Journal of Industrial Ergonomics, 14*, 51–57.

Marras, W. S., & Kim, J. Y. (1993). Anthropometry of industrial populations. *ergonomics, 36(4)*, 371–378.

Marras, W. S., Davis, K., Kirking, B., & Bertsche, P. (1999). A comprehensive analysis of low back disorder risk and spinal loading during the transferring and repositioning of patients using different techniques. *Ergonomics, 42(7)*, 904–926.

McCormick, E. J. (1974). *Human Factor Engineering*, 3rd Ed. New York: McGraw-Hill.

National Institute for Occupational Safety and Health (1989). Criteria for a Recommended Standard: Occupational Exposure to Hand-Arm Vibration, *USD-HHS, PHS, CDC, Division of Standards Development & Technology Transfer*, Publication number 89–106. Cincinnati, OH.

National Institute for Occupational Safety and Health (1994). *Applications Manual for the NIOSH 1991 Revised Lifting Equation*, Publication No., 94-110. Cincinnati, OH,

Putz-Anderson, V. (1988). *Cumulative trauma disorders: A manual for musculoskeletal diseases of the upper limbs*. New York: Taylor & Francis.

Rodgers, S. (Ed.). Eastman Kodak Co. (1986). *Ergonomic design for people at work, Vol. 2.* New York: Van Nostrand Reinhold.

Salvendy, G., & Smith, M. J. (1981). *Machine pacing and occupational stress.* New York: Taylor and Francis.

Silverstein, B. A., Fine, L. J., & Armstrong, T. J. (1986). Carpal tunnel syndrome: Causes and a preventive strategy. *Seminars in Occupational Medicine, 1*(3), 213–221.

Smith, M. J., & Saintfort, P. C. (1988). A balanced theory of job design for stress reduction. *International Journal of Industrial Ergonomics, 4,* 67–79.

Snook, S. H., & Ciriello, V. M. (1991). The design of manual handling tasks: Revised tables of maximum acceptable weights and forces. *Ergonomics, 34,* 1197–1213.

Sommerich, C. M., McGlothlin, J. D., & Marras, W. S. (1993). Occupational risk factors associated with soft tissue disorders of the shoulder: A review of recent investigation of the literature. *Ergonomics, 36*(6), 697–717.

Waters, T. R., Putz-Anderson, V., Garg, A., & Fine, L. (1993). Revised NIOSH equation for the design and evaluation of manual lifting tasks. *Ergonomics, 36*(7), 749–776.

Wilson, J. R., & Corlett, E. N. (1990). *Evaluation of human work.* New York: Taylor & Francis.

Winkel, J., & Westgaard, R. (1992). Occupational and individual risk factors for shoulder-neck complaints: Part II—The scientific basis (literature review) for the guide. *International Journal of Industrial Ergonomics, 10,* 85–104.

CHAPTER 5

Health Care Without Harm:
A Case Study in Advocacy

Charlotte Brody

In nursing school, we learn how to be advocates for our patients. Nurses are taught how to lay out a recommended course of action for patients and how to follow up on that recommendation. But how do we adjust those advocacy skills when the patient is an asthmatic child whose attacks are triggered by air pollution? What is the role of the nurse advocate when the patient is a pregnant womon who is eating mercury-contaminated tuna that can impact the nervous system development of her baby? To solve the environmental health problems described in this book, nurses need to adapt their advocacy skills so they are not only working to change their patients' behaviors, they are working to change the behaviors of the larger society.

Changing society is never easy. Our culture and our political system have the same properties of inertia as does all physical matter. Without an external force, polluting industries will continue to pollute, dangerous pesticides will still be sprayed, and latex gloves will continue to cause allergies. Nurses can be the external force that overcomes inertia and gets society moving toward products and practices that protect human health and the environment.

One example of nursing advocacy for environmental health is Health Care Without Harm (HCWH): The Campaign for Environmentally Responsible Health Care. This international campaign aims to eliminate pollution in health care practices without compromising safety or care. Since its inception, nurses and nursing organizations have been leaders of the HCWH effort. In this chapter, examples from its Campaign will illustrate the six basic steps for all nursing advocacy for environmental health.

STEP ONE: FIGURE OUT WHAT YOU WANT: SET AND CLEARLY STATE YOUR ADVOCACY GOALS

In 1996, the 28 founding organizations of the HCWH coalition agreed to work together to transform the health care industry so it was no longer a source of environmental harm by eliminating the nonessential incineration of medical waste and phasing out the use of polyvinyl chloride plastic (PVC) and mercury. These are very big goals, but because they were clearly stated, the size and scope of HCWH's goals were not overwhelming. The goals spelled out who HCWH was trying to change and what change we were seeking. That clarity has been a big reason for HCWH's growth. In four years, more than 290 nursing, hospital, medical, environmental, health impacted, social justice, labor, and religious organizations in 26 countries have joined the campaign.

THE FIRST STEP IN GOAL SETTING: DESCRIBE THE PROBLEM

How can you determine what you want? Start by understanding the problem you want to address. For the people who started HCWH, the problem in 1996 was that, according to the U.S. Environmental Protection Agency (EPA), medical waste incineration was the leading source of dioxin, a toxic chemical linked to cancer, birth defects, and endometriosis. HCWH's founders learned that medical waste incineration was a large source of mercury pollution as well. Mercury and dioxin were coming out of incinerators' smokestacks because the medical waste being burned included broken mercury-filled thermometers and sphygmomanometers and products made with chlorine, including polyvinyl chloride plastic. The mercury and dioxin from medical waste incinerators lands on grazing land and in water and gets taken up by grazing animals and fish. When we eat fish contaminated by mercury or drink milk contaminated by dioxin we end up with the mercury and dioxin in our bodies. So the problem is mercury and dioxin in our food and in our bodies that comes in part from the purchasing and waste disposal practices of the health care industry. Knowing all of this, the founding members of HCWH could have set a goal of getting mercury and dioxin out of us and out of our children. But that goal does not tell what entity you are trying to change and what change you are seeking.

THE SECOND STEP IN GOAL SETTING: FIND POSSIBLE SOLUTIONS

Before you can decide what change you are seeking, you have to do more than understand the problem. You have to determine what available and achievable solutions exist. The founding members of HCWH learned about Hollie Shaner, a registered nurse in Vermont who had helped her hospital minimize its medical waste through aggressive waste segregation, reuse, and recycling. They learned about hospitals that had found safe and cost-effective ways to handle medical waste without incineration. HCWH researchers found a few hospitals that were phasing out the use of mercury-containing products and a wide array of alternative products that did not contain mercury, PVC, or other toxic chemicals. HCWH developed its campaign around the successful experience of these environmentally innovative, solution-oriented individuals and institutions.

Somewhere, someone is developing innovative solutions for every environmental health problem. European countries often have adopted more environmentally progressive practices than we have. Before you set your goals, do the investigative research work to determine the availability and range of solutions to the problem you want to address. Once you know what is possible, it will be much easier to achieve clarity on developing advocacy goals that set out what you want to achieve.

STEP TWO: DETERMINE WHICH PEOPLE CAN GIVE YOU WHAT YOU WANT

Advocacy goals describe a vision of institutional change: schools with windows that open or drinking water that is free of pesticide runoff from agricultural land upstream. In the second step to nursing advocacy for environmental health, you determine which people have the power to make your vision a reality. These people become your potential focal points or targets.

Brainstorming is one good way of coming up with a list. For HCWH, the list of potential targets includes

- hospital administrators
- hospital purchasing officers
- hospital waste specialists
- religious denominations that run hospitals
- nurses
- physicians
- nursing schools and medical schools
- patients, especially those with environmentally linked disease
- waste handling firms
- U.S. EPA officials who set environmental limits on medical waste incineration

- state officials who administer the regulations on medical waste incinerators
- JCAHO, the entity that accredits hospitals
- the FDA, which approves medical products
- medical device manufacturers
- stockholders of health care organizations and medical device manufacturers
- Medicaid administrators

All of these potential targets are decision makers in health care. All of them have the ability to help eliminate the pollution in health care practices.

STEP THREE: DETERMINE WHAT IT WILL TAKE TO GET WHAT YOU WANT

In every advocacy effort, there are going to be different routes of action to get you to the same goal. You'll always be able to come up with more than one target, more than one set of people who can give you what you want. But choosing which target or targets to focus your efforts on depends on your best assessment of what advocacy actions will be necessary to per-suade each of the possible targets to do what you want them to do. One way to move through step three is to go through your list of possible tar-gets and ask, "How do we convince this target that this advocacy effort is in their self-interest?" For elected officials, the self-interest might mean getting public recognition for doing something good for the community. For a group of parents, it could be an improvement in their children's health. For a corporation it might mean increased sales or preventing a decrease in sales. Once you've attached necessary advocacy actions to each target, you can put your targets in order, with the ones that require the fewest or easiest advocacy actions first.

In HCWH, we determined that medical device manufacturers would make more environmentally safe products when their customers signaled that they wanted to purchase those products. But to do that we needed to have enough resources to move medical device purchasers. That meant, for example, that Becton-Dickenson, the largest manufacturer of mercury fever thermometers, could only become a viable target after HCWH had successfully moved two other targets: health care institutions that used mercury-containing devices and pharmacy retailers that sold mercury fever thermometers. After HCWH received pledges from more than 600 hospi-tals and clinics to phase out the use of mercury and after the United States's largest retailers, including Wal-Mart, K-Mart and Albertson's, announced that they would no longer sell mercury fever thermometers, Becton-Dickenson announced that they would end the production and sale of mercury fever thermometers (*Washington Post*, September 27, 2000).

STEP FOUR: MATCH YOUR RESOURCES TO YOUR TARGETS' NEEDS

Once you've completed step three, you'll have determined what each possible target needs in order to be persuaded to do what you want them to do. Now you have to figure out what you are capable of delivering.

Determine your current capabilities by performing a self-assessment. Doing an accurate self-assessment of an individual or a group can be very difficult. It will be easier if you start with the questions that have quantifiable answers.

- How many people can you identify who are currently committed to solving your advocacy goals?
- How many hours can each of these people spend every month towards reaching these goals?
- What skills/ experience/ connections do each of these people bring to the effort to reach these goals?
- How much money is committed toward achieving these goals?

Once you have the answers to these quantifiable questions, consider:

- How many people can you reasonably say you represent? What basis do you have for that number?
- How well can you explain the problem you want to address?
- How well can you describe your solution?
- Do you have enough information to answer difficult questions?
- Do you have independently verifiable statistics and news stories that help you make your case?
- Do you have written materials that describe the problem and the solution and recruit people to your advocacy effort?

Once you've written down the answers to these questions, you have a description of your current advocacy resources. Now go back and look at the list of targets. Do you have everything you need to perform the advocacy actions necessary to convince the easiest of these targets that your goals are in their self-interest? If you do, then get started advocating! But for almost every advocacy effort to create social change, you'll find that you have to organize.

According to *Webster's Dictionary*, organizing means "uniting in a body or becoming systematically arranged." When HCWN got started in 1996, there were 28 small nonprofit organizations willing to "become systematically arranged" toward the goal of an environmentally responsible health care system. But our self-assessment revealed that we needed the involvement of many more health care professionals, health care institutions, religious organizations, environmental groups, and health-impacted people before HCWH could begin to achieve its goals. So we spent over a year on outreach and educational activities aimed at recruiting enough additional groups into HCWH so we could begin to influence the campaign's targets.

STEP FIVE: ORGANIZE TO GAIN ENOUGH RESOURCES TO MOVE YOUR TARGETS

How do you organize? First, you have to have something to organize around. But you've already got that because you've set your advocacy goals. Second, you need to know who you want to organize. That will come from figuring out what resources you need before you have enough advocacy resources to convince your first target to do what you want it to do. So now that you've determined whom you need to organize, you start organizing by reaching out to those individuals and groups. Organizing is done by talking and listening. Talking and listening doesn't mean giving people a lecture and then listening for their applause. It means respectfully asking people if you can take their time to describe your advocacy effort, listening to the stories they have to tell you in response, finding out what connects your concerns to their past experience and future aspirations, and noting other issues they may bring up in the course of the conversation.

As you talk and listen in your effort to amass the resources you need to achieve your goals, you will learn things that help you refine your advocacy goals. In its first year, as HCWH representatives talked and listened, we learned how hospitals purchase through group purchasing organizations. We learned that among the alternatives to polyvinyl chloride plastic or PVC is latex, a material that causes severe allergies in many health care workers and patients. We learned that medical devices made of PVC also contain a softening plasticizer called DEHP that can leach out of the PVC and into the patient. All of this information was used to refine HCWH's strategic targeting.

STEP SIX: CREATE A STRUCTURE THAT SYSTEMATICALLY ARRANGES PARTICIPANTS TO MAKE CHANGE

You have goals. You have targets and you know what you need them to do to achieve the goals. After assessing your capacities and figuring out what resources you were missing, you have organized and acquired those resources. Now you need a structure that enables the individuals and groups that are part of your advocacy effort to use their skills and expertise most effectively to move targets toward the goals.

While there is no single structure that works best for every advocacy effort, there are some general rules that always apply.

1. Just like targets, participants in advocacy efforts act out of self-interest. That self-interest might be a safer job, or more friends, or greater recognition of their skills. But your advocacy effort will only grow if the individual participants in it feel that they are directly benefiting from their involvement.
2. Give people something they can do. Then thank them for doing it. Many advocacy efforts fail because people who care about the issue are not linked with an effective advocacy action that they can reasonably be expected to take.
3. Don't expect everyone to do the same thing. Create a structure that allows a diverse group of people to use their own skills and experience to win change.

In Health Care Without Harm, some participating organizations implement HCWH goals in their own institution or community. Others are involved in national and international aspects of the campaign. Some member organizations focus their efforts on one aspect of the campaign, such as fighting incineration or helping hospitals phase out the use of mercury. One HCWH member organization may only feel comfortable educating their members about the environmental health problems linked to the health care industry and the possible solutions to these problems, while another member organization may take the lead in working with the international manufacturers of intravenous systems to find alternative materials to PVC. The HCWH campaign works to create printed and web-based materials that clearly spell out what member organizations and their representatives can do and to acknowledge and celebrate the participation of each group.

In Health Care Without Harm's first four years, hundreds of medical waste incinerators have closed, while the market for new incinerators has dried up. Major pharmacy chains in the U.S. (Walmart, K-Mart, Rite Aid,, Albertson's, Walgreens) have agreed to stop selling mercury thermometers at all their outlets. Becton-Dickenson, the largest U.S. manufacturer of thermometers, has announced its decision to end production of mercury containing thermometers. More than 600 hospitals and clinics nationwide have taken the HCWH pledge to go mercury-free; the campaign is working with many of these institutions to implement this pledge. Baxter International, the world's largest manufacturer of IV systems, has agreed to phase out its global line of PVC IV systems over the next several years. Major health care providers and group purchasing organizations (Kaiser Permanente, Universal Health Services, Cardinal) have taken major steps towards the phase-out of PVC products.

These accomplishments move our society towards Health Care Without Harm's goal of eliminating pollution in health care practices without compromising safety or care. But all of HCWH's accomplishments will only be sustained over time if there are hundreds of other equally successful advocacy efforts toward an environmentally healthier world. The model of Health Care Without Harm shows that you can advance positive change by combining the six basic steps for all nursing advocacy with hard work, creative collaboration, and a healthy dose of luck.

REFERENCE

Goldstein, A. Washington Post. September 27, 2000.

PART II

Environmental Health Basics

CHAPTER 6

Toxicology

Barbara Sattler

Toxicology is an essential science to environmental health. A traditional definition of toxicology is the study of poisons or the science that investigates the adverse effects of chemicals on health. The dose–response relationship is a fundamental concept in toxicology, sometimes stated as "the dose makes the poison." Knowledge of the dose–response relationship can establish causality that a chemical has induced certain effects, establish the lowest dose at which the effect occurs (also known as the threshold effect), and determine the rate at which the injury may occur, as depicted by the slope of the dose–response curve.

In toxicology, understanding the host factors is equally important. As noted in chapter 19, on children's environmental health, the embryo, fetus, and child have distinct vulnerabilities to toxic chemicals based on their host factors, including, among others, physiologic immaturity, hand-to-mouth behavior, and higher metabolism. Toxicity refers to the strength of the poison or the ability of the chemical to damage an organ system, to disrupt a biochemical process, or to disturb an enzyme system. Some chemicals are more toxic than others. For example, milligram for milligram, morphine is more toxic than aspirin.

The terms *toxicant, toxin*, and *poison* are often used interchangeably in the literature. A *toxic agent* is anything that can produce an adverse biological effect. It may be chemical, physical, or biological in form. Toxic agents may be chemical (such as cyanide), radiological (such as radon), and biological (such as mold). Elements can be toxic, such as chlorine, lead, mercury, or arsenic. Chemical compounds or mixtures can be toxic. Methylmercury is a mercury compound that is highly toxic. Diesel exhaust is a chemical mixture that contains many toxic elements and chemical compounds.

Nurses and other health care providers do not typically learn toxicology in their basic education. However, all nurses learn basic pharmacology. Toxicology is very similar to pharmacology. The distinction is that pharmacology is the study of the effects of a subset of chemicals called *drugs*. In pharmacology, both the beneficial effects and the unintentional side effects (toxic effects) of the drugs are studied. Toxicologists study only the negative effects of exposures to chemicals, radiation, or biological toxicants. To assist the nurse in understanding the basic principles of toxicology, a side-by-side comparison of pharmacology and toxicology terms and concepts is presented in Table 6.1.

The dose–response curve is the graphic depiction of the dose–response relationship. It is typically a sloping "S-shaped" curve, with increasing doses of the toxic agent on the x-axis and the body response on the y-axis (Fig. 6.1). When toxicity studies are being implemented, the scientist is looking at one specific response at a time, such as changes in a liver enzyme, increase in blood pressure, or changes in cognition. For any given effect, a dose–response curve is created. At the lowest doses no response may be observed. This level is referred to as the "No Observed Effect Level" (NOEL) or sometimes referred to as the "No Observed Adverse Effect Level" (NOEAL). These levels are important when setting health-based standards for environmental pollution such as contaminant levels in our drinking water.

The threshold level refers to the amount of a substance necessary to elicit a response, below which there is no response. There may be evidence of increasing effects as the dose is increased; however at the highest doses the effects may have already been elicited with a lower dose. For carcinogens, there is not a threshold—any amount of a carcinogenic chemical may elicit a response because it can damage the DNA, thus creating the conditions for cancerous proliferation.

Carcinogenicity is a common toxic endpoint that scientists study. However, the Environmental Protection Agency (EPA) has found that of the approximate 3,000 chemicals produced in the United States, at an annual volume of at least one million pounds, only 7% have been fully evaluated for toxicity, and a much smaller percentage has been examined for carcinogenicity (see www.epa.gov). For these reasons, animal studies and in vitro testing have played an increasingly critical role in determining the carcinogenic potential of environmental agents. In addition, the technique of analyzing structure relations for chemical configurations that are similar to known carcinogens allows for the early identification of potential carcinogens that can be further tested.

TABLE 6.1 Comparison of Basic Concepts in Pharmacology and Toxicology

Pharmacology	Toxicology
Pharmacology is the scientific study of the origin, nature, chemistry, effects, and use of drugs.	*Toxicology* is the science that investigates the adverse effects of chemicals on health.
Dose refers to the amount of a drug absorbed from an administration.	*Dose* refers to the amount of a chemical absorbed into the body from a chemical.
A drug can be administered one time, short-term, or long-term.	*Exposure* is the actual contact that a person has with a chemical. Exposure can be one-time, short-term, or long-term.
A *dose–response* curve graphically represents the relationship between the dose of a drug and the response elicited.	A *dose–response curve* describes the relationship of the body's response to different amounts of an agent such as a drug or toxin.
Roots of administration: oral, IM, IV, dermal, topical, etc.	*Routes of entry:* ingestion, inhalation, dermal absorption.
With drugs there are therapeutic responses (desirable) and side effects (undesirable). Beyond the therapeutic dose, a drug may become toxic.	In toxicology, only the toxic effects are of concern. *Toxicity* is the ability of a chemical to damage an organ system, to disrupt a biochemical process, or to disturb an enzyme system.
Potency refers to the relative amount of drug required to produce the desired response.	The *toxicity* of a toxic chemical refers to the relative amount it takes to elicit a toxic effect compared with other chemicals.
Biological monitoring is done for some drugs: clotting time is monitored in patients on anticoagulants like coumadin. Actual drug levels are measures for some drugs, such as digoxin.	*Biological monitoring* is done for some toxic exposures, such as blood lead levels or metabolites of chemicals, such as cotines for environmental tobacco smoke exposures.

B. Sattler, 1998, Curriculum materials for the Environmental Health Faculty Development Workshop.

The International Agency for Research on Cancer (IARC), an agency of the World Health Organization, serves as a clearinghouse for information on research about the human carcinogenicity of agents. In 1969, IARC initiated a program to evaluate the carcinogenic risk of chemicals to humans and to produce monographs on individual chemicals. IARC has established standardized criteria for the classification of chemical carcinogens based on human, animal, and in vitro data. IARC designates chemicals and

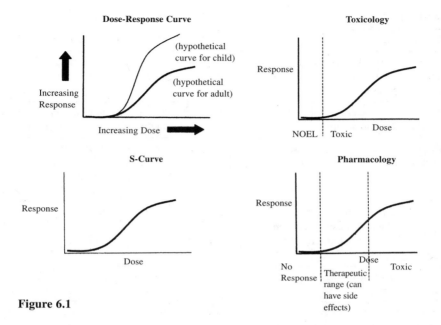

Figure 6.1

processes as human carcinogens (Group 1), probable human carcinogens (Group 2A), and possible human carcinogens (Group 2B). Group 2A chemicals reflect limited evidence in humans and sufficient evidence in animals, and Group 2B chemicals reflect limited evidence in humans without sufficient evidence in animals, or sufficient evidence in animals without any human data. Of the 750 chemicals, industrial processes, and personal habits that IARC has evaluated to date, Group 1 contains 50 and Group 2 contains almost 250. Several other systems for classifying carcinogens exist, including the National Toxicology Program (NTP). The NTP, headquartered in the National Institute of Environmental Health Sciences (NIEHS), develops and maintains the U.S. federal government's official list of known or "anticipated' human carcinogens. This list contains 198 substances. The IARC classifications are taken into account and incorporated into the risk assessments when environmental standards are promulgated. For additional information, IARC's web site is www.iarc.fr.

Virtually all toxicity studies use in vitro models (cell lines) or in vivo models using animals, commonly mice. For ethical reasons, human studies are only sanctioned for therapeutic drug testing. Therefore, the data on which we base our health standards for environmental pollution are derived by extrapolating or making our best estimate about the potential effects on humans after researching the effects on animals. Extrapolation is not an exact science and the policy-making activities are further complicated by the often complex economic and political implications of setting a standard.

It is important to understand some of the complexities that toxicologists face in making extrapolations to humans. For example, when mice are studied, the mice are from a single genetic line. This means that every mouse in the study is genetically identical to the others. The toxicologist first determines the effect that he or she wants to observe, then introduces the toxic chemical. The chemical can be placed in the food or water for ingestion, in the air for inhalation, on the mouse's skin for dermal absorption, in the eyes, or injected intramuscularly or intravenously. The dose is then adjusted up and the observations are made. A dose–response curve is then plotted. During this experiment, it is extremely important to control for all other variables. As such, the air quality and temperature, food and water quantity and quality, exercise/rest cycle, and other variables are all controlled. Also, scientists typically look at adult mice during toxicological experiments and seldom look at mixtures or combinations of mixtures. Once again, the results of the experiments are often extrapolated to predict the human effects. Immediately, one can see the potential for problems with such extrapolation.

Except for identical twins, humans are not genetically identical. They are richly diverse. Their diversity expands far beyond their genetic makeup. They eat differently, in quantity and quality, and they come in many different shapes and sizes—some quite thin and some quite heavy. Some people use pesticides in their homes, some do not; some homes have smokers, others do not. Despite the fact that humans are most likely to be exposed to mixtures of chemicals, an overwhelmingly large portion of the toxicological and occupational research to date deals with single, pure chemicals (Yang and Yang, 1994). Some people are healthy, some are not; some take no medication, some take many. People have vastly different exercise regimes; during exercise metabolism increases. Depending on where they live, people may have few environmental exposures or many. These additional medicines, chemical additives in diet, and/or environmental pollutants may have additive effects, potentiating effects, or antagonistic effects with the toxic chemicals for which standards are set. And, of course, humans come in all ages. These are but a few of the variables that cannot be controlled in human populations that may affect the host–response relationship and therefore the power and precision of extrapolation.

One of the ways extrapolated data are used by the EPA when setting standards, is by creating a reference dose (RfD). A reference dose is the amount of a toxic chemical that is NOT likely to elicit an effect. The reference dose is based on a predicted lifetime exposure by oral delivery (unless otherwise noted). It is measured in milligrams per kilogram of body weight per day. The research on which the reference doses are based involves single chemicals, usually in pure form, and a simple matrix. The actual effect of exposure of populations to complex mixtures, by multiple routes and in multiple matrices, is poorly understood.

It is now possible to identify biochemical and/or cellular changes in humans caused by exposure to an environmental toxin. These changes are called *biomarkers* and are currently used in research studies to identify individuals exposed to specific toxic substances. Advances in the field of biomarker technology may have important implications for the detection, prevention, and treatment of disease. A variety of technical advances have enabled scientists to identify specific changes in humans at the molecular and cellular levels that are secondary to exposure to a particular environmental toxin. Alterations to DNA, changes in protein structure, metabolites in urine or blood and other "footprints" of toxic exposure can now be recognized and are being used as research tools in molecular epidemiology to identify and track toxic exposures (Lubin and Lewis, 1995).

Occupational and environmental health-based standards are set to protect a 70 kg (approximately 160 lb), white, otherwise healthy, middle-aged male. This presents a problem in ensuring protection of the old, young, frail, and unborn. In 1996, Congress recognized the problem inherent in setting standards to protect the healthy middle-aged male when they passed the Food Quality Protection Act (FQPA). This act came on the heels of an Institute of Medicine report that criticized the level of protection offered to children from pesticides on food. Congress called for significant changes in the paradigm for health protection. Table 6.2 includes some of the directives mandated by Congress that are directly related to the toxicology of pesticide-associated pathology (dose, duration, host factors) and the protection of infants and children.

The vast majority of the 72,000 chemicals currently used in commerce (excluding food additives, drugs, cosmetics, and pesticides) have not been tested for their effects on human health.

The effects of drugs and hazardous chemicals can be immediate (acute), long-term, or can present after a latency period, often associated with cancer outcomes. Host factors must be considered when looking at ther-

TABLE 6.2 Food Quality Protection Act of 1996

Health-based standard: A new standard of a reasonable certainty of "no harm" prohibits taking into account economic considerations when children are at risk.

Additional margin of safety: The EPA is required to use an additional ten-fold margin of safety when there are adequate data to assess prenatal and postnatal development risks.

Account for children's diet: Age-appropriate estimates of dietary consumption must be used in establishing allowable levels of pesticides on food to account for children's unique dietary patterns.

Account for all exposures: In establishing acceptable levels of a pesticide in food, the EPA must account for exposures that may occur through other routes, such as drinking water and residential application of the pesticide.

Cumulative impact: The EPA must consider the cumulative impact of all pesticides that may share a common mechanism of action.

Tolerance reassessments: All existing pesticide food standards must be reassessed over a ten-year period to ensure that they meet the new standard to protect children.

Endocrine disruption testing: The EPA must screen and test all pesticides and pesticide ingredients for estrogen effects and other endocrine disruptor activity.

Registration renewal: A 15-year renewal process is required for all pesticides to ensure that they have up-to-date science evaluations over time.

apeutic drugs or hazardous chemicals. Such factors as age, sex, weight, drugs that the person may be taking, or pregnancy status may affect the therapeutic or toxic effect of a drug or a chemical. Medicinal drugs are taken voluntarily and for the most part under the supervision of a licensed health care provider. Hazardous chemical exposures are almost always involuntary. The regulatory process by which a drug comes to the market includes several stages, starting with animal testing and moving slowly and carefully on to human testing. The regulatory process for hazardous chemicals that are not foods, drugs, cosmetics, or pesticides does not require any original toxicological testing. As such, many of our household products, school art supplies, and commercial products have had little or no testing.

The resources for information about drugs include the Physicians Desk Reference (PDR), Poison Control Centers, and the National Library of Medicine's Grateful Med (PubMed). For toxic chemicals, Poison Control Centers can be a good source of information. The National Library of Medicine is excellent and has a substantial holding of information that is accessible via the web in a user-friendly format, including a self-paced toxicology tutorial (see web site: www.toxnet.nlm.nih.gov). The major databases are defined below.

NATIONAL LIBRARY OF MEDICINE

For Toxicology Data
(Factual information on toxicity and other hazards of chemicals)

HSDB	Hazardous Substances Data Bank—Broad scope in human and animal toxicity, safety and handling, environmental fate, and more. Scientifically peer-reviewed.
IRIS	Integrated Risk Information System—Data from the Environmental Protection Agency (EPA) in support of human health risk assessment, focusing on hazard identification and dose–response assessment.
CCRIS	Chemical Carcinogenesis Research Information System—Carcinogenicity, mutagenicity, tumor promotion, and tumor inhibition data provided by the National Cancer Institute (NCI).
GENE-TOX	GENE-TOX—Peer-reviewed mutagenicity test data from the *EPA*.

For Toxicology Literature
(Scientific studies, reports, and other bibliographic material)

TOXLINE	Extensive array of references to literature on biochemical, pharmacological, physiological, and toxicological effects of drugs and other chemicals.
EMIC	Environmental Mutagen Information Center—Current and older literature on agents tested for genotoxic activity.
DART/ETIC	Developmental and Reproductive Toxicology and Environmental Teratology Information Center—Current and older literature on developmental and reproductive toxicology.

For Toxic Release Information (Annual estimated releases of toxic chemicals to the environment—the Environmental Protection Agency's TRI (Toxics Release Inventory)

TRI	Toxics Release Inventory—reporting years 1995–1998.

For Chemical Information (Nomenclature, Identification, Structures)

ChemIDplus	Numerous chemical synonyms, structures, regulatory list information, and links to other databases containing information about the chemicals.
HSDB Structures	2D structural information on the HSDB chemicals.
NCI-3D	2D and 3D information compiled by the National Cancer Institute, and augmented by MDI.

TOXNET is sponsored by the National Library of Medicine, through the Toxicology and Environmental Health Information Program of its Specialized Information Services Division: (www.nlm.nih.gov).

National Library of Medicine Toxline Subfiles (Toxnet, 2000) include:

- Toxicity Bibliography
- Toxicological Aspects of Environmental Health
- International Pharmaceutical Abstracts
- International Labour Office
- Hazardous Materials Technical Center
- Environmental Mutagen Information Center
- Development and Reproductive Toxicology
- Environmental Teratology Information Center
- Toxicology Research Projects
- Pesticides Abstracts
- Toxicology Document and Data Depository
- NIOSHTIC
- Poisonous Plants Bibliography
- Aneuploidy
- Epidemiology
- Epidemiology Information System
- Federal Research in Progress
- Toxic Substances Control Act Test Submissions
- RISKLINE

The National Toxicology Program (NTP) was established by the U.S. Department of Health and Human Services to coordinate toxicology research and testing activities within the Department, to provide information about potentially toxic chemicals to regulatory and research agencies and the public, and to strengthen the science base in toxicology. It has several toxicology activities and is administered by the National Institute of Environmental Health Science (see http://ntp-server.niehs.nih.gov/).

PRECAUTIONARY PRINCIPLE

With thousands upon thousands of chemical compounds now creating a chemical soup in our air and water (in our bodies, in our breast milk), it is increasingly difficult to prove specific hypothesis regarding the relationship of exposure to a singular chemical and disease outcomes in humans. It has been suggested that we adopt a "precautionary approach" when animal research and other indicators demonstrate a possible toxic relationship between a chemical and health effect. See Box 6.1 for the Wingspread Statement on the Precautionary Principle. This "precautionary approach" calls for action to reduce potentially toxic exposure to humans in light of data or other indicators, rather than delaying until more "conclusive" studies are performed. As nurses who are trained in disease prevention, we can appreciate and should advocate for a precautionary approach when it may prevent injuries or illnesses.

Box 6.1 Wingspread Statement on the Precautionary Principle

In 1998, an international group of health and public health professionals, scientists, government officials, lawyers, grass roots activists and labor activists met at a conference center called "Wingspread" in Wisconsin to define the "precautionary principle." The group issued the following consensus statement:

"The release and use of toxic substances, the exploitation of resources, and physical alterations of the environment have had substantial unintended consequences affecting human health and the environment. Some of these concerns are high rates of learning deficiencies, asthma, cancer, birth defects and species extinctions, along with global climate change, stratospheric ozone depletion and worldwide contamination with toxic substances and nuclear materials.

"We believe existing environmental regulations and other decisions, particularly those based on risk assessment, have failed to protect adequately human health and the environment —the larger system of which humans are but a part.

"We believe there is compelling evidence that damage to humans and the worldwide environment is of such magnitude and seriousness that new principles for conducting human activities are necessary.

"While we realize that human activities may involve hazards, people must proceed more carefully than has been the case in recent history. Corporations, government entities, organizations, communities, scientists and other individuals must adopt a precautionary approach to all human endeavors.

"Therefore, it is necessary to implement the Precautionary Principle: When an activity raises threats of harm to human health or the environment, precautionary measures should be taken even if some cause and effect relationships are not fully established scientifically. In this context the proponent of an activity, rather than the public, should bear the burden of proof.

"The process of applying the Precautionary Principle must be open, informed and democratic and must include potentially affected parties. It must also involve an examination of the full range of alternatives, including no action." [End of statement]
(See: http://www.gdrc.org/u-gov/precaution-3.html)

Nurses should be aware of the environmental sciences' underpinning standards, particularly health-based standards. Currently, very few health professionals are involved in any of the environmental standard-making activities. Our voices in these venues would be welcome, particularly as we speak for the protection of our most vulnerable populations. Nurses as advocates have an important role to play in deciding how much predicted cancer, or learning disabilities, or infertility is "acceptable" as we set exposure limits to toxic chemicals in our air, water, and food.

BIBLIOGRAPHY

CEHN. (2001). Basic Toxicology and Risk Assessment Section, Training Manual on Pediatric Environmental Health: Putting it into Practice, www.cehn.org.
Gossel, T. A., & Bricker, J. D. (Eds.). (1990). *Principles of clinical toxicology*, (2nd ed.)
Gosselin, R. E., Smith, R. P., & Hodge, H. C. (1984). eds. *Clinical toxicology of commercial products*. Baltimore, MD: Williams & Wilkins.

Klassssen, C. D. (Ed.). (1996). *Casarett and Doull's Toxicology, the Basic Science of Poisons*, 5th ed. New York: McGraw-Hill.

Loomis, T. A. (1978). *Essentials of toxicology*, 3rd ed. Philadelphia, PA: Lea & Febiger.

Lubin, B., & Lewis, R. (1995). Biomarkers and pediatric environmental health. *Environmental Health Perspectives, 102*(Suppl. 6), 99–104.

McCauley, L. A. (1998). Chemical mixtures in the workplace: Research and practice, (CE Article) *AAOHN Journal, 46*(1).

National Library of Medicine web site (www.nlm.nih.gov).

National Library of Medicine, Specialized Information Services, Toxicology Tutorial web site (http://sis.nlm.nih.gov/toxtutor.cfm).

Stine, K., & Brown, T. M. (Eds.). (1996). *Principles of Toxicology*. Boca Raton, Florida: CRC Press, Inc.

Sullivan, J. B., & Krieger, G. R. (Eds.). (1991). *Hazardous materials toxicology: clinical principles of environmental health*. Baltimore, MD: Williams & Wilkins.

Yang, Shieh-Ching & Yang, Sze-Piao (1994). Respiratory function changes from inhalation of polluted air, Archives of Environmental Health, May/June 1994, Vol. 49 Issue 3, pp. 182–188.

CHAPTER 7

Environmental Epidemiology

Jane Lipscomb

In 1997, the Missoula, Montana City-County Health Department, led by its nurse director, began an investigation of an apparent cluster of birth defects among babies born in Missoula. Three babies whose families lived in the area were born with trisomy 13, a chromosomal abnormality that causes severe multiple organ system abnormalities. At the time of the investigation, two of the babies had died. The Health Department had called for assistance from the Centers for Disease Control and Prevention in its investigation. Statistical evidence from other states suggests that one in 10,000 live births can be expected to have trisomy 13. The three cases reported among the approximately 1,000 births in Missoula in 1997 represent what you might expect to see in 30 years. The only recognized risk factor for trisomy 13 is advanced maternal age (Merriam, 1998). To date, the investigation has not uncovered any environmental cause for the cluster.

Clusters of adverse health events, such as cancer, other chronic diseases, and birth defects, are often reported to health agencies. As this case aptly demonstrates, nurses can play a critical role in a health agency's response to community concern and epidemiologic investigation of such clusters. This is but one example of how nurses can be involved in the field of environmental epidemiology.

Epidemiology is one of the basic sciences of public health and a critical tool in the risk assessment of environmental exposures. As such, epidemiologic studies contribute to our understanding of the environmental determinants of disease. A clear understanding of basic epidemiologic concepts is essential to make full use of epidemiologic studies of the relationship between environmental exposures and health outcomes. The first purpose of this chapter is to define a core set of basic epidemiologic con-

73

cepts and study designs, with an emphasis on disease cluster investigations. The second purpose is to describe how epidemiology has been applied to the study of environmental exposures.

Environmental epidemiology is defined as "the study of the effect on human health of physical, biologic and chemical factors in the external environment. By examining specific populations or communities exposed to different ambient environments, it seeks to clarify the relationship between physical, biologic or chemical factors and human health" (National Research Council, 1991). Health outcomes of interest to the study of environmental epidemiology cover the spectrum of physical and mental illness and range from nonspecific signs and symptoms of disease, such as headaches and mucous membrane irritation, to injuries and chronic diseases, such as cancer. Environmental exposures that are the subject of study include numerous toxic substances such as lead, carbon monoxide, organophosphate pesticides and oxides of nitrogen, and physical agents such as radiation and noise.

The study of workplace exposures is of particular interest within the larger environmental health arena because chemical exposures found in occupational settings are generally at levels that are orders of magnitude higher than those found in the community setting. Therefore, if an association between the chemical and adverse health outcomes exists, it will most likely be uncovered in studies of working populations. On the other hand, community exposures that are generally of much lower concentration or intensity, usually exist 24 hours per day, 7 days per week. In addition, community members include more vulnerable segments of the population such as children, the elderly, and the disabled—groups often not part of the work force. All of these factors are taken into consideration when conducting a risk assessment of community exposures.

BASIC EPIDEMIOLOGIC CONCEPTS

Most if not all epidemiologic studies have as their goal the comparison of illness experience between two or more populations. This comparison, often referred to as a relative risk among exposed compared with unexposed populations, is based on disease frequencies and rates. Common measures of disease frequency include *prevalence* and *incidence*, with both expressed as a *rate*. Prevalence refers to the number of cases present in a population at a certain point or period in time. The number of autistic school-aged children among all school-aged children in Baltimore County, MD, on January 1, 2000, is an example of a prevalence rate. The numerator consists of all cases of disease (or other health cutcome) and the denominator is the population from which the cases were drawn. An incidence rate, by contrast, describes new cases of disease over a specified period of time, for example the number of cases of newly diagnosed breast cancer among women 45 to 54 years of age in Baltimore County, MD, in 2000. Incidence data are critical to the study of causes of disease. Prevalence data are useful for measuring disease burden in a community and projecting health care service needs.

Disease rates are calculated and then compared among differentially exposed groups of individuals to establish associations between exposure and health outcomes. For example, children living in U.S. homes where parents report smoking cigarettes have on average a rate of asthma of 30 per 100 children (30%) compared with a rate of 15 per 100 (15%) among children living in homes where no family member smokes. This particular example includes all children with asthma, not only newly diagnosed cases, and therefore is an example of disease prevalence. The next step in examining the relationship between exposure and disease is the calculation of the ratio of two rates to communicate the importance or magnitude of the risk associated with an exposure under study. For example, the *rate ratio* or *relative risk* of asthma among a hypothetical group of 200 children, half of whom were exposed to environmental tobacco smoke (ETS) is 30 per 100/15 per 100 or 2.0. A rate ratio of 2.0 is interpreted as a twofold or 100% increase in risk. These data are often presented in the form of a "2×2 table" (Table 7.1).

Having neatly assigned these children into categories of ETS exposed and ETS unexposed, it is important to note that *exposure assessment* within environmental epidemiologic studies is subject to imprecision or error.

TABLE 7.1 "2 X 2" Table: Rates and Ratios, Hypothetical Asthma Data

	Asthma	*No Asthma*
Environmental Tobacco Smoke (ETS) exposure	30	70
No ETS exposure	15	85

Prevalence rate (exposed) $= \dfrac{30}{100} = .30$ or 30%

Prevalence rate (unexposed) $= \dfrac{15}{100} = .15$ or 15%

Prevalence rate ratio $= \dfrac{30}{100} / \dfrac{15}{100} = 2.0$

Therefore, in order to collect the most accurate exposure data possible, epidemiologists usually collaborate with industrial hygienists, toxicologists, and/or environmental engineers. Exposure is characterized by the *concentration* and *duration* of exposure in an attempt to approximate the *dose*. Historically, a range of surrogate measures of dose has been used to classify workplace exposures. Figure 7.1 provides a hierarchy of the types of exposure measurement used in epidemiologic studies, ranging from those considered least to most precise.

For example, a very crude measure of a workplace chemical exposure might be obtained from company employment records that indicate that a particular study subject was employed in manufacturing during the period of interest. This type of exposure measurement would only tell us that this individual worked in the facility during the period of interest but would give no estimate of the duration or concentration of exposure to the chemicals under study. A far better measure would be a representative air sample of the chemical under study, taken at the breathing zone of the study subject. However, the most accurate measure of dose would be obtained by taking a biologic sample from the study subject and measuring the level of chemical in the sample such as through blood lead or urine metabolites of organophosphate insecticides. Unfortunately the availability of reliable

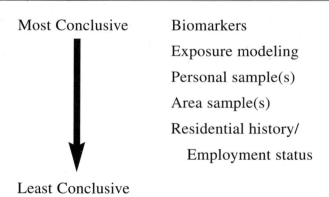

FIGURE 7.1 Exposure assessment.

and standard laboratory tests or biomarkers of exposure is limited to a small number of substances. However, much research and development in the area of chemical biomarkers is currently underway. In those cases where measurements of actual exposure are available from body fluids or from the air, water, or soil, they are reported in parts per million to parts per trillion of contaminant in the appropriate medium.

Most of our knowledge about the toxic effect of chemicals focuses on single chemicals whereas many, if not most, environmental threats consist of a mix of chemicals and, in many cases, a true chemical soup. Understanding the toxicity of mixed chemicals poses an additional challenge to exposure assessment. Understanding whether specific chemicals, when mixed, have an additive, synergistic, or other effect is currently the subject of much interest and inquiry.

Bias, another important concept in environmental epidemiology, is any deviation from truth in the collection, analysis, interpretation, publication, or review of data (Cummings and Lipscomb, 1998). Any bias in the measurement of exposure can result in the misclassification of subjects in the "2 X 2" table and ultimately lead to an incorrect or invalid estimate of the disease risk associated with the exposure under study.

A *confounding factor*, a source of study bias, is a variable that distorts the apparent effect of the risk factor of interest due to its association with both the risk factor and disease. For example, poverty is associated both with deteriorating lead-based paint and is a risk factor for childhood lead poisoning. Thus poverty is a potential confounding factor in any study of the association between lead-paint exposure and lead poisoning. To control for this bias, poverty must be measured and statistically adjusted for during data analysis.

EPIDEMIOLOGIC STUDY DESIGNS

Epidemiologic studies have historically been concerned with the cause of disease epidemics, usually an infectious agent. In recent years, however, epidemiologists have focused on understanding the underlying distribution of and risk factors for chronic diseases, including those that may have environmental causes. Study designs applied to the examination of chronic disease range from cluster investigation to experimental studies. Analytic designs, those that examine causal relationship such as cohort and case-control studies, are frequently used to study environmental exposures. Figure 7.2 lists study designs used to study environmental questions in order of their ability to detect causal relationship between exposures and disease.

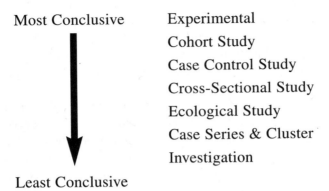

Most Conclusive

Experimental

Cohort Study

Case Control Study

Cross-Sectional Study

Ecological Study

Case Series & Cluster

Investigation

Least Conclusive

FIGURE 7.2 Epidemiology study design

The choice of a study design depends on several factors, including the prevalence of the exposure and the illness in the target population, the latency period between exposure and outcome of interest, and the level of knowledge of the exposure being studied. It is not uncommon for a study hypothesis such as this: "Is there a difference in the cancer incidence rate among pesticide-exposed children compared with unexposed children?" to be examined with the entire range of nonexperimental designs. The following discussion will provide an overview of the major types of study designs and an example of how each design has been applied to the study of an environmental health question.

CLUSTER INVESTIGATION

A *cluster investigation* is the evaluation of a reported excess of disease clustering in space and/or time. It is frequently conducted to study environmental exposures possibly associated with a perceived excess of disease. These investigations are often conducted in response to community concerns about an excess of cancer or birth defects (Brown, 1999; Caldwell, 1990). The well-documented investigation of childhood leukemia associated with contaminated well water in Woburn, MA in the late 1970s, featured in the best-selling novel and motion picture *A Civil Action*, is an example of such an investigation (Harr, 1996). Historically, cluster investigations of environmental exposures have rendered mostly negative or equivocal results. One reason for this is that it is difficult to detect an association between an environmental exposure and cancer among the size population that is often the subject of a cluster investigation, such as a neighborhood or community. This is particularly true if the cancer in question is relatively common. In the limited cases where clusters investigations have yield the most convincing results, the disease in question has been very rare and specific for the putative etiologic exposure. For example, polyvinyl chloride monomer, a chemical used to manufacture polyvinyl chloride (PVC) plastic was linked causally to an angiosarcoma of the liver, an extremely rare cancer, following an investigation of exposed workers (Forman, Bennett, Stafford, and Doll, 1985).

A recent survey of state health departments reported that approximately 1100 cluster investigation requests were made in 1997. Most requests were made by citizens, and no pattern emerged for the types of cancer or hazard suspected (Trumbo, 2000). Although cluster investigations are not a major epidemiologic study design, the frequency of these requests require that nurses play an important role in responding to community members' concerns about possible disease clusters.

Most cluster investigation requests are directed to state health department officials and staff, including public health nurses. As a result, states have taken the lead in conducting and developing methods to conduct such epidemiologic investigations. A number of states have published protocols for responding to these requests. In 1990, the Wisconsin Department of Health and Social Services published a comprehensive protocol for responding to disease cluster reports. Among the 141 cluster investigations they conducted between 1979 and 1990, none required further in-depth epidemiologic investigation beyond the eight stages described below. To determine the parameters of the investigation and if a true cluster exists, it is essential to *circumscribe the cluster*. Because nurses are often the public's first contact with health officials, they are most likely to be involved with the first stage of the study. This includes interviewing the primary informant for key information such as disease outcome, vital status of the cases, number of cases, age and gender of the cases, geographic location, time period during which the cluster was observed, and the suspected cause. This information is usually the basis for determining whether or not the cluster is likely to be associated with an identifiable exposure. If the cases of disease represent multiple diagnoses, it is less likely a cluster will be attributed to an environmental cause (Garfinkel, 1987). Other critical information to consider in determining whether to move beyond this initial stage is the age of the cases. Cancer risk increases with age. Therefore, the observation that many community members have cancer may reflect the increasing age of the population rather than a common environmental exposure. Childhood cancer clusters have been the subject of much concern and investigation because cancer is uncommon among children and therefore a clustering of childhood cancer may suggest an unusual event. In addition, it is important to recognize that the latency or time between the suspected exposure and cancer is usually at least five years and often more than 20 for adult cancers associated with workplace carcinogens. Finally, it is critical to collect information about the perceived length and concentration of exposure. In the event that investigators determine there is sufficient information to warrant further investigations, they should proceed with some or all of the following seven stages.

Case finding or ascertainment refers to a systematic review of various databases to identify all cases of the disease of concern in the prescribed geographical area and time. This step usually involves the review of death certificates, cancer incidence databases and other disease registries, medical records, and/or hospital discharge data. Not all states have a cancer incidence registry and even fewer states monitor birth defects. Where such data do exist, contributing to and ensuring complete reporting of births, cancer, and other chronic disease will contribute to future public health investigations of disease clusters. Nurses are often in a position to contribute their skills and expertise when opportunities for creating, strengthening, or improving such surveillance systems arise.

To assess the risk of an exposed versus an unexposed reference population the exposed population is first characterized by age, race, and gender next an appropriate reference or comparison population is identified and the associated disease rates calculated. The exposed population is usually defined by some geopolitical boundary, such as a census track or county; the reference group is frequently a different county or the state in which the exposed population resides. Next, *statistical tests are employed to analyze disease rates.* A standardized mortality or morbidity ratio (SMR) is often calculated to compare observed disease rates in the exposed population with the rate of disease that would be expected in a demographically similar population and to determine whether a statistical excess of disease exists. An SMR is calculated by comparing the observed disease rate in the study population with the expected rate. The expected rate is derived by applying the rates observed in the reference population to a hypothetical population of the same gender, age, and racial makeup as the study population. *Potential exposure is examined* by a review of existing environmental data, such as air monitoring data near a hazardous waste site (if available) and/or by the collection of additional monitoring data if there is reason to suspect that exposure continues. *Assessing the biologic plausibility* of a portended exposure–disease relationship is a critical step in establishing potential causality. *Determining cluster significance and need for further investigation* and *reporting results* are the final two steps in the Wisconsin protocol. However, regardless of whether the cluster investigation is completed after step 1 or step 8, results should be presented to the community. The nurse should have an active role in the preparation and communication of the study results. For a more thorough discussion of this protocol, see Fiore, Hanrahan, and Anderson (1990).

Because of the various challenges inherent in a cluster investigation, it is essential to communicate study limitation with concerned community members. They should be informed of the limited success of past investigations in identifying environmental causes of disease. Communities should be told that even if an excess number of cases is confirmed, as was the case in Missoula, MT, an environmental cause may not be found. In the event that no environmental cause is linked to a cluster, the community may benefit from the knowledge and reassurance that suspected environmental exposures do not appear to have caused the disease cluster. In addition, previous cluster investigations have provided the necessary justification to establish cancer or birth defect registries where they previously did not exist, to assist in monitoring future disease occurrence. Regardless of the course a cluster investigation takes, community members should be encouraged to be active participants in the process.

The next two study designs are examples of descriptive studies and as such are used to describe the relationship between environmental exposures and health outcomes, whether or not the relationship is causal in nature.

ECOLOGIC STUDY

An *ecologic study* is used in the field of environmental health to generate hypotheses about groups of exposures and health outcomes. The unique feature of an ecologic design, which is also its limiting factor, is that the unit of analysis is the community, rather than the individual. As such, ecologic studies do not allow for the determination of exposure status of individual cases. An ecologic design is frequently used to map cancer density in relation to industrial production and pollution. Griffith, Duncan, Riggan, and Pellom (1989) studied the relationship between hazardous waste sites associated with ground water pollution and cancer mortality for 13 major sites at the county level. The study identified significant associations between excess deaths and county hazardous waste sites for a number of cancers. The authors concluded that more definitive studies are needed to examine the associations reported in this analysis, but that hazardous waste site location may be used as an initial index of possible exposure to toxic chemicals.

CROSS-SECTIONAL STUDY

A cross-sectional study is a descriptive study design in which both exposure and disease are examined at the individual level and at a single point in time. This design is relatively efficient in time and cost while yielding essential descriptive information. Because both exposure and disease are measured at once, a cross-sectional study does not allow us to tell whether the exposure preceded or followed the disease. National surveys, such as the National Health and Nutrition Examination Survey (NHANES), provide critical descriptive health information and are examples of this type of study. Gergen, Fowler, Maurer, Davis, and Overpeck (1998) published data from the Third NHANES (1988 to 1994) that examined the effect of environmental tobacco smoke (ETS) on respiratory health in a national sample of children 2 months through 5 years of age. According to parental reports, approximately 38% of the children were presently exposed to ETS in the home. Nearly 24% of mothers reported smoking during pregnancy. Household exposure to ≥ 20 cigarettes a day or any prenatal smoking was associated with greater than a twofold increase in risk for chronic bronchitis, episodes of wheezing, and asthma.

CASE-CONTROL STUDY

Analytic studies are used to examine causal relationships between environmental exposures and disease. A case-control study, one example of an analytic study design, is the design of choice for studying rare diseases. In a case-control design, study groups are assembled on the basis of the presence or absence of the disease under study. This allows for the examination of multiple risk factors associated with the disease. The case-control study design is efficient in terms of cost and time and is used with increased frequency to study chronic disease. The major limitation of case-control study is the potential for bias in the selection of study subjects and exposure information related to the fact that the exposures under study have preceded the detection of the disease and assignment as a study case. In order to avoid such problems, a detailed study protocol, including a clear and concise case definition, is needed and great attention must be given to the selection of the control group. Numerous examples of case-control studies of environmental health questions are published in the biomedical literature. One example is the work of Pogoda and Preston-Martin (1997) that examined prenatal exposure to household pesticides among mothers of children with brain tumors (cases) and children without tumors (controls) in Los Angeles County, CA. The study found that among all women, the use of chemicals used in flea/tick products increased the risk of pediatric brain tumors by approximately 70%. A significant trend of increased risk with increased exposure was observed for the number of pets treated.

COHORT STUDY

A cohort study, the second type of analytic design, is the choice when studying a rare exposure. A cohort study, sometimes referred to as a prospective study, is a longitudinal study in which groups are assembled on the basis of the presence or absence of the exposure in question. Subjects are followed over time to determine if they develop the disease(s) being studied. The critical distinction and strength of a cohort study is that subjects are assigned to exposure groups prior to the development of the disease(s). As a result, their assignment to an exposure group should not be influenced by whether they have the disease or not. Limitations of a cohort design include the potential loss-to-follow-up of subjects because of the length of time they need to be followed and the cost of the study. Despite these limitations, the cohort study is a highly valued study design, especially critical to the study of rare occupational exposures. A cohort study is designed to mimic an experimental study, had one been feasible. A relevant example of a cohort study involving an environmental exposure is the work of Needleman, Schell, Bellinger, Leviton, and Allred (1990) that examined whether the effects of low-level lead exposure persisted among a cohort of young adults who had initially been studied as primary school children from 1975 through 1978. After 10 years of follow-up, neurobehavioral function was associated with the lead content of teeth shed at ages 6 and 7. Children who originally had dentin lead levels > 20 ppm had a sevenfold increase in their rate of dropping out of high school and a nearly sixfold rate of reading disability.

EXPERIMENTAL STUDY

Finally, the experimental study, or randomized clinical trial, is the gold standard of epidemiologic study designs. Comparability between study groups (those exposed and those unexposed to the treatment under study) is achieved through the random assignment of treatment to individual study subjects. This randomization of treatment leads to study findings that are relatively unbiased by factors that are difficult to completely control for with nonexperimental study designs. Limitations of experimental studies include the fact that ethical considerations often limit their use (i.e., it is unethical to purposefully expose individuals to potentially hazardous substances) and that randomized clinical trials are very costly to conduct. Hovell et al. (1994) provide an informative example of the application of an experimental design to the study of a intervention designed to minimize exposure to an environmental hazard, namely environmental tobacco smoke (ETS). They demonstrated a reduction of ETS exposure among asthmatic children following a behavioral medicine program to reduce asthmatic children's exposure to ETS in the home. Families in the study were randomly assigned to one of the following: a preventive medicine counseling group, a monitoring control group, or a usual treatment control group. Twelve months following the intervention, the experimental/counseling group sustained a 51% decrease in children's exposure to cigarettes in the home from all smokers, compared with a 15% decrease among usual care control subjects.

SUMMARY

Environmental epidemiology is a critical tool in the risk assessment of environmental hazards. Nurses can contribute significantly to this science in a number of roles, including that of study investigator, clinician, community advocate, and risk communicator. Protocols such as the one described to assist in the investigation of disease clusters are available to assist nurses in responding to concerns about possible environmental causes of disease in their community. Nurses' strong communication skills and political astuteness place them in an ideal position to advocate for communities that want to participate fully as subjects of such studies. They are also in an excellent position to enssure that community members' voices are heard and questions are answered, whether the questions are the subject of a disease cluster investigation or an in-depth epidemiologic study.

BIBLIOGRAPHY

Brown, A. M. (1999). Investigating clusters in the workplace and beyond. *Occupational Medicine (Lond) 49*(7), 443–447.

Caldwell, G. G. (1990). Twenty-two years of cancer cluster investigations at the Centers for Disease Control. *American Journal of Epidemiology, 132*(Suppl. 1), S43–47.

Cummings, S., & Lipscomb, J. A. (1998). *Epidemiology* [Television broadcast]. Childrens' Environmental Health Network/Public Health Institute, Emeryville, CA.

Fiore, B. J., Hanrahan, L. P., & Anderson, H. A. (1990). State health department response to disease cluster reports: A protocol for investigation. *American Journal of Epidemiology, 132*, (Suppl. 1):S14–22.

Forman, D., Bennett, B., Stafford, J., & Doll, R. (1985). Exposure to vinyl chloride and angiosarcoma of the liver: A report of the register of cases. *British Journal of Industrial Medicine, 42*, 750–753.

Garfinkel, L. (1987). Cancer clusters. *CA: A cancer Journal for Clinicians, 37*(1), 20–25.

Gergen, P. J., Fowler, J. A., Maurer, K. R., Davis, W. W., & Overpeck, M. D. (1998). The burden of environmental tobacco smoke exposure on the respiratory health of children 2 months through 5 years of age in the United States: Third national health and nutrition examination survey, 1998 to 1994. *Pediatrics, 101*(2), E8.

Griffith, J., Duncan, R., Riggan, W. B., & Pellom, A. C. (1989). Cancer mortality in U.S. counties with hazardous waste sites and ground water pollution. *Archives of Environmental Health, 44*(2), 69–74.

Harr, J. (1996). *A civil action.* Vintage Books, USA.

Hovell, M. F., Meltzer, S. B., Zakarian, J. M., Wahlgren, D. R., Emerson, J. A., Hofstetter, C. R., Leaderer, B. P., Meltzer, E. O., Zeiger, R. S., O'Connor, R. D., et al. (1994). Reduction of environmental tobacco smoke exposure among asthmatic children: A controlled trial. *Chest, 106*(2):440–446.

Merriam, G. (1998, February 28). *Missoulian*, pp. A1, A12.

National Research Council. (1991). *Environmental epidemiology: Public health and hazardous wastes.* Washington, DC: National Academy Press.

Needleman, H. L., Schell, A., Bellinger, D., Leviton, A., & Allred, E. (1990). The long-term effects of exposure to low doses of lead in childhood: An eleven-year follow-up report. *The New England Journal of Medicine, 322*(2), 83–88.

Pogoda, J. M., & Preston-Martin, S. (1997). Household pesticides and risk of pediatric brain tumors. *Environmental Health Perspectives, 105*(11), 1214–1220.

Trumbo, C. W. (2000). Public requests for cancer cluster investigations: A survey of state health departments. *American Journal of Public Health, 90*(8), 1300–1302.

CHAPTER 8

Finding Information About Chemicals in Our Environment

Barbara Sattler

M ost of us have read labels on food packages. We take it for granted that we should have access to the information we seek, such as the ingredients, the nutritional breakdown, and the calorie count. The requirement for food labeling was one of the first major "right-to-know" laws in the U.S. regarding chemicals to which we are exposed. Food labeling laws were passed in response to concerns about the artificial coloring, preservatives, and other additives found in processed foods.

Concerns about chemicals in our environment continued to be raised throughout the 1960s. Rachel Carson's seminal work, *Silent Spring*, brought to light new connections between exposures to man-made chemicals (particularly DDT) and their negative impact in nature. Carson's work helped to launch the modern-day environmental movement. A flurry of environmental and political activism in the 1960s resulted in the 1970 creation of the Environmental Protection Agency (EPA) and the Occupational Safety and Health Administration (WHA), along with a significant number of new regulations about chemical exposures.

By the mid-1970s, many people realized that the occupational and environmental health regulations were still inadequate. There was no legal mechanism for access to basic information, such as the names of the chemicals to which workers were exposed or that were emitted into the air. If you were a worker who developed a rash on your hands from working with a new cleaning solvent and wanted the name of its chemical ingredients in order to discuss the problem with your health care provider, you had no legal access to those names. If you were a school principal whose school was next door to a smoke stack, you would have had no legal right to know the names of the chemicals the stack emitted.

As a result of these legal shortcomings, two sets of sometimes overlapping advocates developed campaigns to address information needs. The campaign to give workers the right to know about the hazardous chemicals with which they work was led primarily by organized labor and public health/occupational health professionals. The push for the right to know about emissions and effluent (pollution discharged into our water ways) was launched primarily by the environmentalist community, with support from the public health community. Both campaigns were adamantly opposed by the chemical manufacturing industry. Despite this opposition, additional "right-to-know" policies have been instituted in recent years.

WORKERS' RIGHT TO KNOW

During the Carter administration, a standard was proposed that would require the labeling of hazardous chemicals in the workplace. This proposed rule was withdrawn when Reagan took office and a strong message was given to organized labor that the labeling standard was not a priority for the Reagan administration. As a result, organized labor worked at the state level. Within a two-year period, half the states had passed worker right-to-know legislation, despite a substantial effort by the chemical industry to defeat these campaigns. However, this resulted in many slightly differing statutes that had different requirements of the chemical manufacturing industry. In response to these sometimes conflicting requirements, the chemical manufacturing industry asked the Reagan administration for a standardized requirement for workplace labeling and access to information on hazardous chemicals that would supersede the states' statutes. The Reagan administration quickly responded and in 1983, the Federal Hazard Communication Standard (worker "Right to Know") was promulgated.

There are several key elements to the standard:

1. Chemical manufacturers must determine whether the chemicals they are producing pose a hazard on the basis of human health threat or physical threat such as flammability or explosiveness.
2. Once chemicals are determined to pose a threat, chemical manufacturers must create a material safety data sheet (MSDS) for each chemical and must distribute it to all downstream users of their product.
3. All hazardous chemicals that are used in the workplace must be labeled and there must be a MSDS for each chemical.
4. Workers must have access to the MSDS.
5. All workers must be trained about the hazardous chemicals with which they work. The training must include a full explanation of the standard

and the hazards, including health hazards of the chemicals that are specific to their workplaces.

6. When new chemicals are introduced or a worker is transferred to a new area, information about any hazards must be provided by the employer.
7. Employers must keep the MSDS in an accessible area of the workplace.
8. Employers must keep a written "Hazard Communication Standard" plan that is accessible to the employees.

In all instances, wherever employees have access to information, a union representing the employees has access to the same information.

Almost 20 years after the promulgation of the standard, problems continue to exist in providing meaningful information to workers about the chemicals with which they work. The first and most important problem is that the MSDS on which much of the information transfer is predicated is an extremely faulty tool. There are approximately 500,000 products that have MSDSs. The problems with MSDSs are many.

READABILITY AND COMPREHENSIBILITY

Regrettably, the average American reads at a sixth-grade reading level. The average MSDS is written at a grade 13 reading level, meaning that one should have a year of college in order to read and fully understand a MSDS. Additionally, when comprehensibility studies have been performed, concerns are raised. When a set of randomly selected MSDSs was reviewed by unionized workers, who spoke English as a first language and had received health and safety training, the workers were unable to comprehend 40% of the information on the MSDS. Given that many American workers do not speak English as a first language and/or have literacy problems, the study results probably reflect a best-case scenario for comprehensibility, and actual comprehensibility is probably significantly worse. This creates a major barrier to realizing the spirit of the worker right-to-know law—providing information with which workers can make informed decisions about their health and safety as they pertain to potentially hazardous chemicals in their workplaces.

FORMAT

When the Hazard Communication Standard was proposed, the chemical manufacturers wanted flexibility in the format for the MSDS. As a result, the Standard did not dictate a format and myriad MSDSs entered the market, all with different formats depending on their manufacturers. One-page and 32-page MSDSs could be found. In addition to size differences, the placement of information varied. On one MSDS the emergency response information might be found on the first page and on another it might be found on the third page. There is also no requirement for how to present units of measure; temperature may be reflected in centigrade or Fahrenheit, weight in metric or U.S. units.

SCIENCE LITERACY

The vast majority of American workplaces do not have a trained health and safety person. The interpretation of information on the MSDS and decisions that may impact health and safety are made by average folks. Although the decisions may be made in good faith, they may have no scientific foundation and risks may be posed. Anatomy and physiology are not taught in standard high-school curricula. More often than not, neither employees nor employers have the scientific background to fully understand the human health effects section of the MSDS, not to mention the information about choosing a NIOSH-approved respirator the conversion of metric to U.S. units.

ACCURACY

When the Occupational Safety and Health Administration commissioned a study to determine the accuracy of the health information on MSDS the results were alarming. Only 11% of the 150 randomly selected MSDSs were accurate on all of the basic health information parameters. Although the chemical manufacturers are responsible for presenting full and accurate information, there has not been a systematic inventory or sanctioning for inaccurate information presented by the manufacturer.

STATE OF THE SCIENCE

Manufacturers of chemicals are not responsible for toxicity testing unless the chemicals or mixtures will be used as food, drugs, or cosmetics. If the chemical will not be used for those purposes, the chemical manufacturer is responsible for reviewing the existing literature and reporting this on the MSDS. Unfortunately, very little research has been done on chemical mixtures so the data is often not available. When a worker experiences a health effect and does not find the health effect listed on the MSDS, he may assume that the chemical could not possibly cause the problem that he is experiencing. But the reality is that the relationship between exposure to that chemical and those symptoms has probably never been explored. The absence of data does not mean the absence of a relationship.

COMPLIANCE ACTIVITIES

The most common violation cited by OSHA is the Hazard Communication Standard. The most common area of noncompliance is the training. Although most workplaces compile the MSDS, most do not provide the required training. When the Government Accounting Office surveyed employers around the country, they discovered that 58% of them were not in compliance and that 30% had never heard of the Hazard Communication Standard.

The labor movement has been consistently supportive of workplace health and safety and has created a number of opportunities for union members to learn about hazardous chemicals exposure. Health and safety committees provide a structure in many unionized workplaces for workers to become better educated about exposure, as well as opportunities to assess information about, discuss, and address unhealthy and/or unsafe conditions.

Occupational health nurses should be actively involved in the implementation of the Hazard Communication Standard in their workplaces. In all workplaces, the Standard should be implemented (hospital settings, clinics, schools, etc.). Nurses can access information using the Standard to help make informed decisions about their health and safety in their individual workplaces. Nurses can also use the Standard to help their patients access information, if a workplace exposure is suspected of contributing to patients' health problems.

COMMUNITY RIGHT TO KNOW

In 1986, when the Superfund legislation was being reauthorized, citizens were looking to expand right-to-know opportunities for community members. (See chapter 16 on hazardous waste for more information on Superfund.) The resulting reauthorization created the 1996 statute Emergency Planning and Community Right to Know Act (EPCRA). This legislation identified a list of 600 chemicals that must be reported to the EPA if they are emitted into the air or water beyond a weight-based action level. This information is to be made available to all citizens. Once reported, this information constitutes the Toxic Release Inventory (TRI), which is publicly available through the EPA. Initially, the EPA provided the information to area libraries, then via CD-ROM; it is now available on the web. The environmental organization Environmental Defense has published these data on a unique, user-friendly website (www.scorecard.org) in which it provides information on the health risks associated with the reported chemicals, information on the chemical-producing entities, and guidance for further action and advocacy.

The Registry for Toxic Effects of Chemicals has toxicity data available on more than 70,000 chemicals and chemical mixtures. Only 600 chemicals are required to be reported under the EPCRA law. The list must be expanded to include a wider range of toxic chemicals and the action level for reporting must be lowered. Nurses can join the environmental and public health advocates who are requesting expansion of the list of reportable chemicals.

The EPCRA requirements mandate that facilities that have MSDSs for chemicals held above certain quantities submit either copies of their MSDSs or a list of MSDS chemicals to the State Emergency Response Commission (SEPRC), the Local Emergency Planning Committee (LEPC), and the local fire department. If a list of MSDSs is submitted, the following information must be included about each chemical: acute health effects, chronic health effects, fire hazards, sudden release of pressure hazard, and reactive hazard (the latter three pieces of information are most important to hazardous materials responders and firefighters). This information is then available to the public from the State and Local Emergency Response Committees.

SERCs and LEPCs are required under the Emergency Planning and Community Right to Know Act. (Since 9/11 access to information is shifting, sometimes making it more difficult for community members to obtain information on chemicals stored or released in their own neighborhoods.

What Are SERCs and LEPCs?

The governor of each state designates a *State Emergency Response Commission (SERC)*. The SERCs, in turn, designate local emergency planning districts and appoint *Local Emergency Planning Committees (LEPCs)* for each district. The SERC supervises and coordinates the activities of the LEPCs, establishes procedures for receiving and processing public requests for information collected under the Emergency Planning and Community Right to Know Act, and reviews local emergency response plans.

The LEPC membership must include, at a minimum, local officials including the police, fire, civil defense, public health, transportation, and environmental professionals, as well as representatives of facilities subject to the emergency planning requirements, community groups, and the media. The LEPCs must develop an emergency response plan, review it at least annually, and provide information about chemicals in the community.

When nurses assess an individual or a community's health status, they should be aware of the potential ambient air exposures and contaminants that may be found in the community's water—both drinking water and recreational water. The community right-to-know laws provide access to some of this information. They also provide an existing infrastructure of public health, environment, and community members who are identifying the chemical hazards in the immediate community and the potential for chemical-related fires, explosions, leaks, and transportation accidents. Every community in the U.S. should have an LEPC. Call the local fire department to find out about your LEPC.

CHEMICAL RISK MANAGEMENT PLANS

When the Clean Air Act was reauthorized in 1990, a new directive required the employers of workplaces in which there are hazardous chemicals to predict the possible ways in which there could be an accidental spill, leak, transportation accident, or other hazardous chemical-related event that would expose workers or the community. Congress required industrial sites that use extremely hazardous substances to disclose worst-case accident scenarios as part of Risk Management Plans (RMP) under the Clean Air Act. These RMPs describe potential hazards, plan emergency response, and assure workers and the public that safe design and operations will prevent an "American Bhopal." In addition to identifying the potential for exposure incidents, employers are supposed to provide a discussion of the methods by which such events are being avoided, as well as the contingencies for response should an accidental release or spill occur.

Through disclosure, Congress intended to create awareness among officials and the general public to save lives, prevent pollution, and protect property from chemical accidents. As Congress directed, the EPA is collecting this information. However, the intended public access and dissemination have been thwarted by a successful industry argument that public accessibility to this information would create a terrorist threat. They argue that publicizing worst-case scenarios will lead terrorists to target their facilities, and that keeping this information off the Internet will keep us safe. Many advocates for public disclosure find this claim nothing less than an industry ploy to prevent access to information about the possible hazardous chemical scenarios in our nation's communities.

DRINKING WATER AND THE RIGHT TO KNOW

Access to information about water is provided under two statutes: the Clean Water Act and the Safe Drinking Water Act. The Clean Water Act was promulgated to protect the nation's waterways and the Safe Drinking Water Act protects drinking water from source water to tap. Through the Safe Drinking Water Act, those who purchase water from a water provider have the right to know what is in their drinking water. Annually, as part of the drinking water right-to-know regulations, the water utility must provide a consumer confidence report listing the contaminants (chemical, biological, and radiological) that have exceeded EPA standards within the last year, the potential health effects, and their probable sources. The EPA requires testing of approximately 80 chemicals and agents. More details of this program can be found in chapter 12, on drinking water.

Industrial contaminants that are released into the water are reportable, based on the chemical and its quantity, under the right-to-know component of the Superfund Amendments and the Reauthorization Act (SARA, 1986). SARA requires polluters to report certain effluent and emissions. This information is available on the EPA web site by zip code at www.epa.gov. These data provide the basis for information on the web site www.scorecard.org, an excellent source for community environmental assessments.

FOOD AND AGRICULTURAL PROCESSES AND THE RIGHT TO KNOW

In 1906, the first Pure Foods Act and Meat Inspection Act began the modern era of American food and consumer protection. In 1938, the Federal Food, Drug and Cosmetic Act replaced the 1906 statute and required a label on processed, packaged food to include the name of the food, its net weight, and the name and address of the manufacturer. On certain products, ingredients were also required. It was not until 1973 that nutritional labeling began and in 1984, sodium content was required to be added to the label.

The latest installment of labeling statutes is the 1990 Nutrition Labeling and Education Act, which requires nutritional labeling for most foods (except meat and poultry) and authorizes the use of nutrient content claims and appropriate FDA-approved claims. Definitions were established for labeling language such as "fat-free," "lite," and "healthy." The health claims that can be used on labels are further regulated. Claims for ten relationships between a nutrient or a food and the risk of a disease or health-related condition are now allowed. The relationships that have been established are

- calcium intake and reduced osteoporosis
- fat intake and risk of cancer
- saturated fat and cholesterol and increased risk for coronary heart disease
- fiber-containing grains and decreased risk of cancer
- fruits, vegetables, and grains (that contain fiber) and decreased risk of heart disease
- sodium and hypertension
- fruits and vegetables and cancer
- folic acid and neural tube defects
- dietary sugar alcohols and dental caries
- soluble fiber from certain foods and heart disease

Under the label's "Nutritional Facts" panel, manufacturers are required to provide information on certain ingredients. The mandatory (underlined) and voluntary components and the order in which they must appear are:

- total calories
- calories from fat
- calories from saturated fat
- total fat
- saturated fat
- polyunsaturated fat
- monounsaturated fat
- cholesterol
- sodium
- potassium
- total carbohydrate
- dietary fiber
- soluble fiber
- insoluble fiber
- sugars
- sugar alcohol
- protein
- vitamin A
- percent of vitamin A present as beta-carotene
- vitamin C

- calcium
- iron
- other essential vitamins and minerals

At the time this book was written, there were no federal laws requiring that the chemicals in animal feed be identified in the food products. For example, when hormones or antibiotics are added to beef, pork, or poultry feed, there is no requirement that this be indicated on the food labels. Several states are entertaining the passage of laws to require reporting of the use of antibiotics or hormones in feed. The U.S. Department of Agriculture, the federal agency responsible for this issue, is currently considering what to do in light of an increasingly concerned citizenry. There are formidable agricultural, chemical, and pharmaceutical industries that are currently opposing such reporting requirements.

Another significant emerging right-to-know issue is genetically engineered (GE) or genetically modified (GM) foods. During the last decade, genes from bacteria, viruses, foreign plants, and animals have been inserted into corn, soybeans, potatoes, tomatoes, squash, papayas, and a host of other species. Already about 50% of the soy produced in the U.S. is genetically modified. There is an emerging literature concerning this issue. An extensive bibliography and resources for activists can be found at the end of the document *50 Harmful Effects of Genetically Modified Foods* (www.peoplesearth.org/50harm.htm).

PESTICIDES IN SCHOOLS AND THE RIGHT TO KNOW

As of 1999, twenty-two states required signs to be posted when pesticides are applied on school grounds and nine states require written notification of school employees and parents when pesticide applications are to be made in schools. The type of notification varies by state. National policies have been proposed but not yet adopted. The National Coalition Against the Misuse of Pesticides (NCAMP) tracks pesticide legislation and published the report, *The Schooling of State Pesticide Laws*, a document that identifies state and local pesticide statutes and ordinances (www.ncamp.org).

When examining each state's pesticide laws, NCAMP looked at five safety measures to determine whether the laws addressed children's health protection. These measures included the presence of restricted spray (buffer) zones to address chemicals drifting into schoolyards from nearby applications, the posting of signs for indoor and outdoor pesticide applications, prior written notification of pesticide use, prohibitions against application of pesticides in certain places and at certain times, and requirements for a strong integrated pest management program to limit the use of certain toxic materials. Thirty states have policies that include at least one of these measures. Some local governments have their own pesticide policies in place for schools (Environmental Health Perspectives [EHP], 1999).

THE RIGHT TO KNOW AND THE RIGHT TO UNDERSTAND

Conceptually, we all understand why it is important to provide information about potentially hazardous chemicals. However, even as we succeed in making increasing amounts of information available, we may not be providing the necessary tools and a context in which workers and community members can sufficiently understand the information. If our goal is to provide information with which to make safe and healthful decisions, we have to look at occupational and environmental health and safety as it is presented in our K–12 and higher educational institutions. We know that nurses receive almost no information on these issues, and unfortunately the same is true for our general citizenry. Occupational and environmental health and safety have not been recognized and valued sufficiently in our curricula, resulting in significant deficits in our ability to translate the risk information into healthy actions. The belief that everything is hazardous and we all have to die from something is an uninformed conviction that can paralyze individuals from engaging in safer and healthier practices and choices in their homes, communities, schools, and workplaces. This deficit in our understanding precludes our ability to consider alternative products, processes, or home/work practices that could help us reduce our exposures to toxic chemicals.

In addition to the educational deficits, there are other issues that may hinder people from acting on information when it is provided. Some are economic. If a mother who is nursing a child discovers that there are contaminants in her water, she may not know the appropriate measures to take to minimize or eliminate the contaminants. Should she use bottled water? Purchase a filter? Should she use tap water to bathe her newborn? Can the contaminant enter the body through the skin? But perhaps more significantly, can she afford the alternatives to tap water?

In non-union workplaces, exercising health and safety rights is not always a simple matter. There is a thin veil of job protection in most private sector jobs and workers are well aware of this fact. Raising health and safety issues and making demands for protection are often sacrificed for job security. These issues raise the question of how we learn about environmental and occupational health and safety, including how we access information and advocate for health and safety. It is not currently contained in K–12 education and there is no other systematic way in which communities learn about these issues. Environmentalist groups, unions, and public health advocacy and education organizations fill some of the gaps, but by increasing the nursing profession's role in this arena, our communities will have another effective resource for information and support. Nurses are uniquely situated to help steer these environmental health questions and help provide answers. But first and foremost, *we* must be educated about the issues.

BIBLIOGRAPHY

Carson, R. ( ). *Silent Spring*.

EHP. (1999). Protecting schools from pesticides, *Environews Forum, Environmental Health Perspectives, 107*, 400.

IFIC. (1998). History of food development. *Food Insight*, July/August.

Kurtzweil, P. (2001). Good reading for good eating. US *Food and Drug Administration* Website: www.vm.cfsan.fda.gov/~dms/fdlaeel2.html#milesto.

National Coalition Against the Misuse of Pesticides. (2001). *The schooling of state pesticide laws* (www.ncamp.org).

CHAPTER 9

Risk Assessment and Risk Management of Environmental Exposures

Jane Lipscomb

The topics of risk assessment and risk management, broadly defined, encompass most if not all of environmental health. The risk assessment side of the equation includes the basic and applied sciences involved in determining the level of the risk posed by a substance or situation. Risk management, on the other hand, involves those actions on the part of the affected individuals, government officials, health professionals, and the public designed to minimize this risk. In addition to the engineering controls described later in this chapter, this includes strategies for risk communication and advocacy described elsewhere in the book.

RISK ASSESSMENT

Risk is the probability of an undesirable health outcome arising from exposure to a hazard. Risk is a function of hazard and dose, with hazard a measure of the intrinsic ability of the stressor to cause harm and dose the amount of the stressor delivered to the person, organism, or ecosystem National Research Council (NRC, 1983). *Risk assessment*, in the context of environmental health, has several different meanings. In its broadest sense, risk assessment is the characterization of the potential adverse health effects of human exposures to environmental hazards (NRC). Risk assessment, in regulatory terms, refers to the use of all available scientific information, usually a combination of epidemiologic, animal toxicologic, and in vitro data, to develop estimates of the risks to the potentially exposed populations. Mathematical models are used to convert these biologic data into regulatory action. Risk assessment allows investigators to extrapolate among different human populations or from laboratory animals to humans. It should be noted that the science of risk assessment is very complex and in a continuous state of flux as science advances (Goldman, 2000).

The process of risk assessment includes the following four steps: hazard identification, dose–response assessment, exposure assessment, and risk characterization.

Hazard identification relies on human epidemiologic data, animal bioassay data, and other supporting data, such as cellular or biochemical information, which are analyzed in a weight-of-the-evidence approach to determine the potential of a substance to cause harm. The amount and quality of these data vary from substance to substance. Human data, the most desirable type, is often limited, so many risk assessments are based primarily on animal data. However, the risks associated with many occupational hazards and several environmental hazards have been described and quantified by epidemiologic study. For example, decades of study of the human health effects of both workplace and community lead exposure has served as a basis for current regulatory actions limiting lead exposure. In the case of the chemical dioxin, a combination of epidemiologic and animal studies has contributed to our understanding of the risk associated with exposure. In other cases, epidemiologic data are nonexistent and hazard identification may rely solely on animal studies. This is the case in those rare instances in which the the EPA, through its "Premanufacture Notification" (PMN) for new chemicals, requires that chemicals be actually tested before they are manufactured. EPA's justification for such a requirement is usually based on the fact that the structure of the new chemical is similar to a previously identified hazardous substance (Goldman, 2000).

Establishing a *dose–response* relationship in human or animal studies, in other words, demonstrating that the risk increases with increasing dose, is a primary criterion for establishing causality. The science behind a dose–response assessment differs for carcinogens and noncarcinogens. Risk assessment of carcinogens has a long history, with several national and international bodies established to evaluate and rate the carcinogenicity of chemicals. Risk assessment of noncarcinogens is a less well-established science. Historically, the assumption on which dose–response assessments have been based stated that for noncancer health effects, a threshold exists below which there is no risk. Conversely, there was no threshold for cancer endpoints. In other words, exposure to any level of a cancer-causing agent was thought to have a biologic effect, and therefore no level of exposure to a carcinogen was considered acceptable. These assumptions are under increased scrutiny as the science of risk assessment advances. Regardless of the health endpoint, quantitative risk assessment, assume that the dose–response curve is linear at low doses and starts at zero. Ideally, dose–response data exist and support the causal link between a hazard and health risk. The absence of a dose– response does not eliminate the possibility of a causal relationship but it does require an alternative explanation.

Third, *exposure assessment* involves the measurement of the amount of the chemical or other harmful substance to which a population is exposed with a goal of estimating dose. Dose is a function of the concentration of the chemical and the duration of exposure. Studies of environmental exposures frequently rely on measurements of the ambient rather than an individual's environment, therefore yielding very nonspecific data regarding individual or even neighborhood exposure. As a consequence, the actual dose of a particular chemical delivered to an individual or population is usually unknown and thus, for regulatory purposes, estimates of reasonable high-end exposures are made. The exception to this is where biologic indices of exposure exist. For example, the availability of indices such as blood lead or organophosphate metabolites in urine greatly enhance this step of the risk assessment process. Unfortunately, standardized biomarkers of exposure are currently available for only a limited number of substances.

Finally, *risk characterization* involves estimating the public health or environmental impact of the problem based on knowledge of characteristics of the population at risk. This step attempts to take into consideration the range of risk profiles in a potentially exposed population including the most vulnerable segments of the population. It is critical that scientific uncertainty be made clear at this stage.

Risk assessment, in general public health terms, has a much broader definition and includes individual and community level assessment, both of which are described elsewhere in this book. In addition to determining the nature and magnitude of the risk associated with a community's exposure to an environmental hazard, an assessment of a community's resources, including its cohesiveness and leadership, should be part of this more comprehensive risk assessment.

RISK MANAGEMENT

Risk management is the part of the equation where nurses can make their most significant contribution. It is the process of evaluating alternative strategies for reducing risk and prioritizing or selecting among them (NRC,

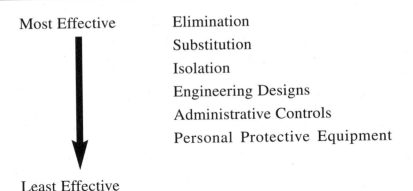

Most Effective   Elimination

Substitution

Isolation

Engineering Designs

Administrative Controls

Personal Protective Equipment

Least Effective

FIGURE 9.1 Industrial hygiene: hierarchy of control.

1983). Risk management strategies often involve policy development, which may include regulatory, legislative, and/or voluntary options, and may be targeted at the local, state, national, or international level. The adoption of any community-centered risk management strategy involves numerous forms of advocacy, discussed elsewhere in the book.

Environmental engineering, although less familiar to nurses, is a critical science in risk management. Engineering and industrial hygiene strategies to control exposure to environmental hazards offer useful models for selecting among alternative management options. The industrial hygiene "hierarchy of controls" model, a framework for the control of occupational hazards (Fig. 9.1, p. xx) describes a range of control measures available to reduce workplace exposures. Control options are ranked beginning with the most effective strategies, those that involve changes to the work process and/or environment, and proceed to those less effective options or quick fixes. Often these quick fixes are employed until more effective controls become available. According to this model, substitution of a hazardous substance with one less hazardous should be considered the first approach to hazard reduction. When substitution is not feasible, isolating the worker/community member from the hazard is a second line of control, followed by such engineering controls as local exhaust ventilation of hazardous fumes or dust from the breathing zone of a worker. Next in the hierarchy are administrative controls that include policies and procedures for limiting exposure to hazards and training of workers. Finally, personal protective equipment, such as respirators, can be used when higher-level controls are unavailable, but they should be viewed as a temporary measure (Smith and Schneider, 2000). The theoretical basis for the "hierarchy of controls" is that it is much more effective to make changes to the environment to reduce exposure, rather than rely on personal behavior change especially involuntary exposure found in the workplace.

A current and relevant example of the application of the hierarchy of controls to reduce needlestick injuries among health care providers can be found in the Needlestick Safety and Prevention Act. Effective April 18, 2001, the Act revised the 1991 OSHA bloodborne pathogen standard to require employers to select safer needle devices as they become available and to involve employees in identifying and choosing the devices. Safer needle devices, a form of engineering control, have been available for more than a decade. However, without the force of the new law, health care workers have been forced to rely on a combination of administrative controls and personal protective equipment namely universal precautions, to protect themselves from the 600,000 to 800,000 needlestick injuries incurred by U.S. health care workers annually (Henry and Campbell, 1995). As a consequence, protection against often deadly needlesticks has been dependent on the "safe practice" of the overworked and overextended nurses working under the most unpredictable of circumstances. This is despite the fact that the technology to allow them to perform their jobs safely and effectively is available. The use of conventional needles in the health care environment has been compared to the use of unguarded machinery decades ago in the industrial workplace. The Needlestick Safety Act is also a clear example of where industry did not act voluntarily to protect workers from the risk of needlestick injuries, and regulatory action was essential to the overall risk management program. Within the context of community exposures to environmental hazards, a similar hierarchy can be described.

Reduction of pollution at its source, also known as source reduction, should clearly be the goal of any environmental risk management strategy. Waste minimization should be viewed as a second line of defense against environmental degradation. Reuse and recycling, although an important and laudable risk management strategy, is further down the list of desirable measures, along with emissions control and, finally, waste clean-up. The Health Care Without Harm campaign, described in chapter 5 of this book, provides an excellent example of the application of this risk management hierarchy to the problem of mercury pollution. The availability and use of mercury thermometers and other mercury containing medical devices are widespread in U.S. hospitals, despite the fact that the negative effects on human health of mercury have been recognized for nearly a century. Acceptable alternatives have been available for decades. One of the primary goals of the HCWH campaign is the replacement of mercury-containing equipment with these widely available substitutes.

Risk management should include the highest level of control feasible, even when such control may force the development of new technology. It should be noted that any successful risk management program will include hazard control at a number of levels. For example, education of all involved parties about the nature of the risk, the costs and benefits of proposed risk management strategies, and how they will be impacted by the various options is an essential part of any program. Nurses should play a central role in such education efforts.

Community members must be active partners in any decision making about risk management options. Community organizing and coalition building are often essential to building a community position on a particular risk management plan. Nurses have a central role to play in this type of community building and often must advocate for community involvement in both the risk assessment and management process. Community-based actions have been responsible for the success of many environmental health protection campaigns. For example, nurses, other health care workers, and their collective bargaining units were solely responsible for the highly successful needlestick prevention campaign that culminated in the passage of the Needlestick Safety and Prevention Act.

Legal remedies, such as recent class-action lawsuits against the lead pigment industry for the public health costs associated with lead poisoning and lead abatement, may be used to manage risk in combination with the above strategies. More nurses are needed to fill the role of technical or clinical experts and/or community advocates in such lawsuits.

The risk management selection process necessarily requires the use of value judgments on such issues as the acceptability of risk and the reasonableness of the costs of controlling the hazard (NRC, 1983). Ultimately, it is the public, as individuals and through our elected officials, who defines what is an acceptable risk relative to environmental hazards. The way we have defined acceptable risk differs based on who is at risk and what is the source of this risk. In the U.S. we strive to control exposures to a level that will have a risk of anywhere from 1 death in 100,000 to one in one million population. The Superfund statute includes an acceptable lifetime cancer risk of 1 in 10,000. By contrast, workplace standards, as determined by the Supreme Court in a controversial and divided majority opinion in an industry challenge to the OSHA benzene standard, argued that OSHA is obligated to regulate only "significant risks" and it offered a sixfold range for guidance as to what constitutes a significant risk. It stated that a risk of death of 1 in 1,000 was clearly significant, whereas a risk of 1 in 1 billion was clearly not so. The implications of the benzene decision for subsequent standards reflect the political and philosophical leaning of a particular OSHA administration (Ashford, 2000). As a case in point, in 1996, OSHA promulgated a standard to protect workers from exposure to 1,3-butadiene, a chemical used in the production of rubber for the tire industry. Butadiene has been association with an increased risk of leukemia among exposed workers. The permissible exposure limit (PEL) established for workplace exposures to 1,3-butadiene was based on a risk of 8 cancer deaths in 1,000 workers (OSHA, 29 CRF–1910.1051).

Finally, an important concept in the management of environmental risks is the Precautionary Principle. Representatives to the 1992 United Nations Conference on Environmental and Development declared that "In order to protect the environment, the precautionary approach shall be widely applied by States according to their capability. Where there are threats of serious or irreversible damage, lack of scientific certainty shall not be used as a reason for postponing cost-effective measures to prevent environmental degradation" (United Nations Conference, 1992).

BIBLIOGRAPHY

Ashford, N. (2000). Government regulations in occupational health and safety. In B. S. Levy, & D. H. Wegman (Eds.), *Occupational health: Recognizing and preventing work-related disease and injury* (pp. 211–236). Philadelphia: Lippincott, Williams & Wilkins.

Goldman L. R. (2000). Environmental health. In B. S. Levy, & D. H. Wegman (Eds.) *Occupational health: Recognizing and preventing work-related disease and injury* (pp. 51–98). Philadelphia: Lippincott, Williams & Wilkins.

Henry K., & Campbell, S. (1995). Needlestick/sharp injuries and HIV exposure among health care workers: National estimate based on U.S. hospitals. *Minnesota Medicine, 78,* 1765–1768.

National Research Council. (1983). *Risk assessment in the federal government: Managing the process.* Washington DC: National Academy Press.

Smith, T. J., & Schneider, T. (2000). Occupational hygiene. In B. S. Levy, & D. H. Wegman (Eds.). *Occupational health: Recognizing and preventing work-related disease and injury* (pp. 161–171). Philadelphia: Lippincott, Williams & Wilkins.

The United Nations Conference on Environment and Development. (1992). *Rio declaration on environment and development, principle 15*. Rio de Janeiro, Brazil: United Nations.

CHAPTER 10

Risk Communication

Barbara Sattler

In health care we are often asked about risk. Questions are posed in terms of "chances": What are the chances that my husband will recover sight after the surgery? What are the chances of developing cancer if you smoke? What people are really asking is: What is the risk of a health outcome based on an exposure: in the first instance the "exposure" is a medical procedure, in the second the "exposure" is the inhalation of cigarette smoke. The answer to these questions is often expressed in math terms: You have a one in a hundred chance that this procedure will not work or a one in a hundred chance of getting cancer if you engage in a certain lifestyle.

A whole field of practice and inquiry has developed around communication that is expressly related to environmental exposures and risk communication. When environmental health outcomes are of concern, risk communication combines both the art of communication and the science that we know, and sometimes even more importantly, the science that we do not yet know. Risk communication involves the "purposeful exchange of information between interested parties about environmental risks" (Environmental Protection Agency, 1990) The National Research Council (1989) has a more comprehensive definition.

> Risk communication is an interactive process of exchange of information and opinion among individuals, groups, and institutions. It involves multiple messages about the nature of risk and other messages, not strictly about risk, that express concerns, opinions, or reactions to risk messages or to legal and institutional arrangements for risk management.

Environmental health risks are often hard to define. The exposures may be difficult to characterize; the exposed population may be very diverse in age, culture, and many other important variables; our exposures will always include multiple chemicals because it is the nature of our "environments" (whereas most scientific investigation is primarily about individual chemicals and rarely chemical mixtures) and because sometimes the science is inconclusive or nonexistent. Risk communication involves a message, a communicator or messenger, an audience / community, and a context.

MESSAGE

In the field of environmental health, we are often armed with insufficient science, particularly human toxicity and/or epidemiological data, to be definitive about health risks associated with an air emission, a contaminant in drinking water, or any other environmental exposure. The pollutant in question may not have been adequately tested and characterized. When toxicity data exist, they are almost always based on animal studies and therefore, to use the data in risk communication, we must explain that they are based on the extrapolation from animal models. As such, we are often making assumptions about the potential effect. This "scientific grayness" should be shared with the audience to whom risks are being communicated. The message in risk communication is based on uncertainty, and because of this and the fact that the context of risk communication is seldom neutral, it is extremely important to help the audience understand the concept of risk and the uncertainty within the full range of sciences. Table 10.1 outlines some risk perception tendencies described by Peter Sandman (1986).

Risks may be perceived as "less" or "more" risky based on the following attributes. Because the context of risk communication is often the presence of a new exposure or new knowledge about the effects of an existing exposure, the community may be anxious and/or angry. It is important to pay as much attention to the "outrage factors," and to the community's concerns as to scientific data (Chess, Hance, and Sandman, 1987).

MESSENGER

For risk communication to succeed the audience must perceive the source (messenger) of the information as trusted and credible. There are a variety of elements outlined in the risk communication literature that affect trust: competency, caring, encouragement of dialogue and participation, honorable and honest behavior, and listening to and acknowledging a com-

TABLE 10.1 Risk Perception Tendencies

Less Risky	More Risky
Voluntary	Involuntary
Familiar	Unfamiliar
Controllable	Uncontrollable
Controlled by self	Controlled by others
Fair not memorable	Memorable
Not dread	Dread
Chronic	Acute
Diffuse in time and space	Focused in time and space
Not fatal	Fatal
Immediate	Delayed
Natural	Artificial
Individual mitigation possible	Individual mitigation impossible
Detectable	Undetectable

munity's outrage. Nurses are considered highly credible and dependable sources of information within the community and fulfill the criteria for trust that is so essential in risk communication.

Nurses also understand the communication process, which is essential for sustaining long-term trust with the community. This process includes cross-cultural competencies, as well as language and literacy issues. Engaging the community in all aspects of communication (no closed meetings), meeting the community's needs for information, providing accurate information, and following up on requests for information that is not readily available will help to ensure a smoother process. Additionally, helping to coordinate multiple agency messages and responses and communication with the media is critical. Community members are more likely to believe what they read in the newspapers or hear on the 5 o'clock news.

AUDIENCE

Audiences bring their own individual biases or perceptions to any forum in which environmental health risks are discussed. Their distrust of the messenger may be based on their feelings about someone from the government, a particular industry, or an environmental organization. An audience may trust or distrust a messenger based on his or her age, race, gender, and so on. There is an excellent body of literature on audience bias and risk perception. A set of key variables has been identified by Chess et al. (1987) that will impact the perception of risk by the audience (see Table 10.2)

The potential impact on health is also important in the perception of the magnitude of the risk. Will an environmental exposure create a risk to children's health? Will the health problem be short-term and reversible? Is cancer the potential health outcome? Are there potential birth defects or other reproductive health threats? These issues must all be considered when engaging in risk communication.

CONTEXT

Risk communication does not occur in a vacuum. It often occurs when there has been a perceived environmental health threat—perhaps be a potentially contaminated water supply, an accidental release of a hazardous chemical, or a newly identified hazardous waste site adjacent to a day care center. The conditions and context will influence the audiences' ability to listen and trust. Additionally, the media can play an important part in a community's understanding and biases regarding environmental risk. It is critical to understand the history of the community and the histories of the individual community leaders. This is where good listening skills can help to facilitate real communication.

The Environmental Protection Agency (EPA) has proposed a code of conduct that will enhance the success of a risk communication initiative. It is a list of basic principles that honors all of the players within a community.

The EPA has created a list of *7 Cardinal Rules for Risk Communication.*

1. Accept and involve the public as a legitimate partner.
2. Plan carefully and evaluate your efforts.
3. Listen to your audience.
4. Be honest, frank, and open.
5. Coordinate and collaborate with other credible sources.
6. Meet the needs of the press.
7. Speak clearly and with compassion.

Risk communication is often the role of the public health nurse, who is called upon to bridge the communication gap between the community and

TABLE 10.2 Variables That Affect Risk Perception

1. *Voluntary risks are accepted more readily that those that are imposed.* When people don't have choices, they become angry. Similarly, when communities feel coerced into accepting risks, they feel furious about the coercion. As a result, they focus on the government's process and pay far less attention to substantive risk issues. Ultimately, they come to see the risk as more risky.

2. *Risks under individual control are accepted more readily than those under government control.* Most people feel safer with risks under their own control. For example most of us feel safer driving than riding as a passenger. Our feeling has nothing to do with the data—our driving record versus the driving records of others. Similarly, people tend to feel more comfortable with environmental risks they can do something about themselves, rather than having to rely on government to protect them.

3. *Risks that seem fair are more acceptable than those that seem unfair.* A coerced risk will always seem unfair. A community that feels stuck with the risk with little benefit will find the risk unfair, and thus more serious. This factor explains, in part, why communities that depend on a particular industry for jobs sometimes see pollution from that industry as less risky.

4. *Risk information that comes from trustworthy sources is more readily believed than information from untrustworthy sources.* If a mechanic with whom you have quarreled in the past says he can't find a problem with a car that seems faulty to you, you will respond quite differently than if a friend delivers the same news. You are more apt to demand justification, rather than ask neutral questions of the mechanic. Unfortunately, ongoing battles with communities erode trust and make the [governmental] agency message far less believable.

5. *Risks that seem ethically objectionable will seem more risky than those that don't.* To many people, pollution is morally wrong. A former EPA official suggested that speaking to some people about an acceptable level of pollution is like talking about an acceptable level of child molester.

6. *Natural risks seem more acceptable than artificial risks.* Natural risks provide no focus for anger: a risk caused by God is more acceptable than one caused by people. For example, consider the difference between the reactions to naturally occurring radon in homes and the reactions to high radon levels caused by uranium mine tailings or industrial sources.

7. *Exotic risks seem more risky than familiar risks.* A cabinet full of household cleansers, for example, seems much less risky than a high-tech chemical facility that makes cleansers.

8. *Risks that are associated with other, memorable events are considered more risky.* Risks that bring to mind Bhopal or Love Canal, for example, are more likely to be feared than those that lack such associations.

The greater the number and seriousness of these factors, the greater the likelihood of public concern about the risk, regardless of the scientific data.

the scientific or technical community. Nurses in clinical settings may be called upon to deliver risk communication, particularly if a patient's family perceives the cause of the family member's illness as an environmental exposure.

BIBLIOGRAPHY

Blake, E. R. (1995). Understanding Outrage: how scientists can help bridge the risk perception gap. *Environmental Health Perspectives 103*(Supp. 6), 123–125.

Chess, C., Hance, B. J., & Sandman, P. M. (1987). Improving dialogue with communities. *A short guide for government risk communication, report to New Jersey Department of Environmental Protection, Office of Science and Research*, (Contract C29444).

Environmental Protection Agency. (1990). *Communicating environmental risks: A guide to practical evaluations. Risk Communication Series* (Publication # EPA 230-01-91-001).

US EPA (1994). Seven Cardinal Rules of Risk Communication. EPA/OPA 87-020 Washington, DC.

Fischoff, B. (2000). Acceptable Risk. *A Conceptual Proposal*, http://www.fplc.edu/RISK/vol5/winter/Fischof.htm.

National Research Council (1989). *Improving risk communication*. Washington, DC: National Academy Press.

Sandman, P. M. (1986). *Explaining environmental risk*. Washington, DC: Environmental Protection Agency.

Sandman, P. M. (1987). Risk communication: Facing public outrage. *Environmental Protection Journal, 13*(9), 21.

CHAPTER 11

Water Pollution

Barbara Sattler

It's interesting to note that the percentage of the water on the earth's surface and the percentage of water in the human body are about the same, around 70%. How critical it is that we keep all of our water healthy! And yet, we continue to contaminate our surface and ground water that, in turn, contaminates our bodies. Chemical plants, pulp mills, and other factories legally dumped over a billion pounds of known toxic chemicals into U.S. rivers, lakes, and coastal waters between 1990 and 1994. Between 1994 and 1995, 45 million Americans drank contaminated water that exceeded the standards for fecal matter, parasites, pathogenic microbes, radiation, heavy metals, and other toxic chemicals.

Drinking water is derived from one of two sources: ground water (aquifers) or surface water (streams, reservoirs, rivers). Well water is drawn from ground water. About half of our nation's drinking water is well water and the other half surface. Both ground water and surface water are vulnerable to contamination from a wide variety of sources.

Water contamination is divided into two large categories: *point source pollutants*, which come from a single identifiable source such as a factory effluent, a sewer overflow pipe, and so on, and *non–point source pollutants*, which come from a great range of exposures such as agricultural runoff of pesticides or fertilizers or from air pollutants that land on the surfaces of great bodies of water.

Point source pollution is often regulated by the Environmental Protection Agency (EPA). If an industry or municipal public works entity such as a wastewater treatment facility intentionally discharges a pollutant into a body of water, it must have a permit from the state regulatory agency. As a society, we have decided that it is acceptable to discharge hazardous chemicals into our waterways, as long as it is within limits. All permits should be publicly accessible for review. The actual permitting process should be a public process in which citizens can learn about the limitations of the permit.

In addition to industrial effluent, there are a variety of sources of pollution to our water. A key mechanism for disposing of liquid hazardous waste is to treat the waste and then dispose of it via deep-well injection. This means that the treated waste is literally injected deep into the earth. Annually, 9 billion gallons of hazardous waste are injected deep into the earth in the U.S. and 2 billion gallons of brine from oil and gas are injected daily (EPA, 2001). The regulations for underground injection require that the operators evaluate the underground geology to ensure that the toxic waste will not find its way to an aquifer for at least 10,000 years. Automotive, industrial, sanitary, and other wastes may be shallow-well injected, resulting in contamination of aquifers.

There are hundreds of thousands of underground storage tanks in the United States, a significant number of which are for gasoline at gas stations. A substantial number of them store fuel oil for residential use. These underground storage tanks are regulated by the EPA. Almost 400,000 of them were found to be leaking by 1997, with the resulting pollution leaching into our ground water. MTBE was a fuel additive to gasoline formulated to increase oxygenation of gas and decrease pollution. It has been listed as a potential human carcinogen (known to cause liver and kidney tumors in mice). During an environmental assessment in Maryland, MTBE was detected in 210 private wells as a result of leaking storage tanks and runoff. MTBE is an extremely persistent pollutant. Annually, approximately 30,000 leaking storage tanks are now reported (EPA, 2001).

Many industries build holding ponds for their toxic wastewater. These ponds may be regulated and permitted, depending on the chemicals involved. Liners may be required to prevent the toxic chemicals from leaching into the ground water, but unfortunately these liners can fail.

There have been a number of transportation of hazardous materials incidents in which rivers and other waterways have been significantly compromised. Inland rail accidents have poured thousands of pounds of pesticides, chlorine, and other chemicals into the water. The most highly visible spills have been the ocean tanker spills of crude oil. All of these incidents are examples of point source pollution.

Old industrial sites, including Brownfields and Superfund sites, may leach any number of chemicals into the ground water or create hazardous runoff into surface waters. The drinking water contaminant of notoriety from the book and motion picture *A Civil Action* (Harr, 1996) was trichloroethylene (TCE), the most common contaminant found in Superfund sites around the country. Other common contaminants in Superfund sites include heavy metals, including lead and polychlorinated biphenyls (PCBs).

In Cape Cod, jet fuel runoff from the Massachusetts Military Reservation has contaminated eight underground streams that provide the drinking water for the citizens of Cape Cod. The Military Reservation is now a designated Superfund site. A similar situation exists in the San Gabriel Valley in California, where the solid rocket fuel perchlorate is found in dangerous quantities in the aquifers from which the area residents derive their drinking water. Perchlorate is used pharmaceutically for people who suffer from hypothyroidism. It enhances thyroid production. Unfortunately, if you have a normal thyroid, you might not want its activity to be increased.

Nonpoint sources of water pollution are sometimes more difficult to identify and control. Rain carries the salt we place on our icy roads to the nearest surface water via the storm management system. Rain similarly carries lawn and agricultural chemicals to our surface waters. In addition, chemicals that are water soluble may be absorbed into the earth and leach into the aquifers. The U.S. Geologic Survey estimates that 42 million American wells are contaminated with volatile organic compounds that are derived from gasoline, solvents, paints, and MTBE (U.S. Water News Online, 1999).

Air pollution from traffic and industrial pollution eventually come to earth. When it descends on our waterways it may stay on the surface or become soluble in the water. Many of the surface contaminants found on the Chesapeake Bay are from the industrial Ohio River Valley, hundreds of miles away. The need for national and global environmental protection policies becomes very apparent when it comes to air and water pollution.

In 1999, 1,000 fairgoers in New York State were infected with *E. coli*. The source was identified as drinking well contamination from animal manure in rain runoff. With increased population comes increased demand for food. In response to this demand, more fertilizers are being used to ratchet up the agricultural output. When fertilizer runoff arrives in waterways, the resultant hypernutrition from the fertilizer chemicals can have an impact on the marine ecology. This "eutrofication" has been associated with algae blooms such as the pfiesteria blooms found on East Coast waterways. In areas where animal fecal matter such as chicken waste runs off, the same phenomenon has been noted. Agricultural runoff (agricultural chemicals—pesticides and fertilizers—and fecal matter) affects 70% of our rivers.

Storm water overflow is a major source of contamination in urban waterways. When storm and sanitary sewer systems are combined (and most are), a summer thunderstorm can send three to four times more water to local wastewater treatment plants than they can handle (EPA, 2000). As a result, and as part of a planned contingency, raw sewage and floating trash are flushed directly into local streams and rivers.

Coastal waters are challenged by beach washups of trash, dredging, and oil spills. In 1989, 10 million gallons of crude oil contaminated nearly 500 miles of once pristine Alaskan shoreline. The cleanup took three years and cost $2.1 billion; yet the effects on wildlife are still being felt.

The U. S. Geologic Service regularly surveys the aquifers and surface waters. The chemicals that we use in our everyday lives are being found in measurable amounts in our nation's water: acetaminophen, caffeine, codeine, cotamine (a metabolite of nicotine, spilled in the urine), 17-b estradiol (estrogen), and sulfamethoxazole (and other antibiotics, particularly in areas where factory farming occurs). We are virtually clueless about the ecological impact these chemicals may have, particularly in combination, let alone the impact they may have on the humans drinking the water. What are the associated risks of a pregnant woman consuming such chemicals during her first trimester? We do not know. Through developmental toxicology and epidemiologic research, we are beginning to understand that embryos and fetuses have developmental stages during which they are exquisitely vulnerable to exposure to certain chemicals.

There are also many naturally occurring chemicals in our water that may create health risks. Arsenic, radon, radium, and heavy metals can be naturally occurring contaminants in water. In Austin, TX, lithium is a naturally occurring contaminant in the drinking water.

The availability of safe drinking water is clearly a public health concern. It is estimated that over 200 million Americans use treated drinking water. The introduction of drinking water chlorination as a standard treatment technique greatly decreased mortality from infectious disease and was a major public health advance in the 20th century. During water treatment, chlorine reacts with naturally occurring organic matter in surface water to produce a number of byproducts, now dubbed disinfectant byproducts (DBPs). Recent studies have shown a relationship between birth outcomes and DBPs. Specifically, risks of stillbirth and spontaneous abortion have been associated with high exposures to trihalomethanes, which are DBPs (Dodds, King, Woolcott, and Pole, 1999). Chloroform, the most prevalent trihalomethane in drinking water, is carcinogenic to rodents. Two other trihalomethanes are associated with intestinal, renal, and liver responses in rodents, as well as liver tumors. The EPA and the National Toxicology Program at the National Institutes of Environmental Health Science have created a research partnership to evaluate the toxicity of DBPs and the EPA is expected to set a final drinking water standard for DBPs by 2003 (National Toxicology Program, 2000).

In the distribution systems that transport source water to our taps, our drinking water is challenged by a number of potential contaminants. Many have been described in this chapter. In our homes, lead pipes and lead solder can provide a source of contamination when the lead leaches into our drinking water. Lead is a serious neurotoxic, reproductive toxic, and hemopoietic toxic chemical. (See the material on lead in chapter 18 of this book for more information.)

Given the critical need that our bodies have for water, it is essential that we protect this vital resource. Nurses have been silent about water quality, yet there are opportunities for participation and input. Each state must have a source water protection plan. The planning process is open to public participation and would be a perfect place for nurses to contribute their special knowledge of the vulnerable populations they serve: pregnant women, the very young and the very old, and the immunocompromised. Nurses' status in the community as trusted communicators enhances their effectiveness in public forums. We should all consider how we can create a nursing platform for public health through more active participation in environmental protection, which ultimately translates to environmental health protection.

BIBLIOGRAPHY

Dodds, L., King, W., Woolcott, C., & Pole, J. (1999). Trihalomethanes in public water supplies and adverse pregnancy outcomes. *Epidemiology, 10*(3), 233–237.

EPA. (2000). *Remember the past, protect the future.* [EPA-902-R-00-001].

EPA (2001). Web site (www.epa.gov).

Harr, J. (1996). *A civil action.* New York: Vintage Books.

National Toxicology Program. (2000). *Safe drinking water program factsheet*, National Toxicology Web site (http://ntp-server.niehs.nih.gov).

U.S. Water News Online (1999). 42 million Americans using groundwater vulnerable to contamination by volatile organic compounds. www.uswaternews.com/archives/arcquality/942mili2.html.

CHAPTER 12

Drinking Water Quality

Brenda Afzal

From earliest times, we and our ancestors have depended on water as a highway, a sewer, a pathway to discovery, a means to empire, an irrigator of crops-in short, as a social as well as a chemical necessity. Chemistry, however, remains the bottom line: whatever else we do with water, we must also drink it.

Charles J Hitch

HISTORICAL OVERVIEW

The post-World War II growth in agricultural and industrial development and the production of man-made chemicals provided an economic boom in the United States. Unfortunately, it also led to pollution of the nation's water. Rachel Carson first brought the nation's attention to the issue of pollution in her book *Silent Spring* (1972). She reported on widespread poisoning of our nation's waterways from toxic industrial chemicals and agricultural and sewage runoff. Many once pristine waterways had become unsafe for swimming and, worse, unsafe for drinking.

Early concern for drinking water quality centered on its aesthetic qualities. There was little understanding of the relationship between drinking water and disease until the mid nineteenth century when Dr. John Snow, a British physician, correlated an outbreak of cholera in London to drinking water drawn from a contaminated source. Although this association was made before the recognition that microbes cause disease, it did imply that water was a medium for the transmission of disease. The discovery of the germ theory of disease by Dr. Louis Pasteur, late in the nineteenth century, helped to explain why water sometimes made people sick. Bacterial pathogens would remain the focus of concern during most of the twentieth century.

SCOPE OF THE PROBLEM

The Clean Water Act is a 1977 amendment to the Federal Water Pollution Control Act of 1972. The Clean Water Act's primary objective is to restore and maintain the integrity of the nation's waters. This objective translates into two fundamental national goals: eliminate the discharge of pollutants into the nation's waters, and achieve water quality levels that are fishable and swimmable. "Each year in the U.S., millions of pounds of industrial and agricultural chemicals are released into the environment, either through intentional or uncontrolled discharges. Ground water and surface water bodies that serve as our drinking water sources are vulnerable to contamination by these chemicals as a result of runoff of agricultural and household chemicals, industrial waste discharges, and uncontrolled releases from sources such as landfills and leaking underground storage tanks" (Physicians for Social Responsibility, 2000). Public water systems are increasingly challenged to remove chemical contaminants. A report by the U.S. Public Interest Research Group Education Fund (2000) indicated that in the 20 years since the Clean Water Act was instituted, there had been 220,000,000 pounds of toxic chemicals dumped directly into our nation's waterways, indicating that we have not yet met our clean water goals.

Agricultural runoff is also an enormous source of pollution, causing 70% of our rivers and streams to be affected by nutrient and animal waste runoff (U.S. Environmental Protection Agency, 1998). Waste generated from Concentrated Animal Feeding Operations (CAFOs), sometimes referred to as factory farms, has created a disastrous source of water pollution producing "130 times the waste generated by humans in this country each year" (Minority Staff of the U.S. Senate Committee on Agriculture, Nutrition and Forestry, 1997, p. 3).

Water chlorination was first used to disinfect water in the United States by the New Jersey City Water Works. As water suppliers across the country added chlorine to water drawn from surface water sources, waterborne disease outbreaks dropped dramatically. However, in the 1970s, by-products of chlorination were identified in drinking water. When chlorine is used to disinfect public drinking water, it can combine with organic material in the water distribution system, forming organic chlorinated compounds. These compounds are referred to as disinfectant byproducts (BPs). Several epidemiological studies indicate that there may be an increased risk of reproductive and developmental effects to the fetuses of pregnant women exposed to high levels of these DPWs (King, Dodds, & Allen, 2000; Moline et al., 2000; Swan et al., 1998). In addition, studies have also associated the ingestion of certain types of DBPs to bladder and colorectal cancer (Cantor et al., 1998; King and Marret, 1996; McGeehin, Reif, Beecher, and Mangione, 1993).

The Food Quality Protection Act mandates the EPA to add the contribution of pesticide residues in drinking water to the total dietary exposure to pesticide residues. Although pesticide residues in drinking water are not thought to be a primary source of pesticide poisoning, the presence of pesticides in drinking water can pose a health threat. A report by the Greater Boston Physicians for Social Responsibility (2000) describes the toxic threat that exposure to pesticides from water, air, and soil has on a child's neurological development. The report describes a recent study of preschool children (Guillette et al., 1998) that revealed that children who sustained heavy pesticide exposures (from multiple sources) had less stamina, decreased gross motor coordination, impaired fine hand-eye coordination, decreased 30-minute memory, less ability to draw a person (Figs. 12.1 and 12.2), and increased aggressiveness, than those without exposures.

A 1999 publication (American Society for Microbiology) estimated that 900,000 people suffer annually from waterborne infections and 900 die. Reports and estimates vary on the incidence of waterborne microbial disease occurring in the United States, probably because not all outbreaks are "recognized, investigated, [or] reported" (Centers for Disease Control, 2000, p. 2). Although waterborne diseases are reportable, few health care practitioners recognize the possibility of a waterborne etiology, and therefore there is significant underreporting.

"The largest outbreak reported in the U.S. since health officials began tracking waterborne disease in 1920 occurred in Milwaukee, Wisconsin in 1993. After drinking water contaminated with a single-celled parasite *Cryptosporidium parvum*, over 400,000 people suffered from gastrointestinal illness and it is estimated that over 50 people died" (U.S. EPA, 1999b, p. 30). Table 12.1 gives examples of other significant waterborne disease outbreaks that have occurred in U.S. community water systems.

WHERE DOES DRINKING WATER COME FROM?

There are more than 170,000 public water systems in the United States serving the population (United States Environmental Protection Agency, 1999a). Roughly 80% of the United States public water systems obtain water from ground water sources. Ground water refers to water that is held in rock (aquifers) beneath the surface of the earth. The remaining 20% of public water systems obtain water from surface sources such as lakes,

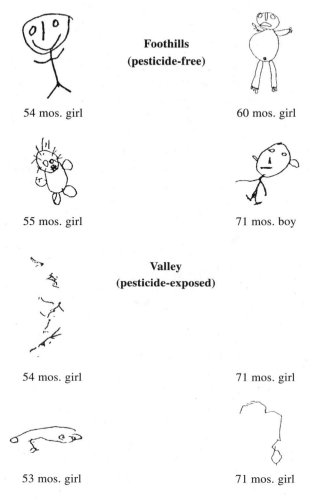

Foothills
(pesticide-free)

54 mos. girl

60 mos. girl

55 mos. girl

71 mos. boy

Valley
(pesticide-exposed)

54 mos. girl

71 mos. girl

53 mos. girl

71 mos. girl

Figure 12.1 Illustrations are those by Mexican Yaqui Indian children drawn during a study of the effects of pesticide exposure on neurological development. The study was conducted by Elizabeth A. Guillette, PhD, University of Arizona. Originally published in the Journal of Environmental Health Perspective.

rivers, and reservoirs. Groundwater moves from high elevation to low elevation or from high-pressure areas to low-pressure areas. The rate of travel varies but it flows at a much slower rate than surface water. It was once thought that groundwater was pure and free of contamination. We now understand that as water seeps into aquifers from the surface of the earth, it may pick up both natural and man-made contaminants along the way.

Table 12.1 Waterborne disease outbreaks in the U.S.

Year	State	Cause of Disease	# of People Affected
1985	MA	Giardia lambia	703 illnesses
1987	GA	Cryptosporidium parvum	13,000 illnesses
1987	PR	Shigella sonnei	1,800 illnesses
1989	MO	E Coli)157	243 illnesses, 4 deaths
1991	PR	Unknown	9,847 illnesses
1993	MO	Salmonella typhimurium	650 illnesses, 7 deaths
1993	WI	Cryptosporidium parvum	400,000 illnesses, 50 + deaths

(Adapted from U.S. EPA, 1999b, p.30) PR=Puerto Rico

DRINKING WATER CONTAMINANTS

In writing the Safe Drinking Water Act (SDWA), Congress gave the EPA a mandate to regulate contaminants in public drinking water that are known to, or are likely to, pose a risk to public health. The EPA does not have the authority to regulate private drinking water systems. It regulates contaminants by setting standards for "finished" drinking water that flows from treatment facilities to customers. Currently, more than 80 contaminants are regulated. A 1996 amendment requires the EPA to "review and revise," if necessary, the safe drinking water standards. Some of the current drinking water standards were set decades ago and in light of new scientific evidence there is concern that they may not be protective of public health.

Contaminants are classified as inorganic or organic chemicals, radionuclides, and microorganisms. Inorganic chemicals are mineral based and do not contain carbon. They may occur naturally in the watershed or enter the watershed from farming or industrial discharge. Examples of inorganic chemicals are lead, nitrates, arsenic and asbestos. Organic chemicals contain carbon and can gain access to the watershed from agricultural and industrial runoff. Some organic chemical contaminants are referred to as volatile organic chemicals (VOCs) or synthetic organic chemicals (SOCs). VOCs are persistent in the environment and have been associated with some types of cancer as well as negative neurological and reproductive affects. Examples of VOCs are gasoline, degreasing and dry-cleaning solvents. There are 34 standards for SOCs; many are pesticides.

Microbial contaminants found in water may be bacteria, viruses, or parasites. Disinfection and filtration methods used by public water suppliers have decreased the threat from many pathogens for healthy individuals. However, vulnerable populations are at greater risk. The infectivity of microbes may be higher for individuals with weakened immune systems. Disease outbreaks from these pathogens are usually a result of a water system treatment failure or from drinking from a contaminated water source.

Radionuclides emit ionizing radiation. Lifetime exposure to radiation at levels over the EPA standard from a drinking water source results in an increased risk of some types of cancer. The EPA currently regulates radium 226 and 228, as well as gross alpha particle activity. Drinking water standards for radon and naturally occurring uranium are expected soon.

DRINKING WATER STANDARDS

There are national primary and secondary standards for drinking water. National Primary Drinking Water Standards (NPDWSs) are legally enforceable standards limiting the amount of contaminants that can be detected in drinking water. There are two types of enforceable NPDWSs: Maximum Contaminant Levels (MCLs) and Treatment Techniques (TTs). The MCL indicates the highest level of a regulated contaminant that is allowed in finished drinking water. For some contaminants for which there is no measuring method that is economically or technically achievable, a TT is set. TTs set a specific procedure or technology that must be used by public water systems to control a regulated contaminant. An example of a TT is the Surface Water Treatment Rule that provides for disinfection and filtration of drinking water.

National Secondary Drinking Water Standards (NSDWSs) are not enforceable. The EPA recommends them to public water systems to control cosmetic and aesthetic effects of drinking water. Although NSDWs are not federally enforceable, some states have chosen to adopt them as enforceable standards.

DRINKING WATER LAWS AND REGULATIONS

The Public Health Service set the first federal drinking water standards for contaminants in 1914. There were 14 standards for bacterial contaminants regulating systems that provided water to interstate carriers. By 1964, the Public Health Service regulated a total of 28 contaminants.

Public concern about the poor state of our nation's waterways in the 1960s and 1970s compelled the federal government to investigate drinking water quality in the United States. The results of the investigation indicated that our worst fears were true. Public health standards were being met by only 60% of the water systems surveyed (United States Environmental Protection Agency, 1999b). There were serious issues concerning the disinfecting process, with small water systems having many deficiencies. One study of the Mississippi River (Industrial Pollution of the Lower Mississippi River, 1972) showed that water taken from the river, which had passed through a water treatment facility, still contained 36 potentially hazardous chemicals. These concerns and others related to environmental health fostered debates in Congress that led to two landmark environmental acts of legislation, the Federal Water Pollution Control Act of 1972 and the Safe Drinking Water Act (SDWA) of 1974. The Environmental Protection Agency administers both.

The purpose of the Clean Water Act (CWA) of 1977, an amendment to the Federal Water Pollution Control Act, was to restore and maintain the chemical, physical, and biological integrity of the nation's waters. The SDWA attempts to control drinking water contamination through the use of a multiple barrier approach. This approach includes source water and drinking water assessment and protection, wellhead protection, qualification of water system operators, ensuring the integrity of distribution systems, and public notification of drinking water quality.

NURSING AND WATER QUALITY

Historically, environmental health has been a focus for nursing. Lillian Wald, an early public health nursing advocate, and Florence Nightingale voiced clear concerns for the environment in which individuals and communities live and work.

> In watching diseases, both in private homes and in public hospitals, the thing which strikes the experienced observer most forcibly is this, that the symptoms or the sufferings generally considered to be inevitable and incident to the disease are very often not symptoms of the disease at all, but of something quite different—of the want of fresh air, or of light, or of warmth, or of quiet, or of cleanliness, or of punctuality and care in the administration of diet, of each or of all of these [Nightingale, 1860, p. 8].

The traditional role of the nurse as an investigator, educator, advocate, communicator, and leader gives an unmistakable mandate in environmental health matters. The Institute of Medicine's report *Nursing, Health, and the Environment* (1995) asserts the need for nurses to understand the basic and applied principles of environmental health. As one of the most trusted sources of drinking water information, nurses must be able to field questions and guide vulnerable populations to informed decisions about water quality. A valuable tool to assist nurses in this process is the Consumer Confidence Report.

CONSUMER CONFIDENCE REPORTS

A 1996 amendment to the Safe Drinking Water Act allows consumers and their health care providers to have access to information concerning the quality of their drinking water. This amendment requires public water system providers to produce and make available to consumers a Right to Know or Consumer Confidence Report (CCR). The purpose of these reports is to help consumers make informed decisions about their drinking water. These reports also provide an opportunity to educate consumers on basic water quality issues and the challenges of delivering safe drinking water. The first reports were required to be published by October 19, 1999; thereafter, CCRs must be published annually by July 1. Every community water system that provides drinking water to 25 or more of the same people year-round must publish a CCR. It is hoped that these reports will help stimulate concern for drinking water quality among consumers and motivate them to learn about and be involved in source water protection. Table 12.2 outlines the basic CCR report requirements.

The EPA has an online website where many local CCRs can be found www.epa.gov/safewater/dwinfo.htm. Although most states have some regulations regarding the water testing of new private wells there are seldom requirements for periodic retesting. The right-to-know statutes do not apply to personal wells.

A "report card" grading the early attempts by water utilities to produce CCRs (The Campaign for Safe and Affordable Drinking Water, 2000) indicated that 44% of the reports received a grade of D or F. Nurses, in their roles as advocates and educators, should assess their communities' reports, and if they have recommendations for improving the CCR they should contact the water provider.

WHEN DO YOU RECOMMEND AN ALTERNATIVE SOURCE OF TAP WATER?

A variety of issues may indicate the need for an alternative source of drinking water for individuals or communities. Alternative sources of drinking

TABLE 12.2 Basic Consumer Confidence Report Requirements

Water System Information
- Name/phone number of contact person
- Information on public participation opportunities
- Information for nonEnglish speaking populations, if applicable

Sources of Water
- Type, name, and location of water sources
- Availability of source water assessment
- Information on significant sources of contamination, if available

Definitions: MCL, MCLG, others as needed

Detected Contaminants
- Table summarizing data on detected regulated & unregulated contaminants
- Known or likely source of each detected contaminant
- Health effects language and explanation [for MCL violations]
- Information on *Cryptosporidium*, radon, and other contaminants, if applicable

Compliance With Other Drinking Water Regulations

- Explanation of violations, potential health effects, and steps taken to correct the violations
- Explanation of variance/exemption, if applicable required educational information
- Explanation of contaminants and their presence in drinking water
- Warning for vulnerable populations about *Cryptosporidium*
- Informational statements on arsenic, nitrate, and lead, if necessary

From Preparing your drinking water consumer confidence report: Guidance for water suppliers. (EPA 81 6-R-99-002) March 1 999c.

water may be necessary for individuals with special vulnerabilities such as infants and children, the immunosuppressed, pregnant women, and the elderly. Individuals who are known to be immunocompromised should err on the side of safety and seek an alternative source of drinking water while a risk of infection is present. Exposure to a small dose of some microbes may be very serious for such individuals. On occasion, water utilities will issue a "boil water advisory" via media (television, radio, and newspapers) when there is an indication that the water they deliver to homes may have a risk of microbial contamination. All individuals, not just special populations, should use an alternative source of drinking water during a boil water advisory.

Children under 6 months of age who are exposed to elevated levels of nitrates in drinking water may have an increased risk of developing methemoglobinemia, which can develop when the immature infant gut converts nitrates to nitrites. Nitrites oxidize hemoglobin thus reducing its ability to carry oxygen. There is a 7 to 8% fatality rate for infants who develop this disease (Physicians for Social Responsibility, 2000). Although any part of the country can have elevated levels of nitrates, agricultural areas have a higher risk of contamination because of agricultural chemical contamination. Parents of newborns in areas that are at risk for nitrate contamination should consider several options. Never boil infants' water. If nitrates are present, boiling the water will concentrate them. If the source of drinking water is a private well, the well water should be tested for nitrate levels. Parents should be made aware that seasonal variations in nitrate levels, which cause spikes in levels, are possible. If it is confirmed that the drinking water is contaminated with nitrates, or that there is a possibility of contamination, an alternative source of drinking water should be obtained.

WHAT ARE THE ALTERNATIVES TO DRINKING STRAIGHT FROM THE TAP?

Tap water can be altered by boiling it or by the use of a filtering device. Bottled water can be used when tap water is deemed unsuitable for use.

BOILING WATER

Boiling water is an inexpensive, short-term method used for microbial disinfection. Bringing water to a full rolling boil for one minute will kill most microbes. This method may be used in response to a water advisory that is issued due to microbial contamination. If this method is used, there are factors that should be considered. If metals are present, boiling water will concentrate them and if volatile chemicals are present they will vaporize into the air creating an additional route of absorption. Additionally, people using this method should be cautioned to use boiled water for everything, including food preparation and brushing teeth.

BOTTLED WATER

The Food and Drug Administration (FDA) (not the EPA) is responsible for good manufacturing practices for bottled water. They assess whether the water comes from an approved source (i.e., if the labeling says spring water then the source must satisfy the FDA's definition of spring water), and that it is manufactured under safe and sanitary conditions and has been responsibly tested for contaminants. Whenever the EPA adopts a standard for drinking water, the FDA is required to adopt the same standard or give a reason why not. The FDA does not have jurisdiction over intrastate commerce of bottled water, meaning water that is bottled and sold in the same state. This exempts roughly 60% to 70% of bottled water from FDA regulation. FDA regulations do not apply to carbonated water. Some states (MA, NY, CA, for example) have bottled water standards that exceed FDA standards. Water that meets these states' standards will so indicate on the label by giving a certification number from the state.

More than half of all Americans drink bottled water; about a third of the public consumes it regularly. The Natural Resource Defense Counsel (NROC) (1999) did a four-year study to evaluate the quality of bottled water and determined that bottled water regulations are inadequate to assure consumers of safety. At least one-third of the bottled waters tested violated a state standard or guideline for microbials. Exclusively drinking bottled water as an alternative to tap water is very expensive. According to the NRDC, people spend from 240 to 10,000 times more per gallon of bottled water than they typically would for the same amount of tap water. Clearly, the use of bottled water as a source of "safe" drinking water and as a long-time replacement for tap water for vulnerable populations is prohibitively expensive and, equally important, lacks a guarantee of purity.

So what can we recommend? NSF International (NSF) is an organization that tests and verifies that bottled water products meet specified standards for microbial, heavy metal, and mineral reduction. If the bottled water manufacturer meets these standards the label will indicate that the bottled water manufacturing process meets the certification requirements. Examine the bottle's label for either the certification from the NSF or for some indication that the bottler has attempted a purification process such as reverse osmosis or submicrobial filtration for less than one micron. These processes will offer some assurances regarding microbial and heavy metal (lead and arsenic) contamination but the process does not remove organic and inorganic chemicals or radionuclides. If there is a long-term need for an alternative source of tap water that is pure (98%), a home distilling filtration unit should be considered.

WATER TREATMENT UNITS

Many people who are concerned with the aesthetic qualities of their drinking water and those concerned with its possible contamination are turning to water treatment units (filtration systems) as a solution to their concerns. Water treatment units range from the low-priced carafe models to expensive reverse-osmosis models. There is no individual unit that removes all types of contaminants completely. Therefore, it is important to select a filter that meets an identified need or concern.

An early step in the process of choosing a water treatment device is to access the CCR for the utility that provides the tap water. The CCR will list contaminants that have been found at levels exceeding EPA regulations. The local health department or department of the environment can be very helpful in identifying contaminants that are known to exist in the area of concern. In addition, you may choose to test the water in order to determine what contaminants are present. If drinking water is derived from well water, the department of health or environment may be able to give you some indication of contaminants that have been identified in the areas aquifers. Water testing for some contaminants can be expensive. Having done some preliminary research into known contaminants will help to focus the testing, thus reducing the cost. A list of certified labs can usually be obtained from the state department of the environment or the state health department.

Once you have identified the contaminant(s) of concern, the search for a water treatment unit to remove that contaminant can begin. There are two basic types of filtration systems: point-of-entry (POE) and point-of-use (POU) systems. A POE system treats all water entering a house; it is installed between the water meter and the house plumbing system. POU systems include personal water bottles/carafes, faucet mounts, countertop manual fill systems, counter top filters connected to the sink faucet, and plumbed-in systems that are directly connected to the existing water pipe of a sink.

There are a variety of technologies available to remove contaminants. They include but are not limited to adsorption, softeners, ultraviolet technology, reverse osmosis, and distillation. The type of technology selected should meet the identified concern. For example, if a parent is concerned only about elevated lead levels in tap water, a water carafe or an inexpensive faucet filter could be used. A study by Consumer Reports (Fit to drink, 1999) indicated that most simple systems effectively remove lead. However, if the concern is microbial contamination for a vulnerable individual, a distillation or POE reverse osmosis system should be considered.

NSF International tests and verifies that water treatment devices meet specified standards. They do not recommend, rate, or compare products. NSF has several standards for drinking water treatment units. If NSF certifies a product it must meet five requirements. The contaminant reduction claims must be true; the system does not add anything harmful to the water;

the system is structurally sound; the advertising, literature and labeling are not misleading; and the materials and manufacturing processes used do not change. You will find additional information about water treatment devices including types of treatment technology (see Table 12.3), performance claims, and categories of contaminants from NSF's helpful website located at http://www.NSF.org.

COST OF WATER TREATMENT DEVICES

Cost is a consideration when purchasing a water treatment device. A report published in *Consumer Digest* (Wasik, 1996) offered some basic information about cost. The report suggested that initial cost of the water treatment unit as well as the cost and frequency of replacement filters should be considered. Of the filters that the report evaluated, researchers found

TABLE 12.3 Types of Treatment Technology

Water treatment units use diverse types of technology to remove contaminants from drinking water. These technologies include:

1. *Adsorption* A physical process in which liquids, gases, dissolved or suspended matter adhere to the surface or pore of some type of absorbent medium, such as carbon filters.

2. *Softeners* Most softeners use a cation exchange resin to reduce the hardness (hardness meaning the amount of calcium and magnesium) in water. Calcium or magnesium is replaced with sodium or potassium ions. This technology is effective in removing radium from drinking water although it will raise the sodium content of the water in doing so.

3. *Ultraviolet Treatment* This treatment is used to disinfect water or reduce amount of heterotrophic bacteria.

4. *Reverse Osmosis* A process that reverses the flow of water in a natural process of osmosis so that water passes from a more concentrated solution to a more dilute solution through a semi-permeable membrane. This process removes most microbial contaminants as well as minerals. Most of these systems also use a pre and post filter along with the membrane to remove VOCs, SOCs and Radon.

5. *Distillers* Distilling systems heat water to a boiling point, collect the water vapor as it condenses, leaving many of the contaminants behind, particularly heavy metals. Unfortunately, some contaminants, such as volatile organics may carry over with the vapor. If combined with activated carbon filtration, additional contaminants such as volatile organics and radon can be removed. Home distillation units can cost from a few hundred dollars to over $1000.

Adapted from NSF International [Online] Available: www.nsf.org/consumer.html

that filters that attach to the faucet are compact, inexpensive, and are easy to install. Drinking water carafes are also inexpensive, ranging from $10 to 30, but they filter small quantities of water and their filters are expensive ($28 to $78 a year) to replace. Faucets with built-in filters are more expensive ($150 to 295) and they did not perform as well as the less expensive models tested. Point-of-entry systems are the most expensive but they do more. The cost of replacing the filters that do the clean-up work should be factored into the cost of any filtering device.

SUMMARY

The safety of drinking water cannot be assumed. It depends on a variety of issues. It may depend on the water utility's ability to mediate the source water it is using. It may depend on funding allocations to research current and emerging water quality issues. It may depend on the political will of community leaders to regulate pollution sources. It may depend on who you are and where you live. In the end, the safety of the nation's drinking water may depend on individuals and communities advocating for their right to safe drinking water.

BIBLIOGRAPHY

American Society for Microbiology. (1999). *Microbial pollutants in our nation's water*. Washington, DC: Author.

Barwick, R., Levy, D., Craun, G., Beach, M., & Calderon, R. (2000, May 26). Surveillance for waterborne-disease outbreaks: United States, 1997–1998. *MMWR Surveillance Summary 49*(SS04), 1–35.

Cantor, K., Lynch, C., Hildesheim, M., Dosemeci, M., Lubin, J., Alvavanja, M., & Craun, G. (1998). Drinking water source and chlorination by-products I. Risk of bladder cancer. *Epidemiology, 9*, 21–28.

Carson, R. (1972). *Silent Spring*. Boston: Houghton Mifflin.

Fit to drink: Devices that help keep water in good taste and you in good health. (1999, October). *Consumer Reports, 64*(10): 52–55.

Industrial pollution of the lower Mississippi River in Louisiana. (1972). EPA Region VI, Surveillance and Analysis Division.

Institute of Medicine. (1995). *Nursing, health, and the environment*. Washington, DC: National Academy Press.

Guillette, E., Meza, M., Aquilar, M., Soto, A., & Garcia, I. (1998). An Anthropological approach to the evaluation of preschool children exposed to pesticides in Mexico. *Environmental Health Perspectives, 106*(6), 347–353.

King, W., & Mareet, L. (1996). Case-control study of bladder cancer and chlorination byproducts in treated water. *Cancer Causes and Control, 7*, 596–604.

King, W., Dodds, L. & Allen, A. (2000). Relation between stillbirth and specific chlorination byproducts in public water supplies. *Environmental Health Perspectives, 108*(9), 883–886.

Marks, R. & Knuffke, R. (1998, December). *America's animal factories: How states fail to prevent pollution from livestock waste.* Natural Resource Defense Council & Clean Water Network.

McGeehin, M., Reif, J., Beecher, J., & Mangione, E. (1993). Case-control study of bladder cancer and water disinfection methods in Colorado. *American Journal of Epidemiology, 138*, 492–501.

Minority Staff of the U.S. Senate Committee on Agriculture, Nutrition and Forestry, *Animal waste pollution in America: An emerging national problem.* (1997, December). Washington, D.C: Author.

Moline, J., Golden, A., Bar-Chama, N., Smith, E., Rauch, M., Chapin, R., Perreault, S., Schrader, S., Suk, W., & Landrigan, P. (2000). Exposure to hazardous substances and male reproductive health: A research framework. *Environmental Health Perspectives, 108*(9), 803–813.

Natural Resource Defense Council. (1999, February). Bottled water: Pure drink or pure hype. New York: Author.

Nightingale, F. 1860. *Notes on nursing: What it is and what it is not.* New York: D. Appleton. Reprinted, 1969. New York: Dover.

Physicians for Social Responsibility. (2000). *Drinking water and disease: What health care providers should know.* Washington, DC: Author.

Swan, S., Waller, K., Hopkins, B., Windham, G., Fenster, L., Schaefer, C., & Neutra, R. (1998). A prospective study of spontaneous abortion: Relation to amount and source of drinking water consumed in early pregnancy. *Epidemiology, 9*(2), 126–133.

The Campaign for Safe and Affordable Drinking Water. (2000, March). *Measuring up: Grading the first round of drinking water right to know reports.* Washington, DC: Author.

United States Environmental Protection Agency. (1998). *The challenge ahead.* (EPA-903-R-99-005). Washington, DC: U.S. Government Printing Office.

United States Environmental Protection Agency. (1999a). *Safe Drinking Water Act, Section 1429 ground water report to Congress.* (EPA Publication No. 816-R-99-016). Washington, DC: Author.

United States Environmental Protection Agency. (1999b). *25 Years of the safe drinking water act: History and trends.* (EPA Publication No. 816-R-99-007). Washington, DC: Author.

United States Environmental Protection Agency. (1999c, March). *Preparing your drinking water consumer confidence report: Guidance for water suppliers.* (EPA Publication No. 816-R-99-002). Washington, DC: Author.

U.S. Public Interest Research Group Education Fund. (2000, February). *Poisoning our water: How the government permits pollution.* Washington, DC: Author.

Wasik, J. F. (1996, May/June). Special report: How safe is your water? *Consumers Digest.*

CHAPTER 13

Air Pollution

Barbara Sattler

BACKGROUND

In the 1960s, there were a number of visible signs that pollution urgently needed to be addressed. One of these signs was the brown air that was engulfing so many of our nation's cities. In 1970, the Environmental Protection Agency (EPA) was established and significant amendments to the 1963 Clean Air Act (CAA) were made, setting the stage for a new era of "command and control" policies to try to turn the tide on what was the increasingly threatened state of our air. The policies that have been developed over the years have attempted to address air pollution in a comprehensive manner by reducing air pollutants from their many sources: mobile sources (automobiles and trucks), fixed site facilities (factories, waste treatment facilities, power plants), and through consumer products such as refrigerants in refrigerators, aerosol spray cans, and other products that threaten air quality. We are also developing a better understanding of the association between poor air quality and human and ecological health.

The results of the CAA are noted in some improvements in air quality, although these improvements are neither uniform for all forms of air pollution nor consistent globally. Ground-level ozone continues to persist at unhealthy levels in many areas, as do sulfur dioxide and mercury from coal-fired power plants. Sulfur dioxide continues to be a major contributor to acid rain. Although visibility has improved over many U.S. cities, it is worsening in many third world cities. Airborne persistent organic pollutants (POPs) are not deterred by national boundaries and are carried and deposited based on dominant weather patterns.

The CAA required that a set of standards be created that would protect sensitive populations, such as people who suffer with asthma. These health-based standards are the National Ambient Air Quality Standards (NAAQS). In 1996, 46 million Americans still lived in areas where the air did not meet the NAAQS, evidence of our need for continued air quality vigilance. When the CAA was amended in 1990, Congress additionally mandated the EPA to regulate "hazardous air pollutants" (HAPs) or air toxics, those chemicals known or suspected to cause serious health problems. The amendments named 189 toxic air pollutants for which standards must be created, many of which are carcinogens, mutagens, and/or reproductive toxins, including beryllium, mercury, asbestos, vinyl chloride benzene, arsenic, and radionuclides. Such toxic air pollutants may be gases, metals and other fine particles, and gases absorbed onto fine particles. Congress also tightened controls on contributors to acid rain, increased measures for controlling airborne carcinogens, created cleanup schedules for cities that were not complying with the NAAQS, and tightened standards for auto emissions.

Air pollution sources are described by the location from which they emanate and by the patterns of their releases. Point source refers to a specific location such as a smoke stack. Area sources refer to pollutants that come from a range of smaller generators such as dry cleaners (perchlorethylene), automobiles, gas stations (benzene), and wood stoves. Routine releases occur "continuously," certain production activities cause the release of intermittent emissions known as "batches," and "accidental" releases occur during explosions, equipment failure, or transportation accidents. Traffic-related pollution may be referred to as a mobile source!

AIR QUALITY INDICATORS

The EPA uses six "criteria pollutants" as indicators of air quality and has set standards for each of these under the NAAQS. When an area does not meet these standards, it is designated as a nonattainment area and must develop and implement a plan for attainment. The six criteria pollutants are ozone, carbon monoxide, sulfur dioxide, nitrogen dioxide, particulate matter, and lead.

OZONE

Ozone, an odorless, colorless gas, made up of three atoms of oxygen, is the major component in smog. There is "good" ozone and "bad" ozone depending on its location. The "good" ozone is in the upper atmosphere and provides a shield from harmful ultraviolet radiation. (This ozone shield is being seriously threatened by various global warming processes.) The "bad" ozone is at ground level where it poses a significant threat to human health by damaging lung tissue, reducing lung function, and sensitizing the lung to other irritants, causing a range of symptoms including coughing, sneezing, pulmonary congestion, and chest pain.

Ozone is created by a complex set of Volitile Organic compounds (VOCs) and oxides of nitrogen in the presence of sunlight. These chemical reactions are affected by sunlight and heat, resulting in greater production of ozone in warmer seasons. Volatile organic compounds are emitted by a wide range of polluting sources, including dry cleaners, cars, chemical manufacturers, paint shops, and many others.

CARBON MONOXIDE

Carbon monoxide is a colorless, odorless, and poisonous gas produced during the burning of fossil fuels (coal and oil). The vast majority of carbon monoxide is produced by automobiles. However, incinerators, wood-burning stoves, and other industrial sources also contribute. Carbon monoxide binds with human hemoglobin in a way that precludes the binding of oxygen. This results in anoxia. The most sensitive populations to carbon monoxide poisoning are people with cardiovascular diseases and chronic obstructive pulmonary disease (COPD) and smokers. There is some evidence that carbon monoxide exposure may actually accelerate atherosclerosis. Flu-like symptoms such as headache and fatigue are associated with low-level exposures. Neurologic manifestations include changes in auditory and visual perception, psychomotor function, and dexterity.

SULFUR DIOXIDE

Sulfur dioxide is a gas that is formed during the combustion of fossil fuels, during an array of industrial processes, and during the production of energy from coal, oil, and biomass. It is a major contributor to acid rain. Sulfur dioxide is also associated with a constellation of health effects, including respiratory illness, alterations in pulmonary function, aggravation of existing cardiovascular diseases, and exacerbations in asthma.

NITROGEN DIOXIDE

Nitrogen dioxide is also created by the combustion of fossil fuels and affects the lungs as well as immune function. Low-level exposures are associated with specific lung changes such as impaired mucociliary clearance, particle transport, macrophage function, and local immunity. In very high concentrations, lung injury can be severe, resulting in pulmonary edema and bronchopneumonia. Moderate exposures have been associated with acute respiratory infection, sore throat, and colds. Nitrogen dioxide also exacerbates asthma.

PARTICULATE MATTER

Particulate matter is a classification of liquid and solid aerosols that includes emissions from fuel combustion (coal, oil, biomass), transportation, and high temperature industrial processes, including incineration. It includes dust, dirt, soot, smoke, and liquid droplets. Smaller particles include viruses and some bacteria, but most are sulfate and nitrate aerosols and other combustion-derived atmospheric reaction products. The larger particles include pollen, spores, crustal dust, and other mechanically generated dusts. The size of the particle determines the deposition site in the airways. The smaller particles can penetrate deep into the lung tissue, whereas the larger ones will be deposited in the nasal-tracheal area. There is much scientific study regarding differentiation of health effects based on particle size.

Acute signs and symptoms of particulate exposure include restricted activity, respiratory illnesses, and exacerbations of asthma and COPD. Clinical observations associated with particulate matter have included increased numbers of lung- and cardiac-related admissions to hospital emergency rooms. Communities with higher exposures to fine particulate have been noted to have a higher incidence of lung cancer, when adjusted for cigarette smoking and other risk factors. The World Health Organization estimates that globally, about 460,000 excess deaths are attributed to suspended particulate matter.

The first standards for particulate matter were set in 1971. Total suspended particulate (TSP) was the term referring to particles suspended in the air. Since 1987, the EPA has used the indicator PM-10, which includes those particles with aerodynamic diameter smaller than 10 micrometers. These smaller particles are likely to be responsible for most of the adverse health effects of particulate matter because of their ability to reach the lower regions of the respiratory tract. In 1997, the EPA added two new PM 2.5 standards.

DETERMINING HEALTH RISKS

The processes by which health risks are determined, which are then translated into policy, are a combination of science, economics, and politics. A four-step risk assessment is applied in which a hazard identification begins the process. A hazard is identified when animal or human studies indicate that a health risk is created by a specific exposure. The weight of evidence is based in part on the research methodologies—human studies carry more weight than animal studies, occupational exposures usually represent less confounding variables than environmental studies. Once a health hazard has been determined, an exposure assessment is made.

The exposure assessment estimates what people are exposed to during a specified time period. For example, is the source of the exposure a factory smokestack that operates during the day or does the exposure derive from automobile traffic? Air quality monitoring is combined with computer modeling to determine the "fate and transport" of air pollution, or the mapping of the travel and/or landing of an air pollutant. This will also help to determine who and how many will be exposed. Then an estimate is made of the amount inhaled by individuals, by estimating breathing rates and life span exposures.

The next step is the dose–response estimate. Included in this part of the assessment is an understanding of the routes of entry of a pollutant into the body; the effects that the chemical will have on individual cells, tissues, organs and organ systems within the body; and the mechanism of excretion. The dose–response relationship describes the association between exposure and the observed health effect.

When the EPA is developing its air and other standards, it assumes that there is no exposure for which there is zero risk to a carcinogen and that the relationship is a straight line, meaning that for each unit of increase in dose (exposure) there is an increase in cancer response. For noncarcinogens, the EPA typically assumes that at low doses for which no adverse health effects are noted, the body's natural protective mechanisms repair any damage caused by the pollutant. Even with additional protection factors, weaknesses in the protection offered by this policy may occur in protecting the fetus, very young children, the elderly, and other highly vulnerable populations.

The final step in risk assessment is risk characterization. This step synthesizes the information derived from the previous steps. Combining the results of the exposure assessment and the dose–response assessment gives an estimate of the increased lifetime risk of cancer for an individual exposed to maximum long-term concentration. Public health agencies concerned with air quality perform risk assessment to determine the increased risk of illnesses from a specific human exposure.

maximum lifetime exposure × dose–response relationship
= maximum individual lifetime risk

People with asthma, COPD, and cardiovascular diseases may need to change their outdoor behavior when air pollution is severe and reduce their overall time outside. Even for otherwise healthy people who work outdoors, the American Conference of Industrial Hygienists suggests that their duration and workload be reduced during high ozone days. Many newspapers and television weather reports will include ozone alerts. It is also recommended that children not play sports outdoors during the middle of the day on high ozone days.

As the public becomes increasingly concerned about air quality, primary care providers will need to be prepared to answer their patients' questions, as well as to determine what air pollutants in their area may be affecting their patients' health. To do the latter, they will need to know where to go to find out what the air pollutants are. There are several sources of information.

ACCESSING INFORMATION ABOUT AIR POLLUTANTS

The EPA developed the Air Quality Index (AQI), formerly the Pollutants Standards Index (PSI), that allows for a conversion of individual pollutant concentrations to a scale describing good, moderate, unhealthy, very unhealthy, and hazardous air quality. The AQI scale ranges from 0–500, with 100 representing the national ambient air quality standard for that pollutant. When the pollutant levels are high, states are required to report the AQI to the public in metropolitan areas (populations greater than 350,000) in the local media (newspaper or local television or radio). The public can also call state hotlines to obtain daily air quality readings. This information can be helpful in evaluating possible respiratory effects in our patients.

For more specific information about hazardous chemicals released into the air in your area, the Toxic Release Inventory (TRI) will be helpful. The TRI is a compendium of chemicals that are intentionally released into the air and water by companies and facilities and reported to the EPA. (There is more information on this subject in chapter 8 on the Right to Know.) In addition to the TRI, there is a National Toxic Inventory, maintained by the EPA, which will provide information on small point sources that may not be covered by the TRI requirements, but that accounts for over 30% of the toxic emissions in the U.S. Under "EnviroFacts," on the EPA's website, TRI and the National Toxic Inventory can be accessed by zip code. (see www.epa.org.)

AIR QUALITY THREATS

In agricultural areas, where aerial pesticide applications are made, pesticides may drift, volatilize, and disperse downwind. Ground water, surface water, soil, and food may become contaminated. The indoor air is also likely to become contaminated with the pesticide drift. General population exposure has been well documented, with residues of pesticides and metabolites found in blood, urine, breast milk, fat tissue, and other tissues. Health practitioners should factor such potential exposures into their patient and community assessments.

Incinerators pose a threat to air quality, releasing a range of pollutants depending on the waste stream composition. They will typically include the metals (mercury, lead, arsenic, cadmium, chromium, manganese, nickel, antimony, selenium, zinc, and vanadium); PCBs, furans, polycyclic aromatic hydrocarbons, and acid gases and oxides of nitrogen, sulfur, and carbon. Proximity to incinerators is associated with increased local soil lead levels.

A particular concern arising from our poor air quality is global warming, a change in our global climate resulting from the changes in industrial and agricultural processes that, in turn, have changed the gases in our atmosphere. So-called greenhouse gases are those gases (both naturally occurring and man-made) that are capable of adsorbing heat in the atmosphere. The naturally occurring greenhouse gases are water vapor, carbon dioxide, methane, nitrous oxide, and ozone. Man-made contributions to these gases include carbon dioxide, methane, nitrous oxide, and several very powerful greenhouse gases: hydrofluorocarbons (HFCs), perfluorocarbons (PFCs), and sulfur hexafluoride (SF6), which are generated by industrial processes.

The resulting climate changes occurring from the extraordinary addition of man-made, greenhouse gases are rising temperatures (.5–1 degree since the nineteenth century) and a rise in the sea level (4–8 inches in the last century). Alterations in forests, crop yield, and water supplies are predicted. There is nothing that will reverse this trajectory in the near future, and only a global strategy will succeed in addressing the long-term trends. Because of the inevitability of the warming processes and the potential public health ramifications of global warming, health professionals should be educating themselves and weighing in on this very important issue.

CONCLUSION

Good air quality is essential for good health, both in the short term and for future generations. Clinical care practitioners must incorporate an understanding of the air quality in their areas when doing their health assessments and making differential diagnoses. Community and public health professionals must understand the community-wide risks that compromised air quality can increase and the mechanisms by which air quality can be improved. We are a society reliant on fossil fuel and individualized transportation. Our dependence on these two factors and others that affect air quality should be part of our public health discourse and policy decisions. If we choose to ignore these issues, we will continue to see upward trends in negative health effects associated with environmental degradation. Once again, nurses are in a unique position to raise awareness and educate patients, communities, and fellow health professionals to become more involved in this important environmental health issue.

CHAPTER 14

How Food Production Can Affect Safe Consumption

Jackie Hunt Christensen

This chapter does not discuss nutrition and its role in human health. Instead, it examines some of the ways food production methods can influence human health, and some of the relevant diseases or conditions that nurses may face in their work. Because of the scope of this topic, descriptions will be brief and the reader is encouraged to turn to the resources at the end of the chapter or contact the author for more information.

If asked, "Where does your food come from?" the average consumer, particularly the urban consumer, would respond, "the grocery store" or "the supermarket." As food production and processing become more global and crops such as corn are rarely eaten in their natural state but more often in the form of high fructose corn syrup, this should come as no surprise.

Yet food production—not only where it is grown or raised, but how it is processed—can have a great impact on the types of health problems that patients present in a clinical setting. These problems can go beyond the acute episodes of food poisoning that appear in the emergency rooms. What people eat can play an important role in chronic diseases such as cancer, diabetes and heart disease. Healthy food is critical for the growth and development of healthy children.

FOODBORNE ILLNESS: "IT MUST HAVE BEEN SOMETHING I ATE"

Factors related to adverse health impacts can be categorized in several ways: pathological or chemical, acute or chronic, even intentional versus accidental. The pathological and the acute tend to occur together. ER nurses are frequently faced with patients complaining of nausea, vomiting, and/or diarrhea that may be caused by "something I ate."

According to a 1999 report by the Centers for Disease Control and Prevention, approximately 5,200 Americans die each year from foodborne illnesses. More than 76 million U.S. residents develop some type of food-related illness annually (Raloff, 1999). However, most people would be unlikely to suspect an environmental link to their illness. Certainly, pathogens can and do often enter the food system through poor hygiene in processing plants, restaurants, and even home kitchens.

Pathogens may enter the food long before it gets to a processor or a supermarket. There are several ways in which this may occur.

1. *Through the use of uncomposted animal manure as a fertilizer.* Composting manure or food waste brings it to a temperature at which most pathogens should be killed.
2. *Through exposure to untreated animal manure as a result of improper manure management.* For example, large-scale confined animal feeding operations (CAFOs) may contain literally thousands of hogs or poultry on one farm. Waste from these animals is generally stored in lagoons or pits, many of which are unlined. During periods of heavy rain, these lagoons can overflow into surrounding fields and water supplies. Manure may also be land-applied as fertilizer, but at rates higher than the soil can accommodate. This can lead to runoff that affects areas beyond the application site.
3. *Through land application of sewage sludge* (sometimes called biosolids) *as a fertilizer.* Sewage sludge is the semisolid material that remains after wastewater, grit, and heavy items have been screened out of the sewage treatment system. Other pathogens, such as those that cause hepatitis A, typhoid, cholera, polio, and amoebic dysentery have been found in sludge (Mackenzie, 1998). Microbiologist and EPA whistle-blower, Dr. David Lewis, has found extremely high levels of *E. coli O157:H7* and *salmonella* on farmland near Kansas City more than five years after the sludge applications are believed to have taken place (Lewis, 1999).

Unfortunately, tracking exposure to pathogens from one of these sources can be very difficult, particularly if the patient lives in an urban area. In rural settings, patients will generally be aware that they live near a large feedlot because of the odors associated with those types of facilities.

WHAT NURSES CAN DO TO BECOME MORE INFORMED ABOUT PATHOGENS IN FOOD

Here are some questions that nurses can use to think about their own exposure to foodborne pathogens other than from meals outside the home or from kitchen practices. These questions can be added to existing interview procedures in order to identify possible exposure to pathogens from animal waste or sludge.

1. *Do you grow any of your own food?* If yes, *do you use any substances to help the plants grow?* (Or *Do you add anything to the soil to improve plant growth?*) Responses that mention manure, biosolids, sludge, or commercially available sludge products such as Milorganite(r) indicate potential sources of pathogens.
2. If yes, *do you live near any large cattle or hog feedlots or poultry operations?* If yes, *has there been any flooding recently that could have exposed your garden to runoff from nearby farms?* (If patients live in a rural area, even if they do not know of existing livestock operations, such runoff is a possible source of contamination.)
3. *Have you eaten any raw fruits or vegetables in the past 14 days?* If yes, *do you know if any of that produce had been grown using sewage sludge or animal manure as fertilizer?*

Many agricultural and community groups oppose the land application of sewage sludge on agricultural land, despite EPA regulations, because of concerns about pathogens, toxic chemicals, and radioactivity, and because of the lack of enforcement mechanisms in the rules. Concerned clinicians can check the end of this section for contact information at the EPA and grassroots groups working on this issue. Similarly, many communities near large CAFOs have concerns about pathogens in waste, odors, hydrogen sulfide, and so on. One new issue that is emerging from the discussions around CAFOS is antibiotic resistance.

How do "factory farms" and antibiotic resistance relate to one another? For decades, some conventional livestock farmers have used subtherapeutic levels of antibiotics in feed to promote faster growth and to convert "feed to flesh" more quickly. In this context, subtherapeutic means "the use of an antibiotic as a feed additive at less than 200 grams per ton of feed . . . at dosages below those required to treat established infections" (Halverson, 2000, p. 33). This extra growth or weight can cut feed and shelter costs to producers while also getting the animals to market faster. The practice is most often used in large feedlot settings, where a producer may house thousands of hogs, chickens, or turkeys. The stress of confinement, combined with very limited space and the large numbers of animals, also increases the likelihood that antibiotics will need to be used to control disease. The practice has become so common that animal agriculture use accounts for 40% of antibiotics manufactured in the U.S. (Levy, 1998). Eighty percent of this use is to promote growth and control but not to treat disease (Halverson, 2000).

However, the drugs and their effects go beyond the animals ingesting them. Antibiotic residues can sometimes remain in the animal, and thus in the food it produces for human consumption. Antibiotic residues and/or the disease-resistant microbes they produce can also contaminate water and supplies if the manure is not properly stored or managed. This use of antibiotics in animal agriculture can affect food safety, and thus health, in several ways. Because both antibiotic residues and drug-resistant pathogens are excreted in animal waste, the resistant pathogens spread.

Stressed animals shed more pathogens in their feces than unstressed animals. The pathogenic bacteria that survive the gut and are excreted in the feces are the antibiotic-resistant ones. These bacteria end up in airborne dust, on the floors, and in the liquid manure storage where they are preserved until they are spread, along with the manure, on the fields where they can be detected both in soil and water. Once on the fields, antibiotic-resistant bacterial pathogens, as well as parasites in the feces, can persist and infect wildlife and livestock that ingest them. These resistant pathogens may pass through several "vectors" before multiplying to an infectious dose for the next host. [Halverson, 2000a, p. 33]

For clinicians, this will mean an increase in the number of patients presenting with resistant infections.

More important, the use of antibiotics in agriculture may remove, or at least affect, a critical line of defense against infectious diseases for nurses and physicians. Eleven of the antibiotics used subtherapeutically in agriculture, including penicillin and the tetracyclines, are identical to those used to treat human patients.

In the United States, nearly 30 antibiotics and chemotherapeutics are approved for use in farm animals as subtherapeutic feed additives to promote growth and increase the efficiency with which animals convert feed to flesh. . . . Feed additives also include the so-called antibiotics of last resort for treatment of human diseases, such as vancomycin. [Halverson, 2000b, p. 32]

Last, faced with increasing cases of drug-resistant pathogens, many of which are contracted from food, many nurses and physicians have ordered antibiotics to treat indeterminate food-related illness. In the case of children with *E. coli O157: H7*, this can be dangerous or even fatal. The drugs can actually cause hemolytic urinary syndrome, which can lead to kidney failure and death. In this way, the indirect misuse or inappropriate use of antibiotics (e.g., fostering resistant strains of *E. coli O157: H7* to persist in livestock and poultry) may jeopardize the health and well-being of many children.

There are other issues associated with antibiotic resistance that relate to health care practices. Those issues cannot be addressed here, but it is clear that subtherapeutic antibiotic use in agriculture complicates matters considerably and needs more attention.

WHAT NURSES CAN DO TO BECOME MORE INFORMED ABOUT ANTIBIOTICS AND FOOD

1. Consult the growing number of resources about antibiotic use in agriculture.
2. Investigate whether your onsite cafeteria has committed to purchase meat and dairy products from producers that have pledged not to use antibiotics for growth purposes.
3. Convene discussion groups among staff, particularly in ER and gastroenterology departments, to compare anecdotal data about potential environmental vectors for foodborne illness.

THESE REALLY STICK WITH YOU: HEAVY METALS AND PERSISTENT BIOACCUMULATIVE TOXINS

While pathogens bring on urgent illnesses, often with immediate and obvious symptoms, certain chemical pollutants can lurk silently in food without any apparent harm.

Although not traditionally considered when collecting information to make a diagnosis, even anecdotal information from patients can provide insight to possible long-term health. As more health care systems move to provide preventive care, this type of information may offer insights for the clinician and the patient about potential health risks from dietary intake. In fact, nurses can gain important anecdotal information to predict health problems by asking follow-up questions to those they may already routinely ask about dietary fat intake or the amount of saturated fat patients consume.

Some researchers have speculated that it is not only the *amount* of fat in the diet but also the *type* of fat one eats that determines the likelihood of developing cancer or heart disease. Many chemicals that are either used intentionally in food production or released to the environment, where they enter the food chain, do not degrade easily and are lipophilic (fat-loving). Animals raised for food production pass on some of their body burden of pollutants along with their nutrient value. These chemicals may actually play more of a role in the cause of a disease than the fat itself.

Food is actually the primary means of exposure to many chemicals such as pesticides, dioxin, mercury, and lead. Many of these compounds are stored in fat and build up in the food chain. Patients do not have to work in the agricultural industry to be exposed to these compounds, although conventional farmers and farm workers experience both occupational and dietary exposure.

Exposures from food can be further divided into the categories of agricultural input, pollutants applied or used knowingly by the food producer, and environmental input, pollutants that enter the food chain without the knowledge or control of the producer. Agricultural input includes pesticides and fertilizers that are intentionally used in conventional agriculture and that may leave residues in the food.

Pesticides are probably the best-recognized agricultural input with food implications, although the intent is to control a pest, not adulterate the food. The term *pesticide* encompasses all chemicals that are used to control weeds; kill insects, rodents, or other animals that damage crops in the field; keep away fungi; and keep pests away from harvested crops. Given the diversity of uses for pesticides, many food crops are treated with several chemicals as they are grown and processed. Many of these chemicals leave residues on the skin or exterior of the fruit or vegetable; others become part of the plant as it grows. Chemicals with biocidal properties are used to raise livestock as well.

Various pesticides have been associated with a wide array of effects. Cancer is certainly one with which many nurses are familiar. However, there are many others, some of which are just beginning to be linked to pesticides. These include hormone disruption, in which chemicals are suspected of mimicking, blocking, or changing the actions of hormones that naturally occur in the human body; birth defects; and neurological effects.

This is not surprising, as many pesticides work by interfering with the nervous system of the intended insects. The problem is that the chemicals cannot discern the nervous system of the "enemy" or pest from that of an animal or a person.

Children are especially at risk from pesticide residues because they eat more fruits and vegetables than adults do and thus are at higher risk for greater exposure. This increased risk was substantiated in *Pesticides in the Diets of Infants and Children*, a 1993 report by the National Academy of Sciences (NAS), as well as by the World Health Organization, the EPA and three separate, earlier committees of the National Academy of Sciences (EWG, 2000). The NAS study included in its report concern about neurological effects of pesticides on children.

Parents can reduce health risks to their children by feeding them fruits and vegetables with consistently low pesticide residues (see Table 14.1).

Children need to be protected not only from cancer, but also from chemicals that affect the development of their nervous system, reproductive system, and growth. It is also important to note that such protection, in order to be truly effective, must begin before birth. Pregnant women should also

TABLE 14.1

C. SpannerPANNER Most Contaminated Foods		C. Spanner Least Contaminated Foods	
Rank	Food	Rank	Food
1	Apples	1	Corn
2	Spinach	2	Cauliflower
3	Peaches	3	Sweet Peas
4	Pears	4	Asparagus
5	Strawberries	5	Broccoli
6	Grapes—Chile	6	Pineapple
7	Potatoes	7	Onions
8	Red Raspberries	8	Bananas
9	Celery	9	Watermelon
10	Green Beans	10	Cherries—Chile

Source: Reprinted with permission of the publisher, from Environmental Working Group. *How Bout' Them Apples? Pesticides in Children's Food Ten Years After Alar*. Environmental Working Group: Washington, DC, 1999. Compiled from USDA and FDA pesticide residue data 1992–1997.

be mindful of the exposure of the developing fetus to these chemicals.

In 1998, Congress passed the Food Quality Protection Act (FQPA), which gave the EPA a statutory mandate to establish standards to protect infants and young children from pesticides in food and in the environment. However, the first exemption to the FQPA was made only three weeks after its passage. Exemptions continue to be made, using economic losses to the food producers as justification for allowing pesticides that are known to be hazardous to humans or those with no data.

WHAT NURSES CAN DO TO LEARN MORE ABOUT PESTICIDES IN FOOD

Nurses should by no means discourage consumption of fruits and vegetables, nor should they restrict their own. Instead, here are some suggestions that they can try in their own homes or consider when discussing dietary issues with parents or caregivers.

1. *Eat a variety of fruits and vegetables, particularly those with the least pesticides* (using information such as Table 14.1).
2. *Thoroughly rinse and peel the skin from conventionally grown fruits and vegetables.* Soaps or chemical rinses are not necessary. This process will reduce, but not entirely eliminate, pesticides, fungicides and other chemicals used in their production.
3. *Buy organic food when possible.* Organic foods (those produced under very specific production requirements, which prohibit synthetic pesticides or fertilizers, among other things) are more expensive, but may be an option for some clients. Organic foods may not be pesticide-free, as there may be residues in the soil or drift from nearby conventional farms, but chemical pesticides are not allowed on farms that have been certified as organic.
4. *Join a community-supported agriculture (CSA) farm as a way to learn how food is grown locally.* Near many metropolitan areas, small farmers sell "shares" of the coming season's harvest prior to growing it. Many of these CSAs produce organic or minimally treated food and offer members (those who buy shares) an opportunity to visit and/or work on the farm. This gives consumers a more active role in their food choices and provides additional insight into their production.

Fertilizer products are used intentionally to augment nutrients in the soil that crops need in order to grow. However, some of them contain "tag-along toxins." These may be heavy metals, such as lead, cadmium or mercury, or chemical pollutants such as dioxin or polychlorinated biphenyls. Sewage sludge also contains heavy metals, which treatment systems are not equipped to handle. Some fertilizer products are made with waste materials from industrial processes such as steel smelting or cement kilns. These materials are used for the calcium, zinc, or other nutrients plants require. Unfortunately, other metals or chemicals "tag along" so that farmers are unknowingly applying poisons like arsenic, lead, or cadmium. (Cadmium may also be present in phosphate fertilizers, when the phosphate is mined.)

When sludge or waste-derived fertilizer is used on farmland, the food crops or grazing fodder may absorb the heavy metals. Some crops are more likely to absorb a particular metal than others are. There may even be variances within crops. Spinach can absorb mercury (U.S. Environmental Protection Agency, 1997). Many plants, including tobacco, wheat, corn, and leafy vegetables like lettuce and spinach, readily absorb cadmium. Even plants that do not absorb significant amounts of cadmium can contribute a notable amount to the diet (McBride, 1998). Grazing animals can also ingest the pollutants, as they tend to consume a great deal of soil as they graze.

WHAT NURSES CAN DO TO LEARN MORE ABOUT HEAVY METALS IN FERTILIZERS

1. Become an informed gardener; read labels on fertilizer products for home use. Some products, even if they are derived from natural materials, can be dangerous.
2. Check to see if your state has or is considering regulations on heavy metals in fertilizers.

STEALTH POLLUTANTS: DIOXIN AND MERCURY

Unlike chemical contaminants in fertilizer or pesticides that are toxic outright, some pollutants "sneak" into food. Dioxin and mercury are two such contaminants. (Lead, cadmium, and other heavy metals can enter the food chain from airborne sources as well as from farm inputs.)

Dioxin

Dioxin is the unwanted byproduct of numerous industrial processes that involve chlorine, organic (carbon-containing) material, and combustion (trash incinerators, medical waste incinerators, cement kilns that burn hazardous waste), or a chemical reaction (bleaching paper white with chlorinated compounds, making pesticides, or manufacturing the building blocks of polyvinyl chloride plastic). Dioxin is considered to be one of the most toxic compounds ever studied, and it is widespread in the environment.

About 95% of the average person's dioxin exposure comes from food, particularly meat, fish, and dairy products. Dioxin may travel more than 1000 miles from the incinerator or other facility that generated it, so you don't have to live near an incinerator. It falls to the ground with rain or dust, landing on pastures or grazing lands, where it is eaten by cattle or other grazing animals. Dioxin is fat-soluble and does not break down easily, so it builds up in animal fat. When people drink milk or eat cheese or a hamburger, they are also eating dioxin.

Breast milk, because of its high fat content, is the absolute pinnacle of dioxin exposure. Nursing infants may consume 50 times more dioxin per day than adults. This has been calculated to amount to about 10–12% of an individual's total lifetime exposure (Center for Health, Environment and Justice, 1999).

The International Agency for Research on Cancer and the U.S. EPA have named dioxin as a known human carcinogen (IARC, 1997; Skrzycki and Warrick, 2000). Dioxin has been linked to cancers of the lung, stomach, soft tissue, and liver; endometriosis; infertility; birth defects, learning disabilities; immune system suppression; and altered glucose tolerance (CHEJ, 1999).

One of the most disturbing things about dioxin is that most people already have nearly the amount of dioxin in their bodies that causes health problems in lab animals. Some people have already passed that threshold.

There is no way to remove dioxin from food once it is there. Although animal products constitute the overwhelming majority of exposure, some dioxin will be ingested with fruits and vegetables. Even organic milk products and meat contain dioxin. However, there are alternative industrial processes already available for most of the sources of dioxin emissions.

WHAT NURSES CAN DO TO LEARN MORE ABOUT HOW TO STOP DIOXIN EXPOSURE

1. Do a "waste audit" of what is truly infectious waste in your facility and what is not. Then learn what happens to those waste streams. If any of the wastes are being incinerated, it is likely that dioxin is being formed. Other pollutants will also be released and will most likely enter the food chain at some point.

2. At home and in the workplace, look for paper products that are unbleached (brown) or not bleached with chlorine (labeled "Process-Chlorine-Free" or "Totally Chlorine-Free").
3. Contact the Health Care Without Harm campaign (see "Resources").

Mercury

Mercury is an element that occurs naturally in the environment. However, the widespread wholesale distribution of mercury is due to anthropogenic activities. Coal-burning power plants are the largest source of mercury emissions, but medical waste incinerators account for 10% of mercury air emissions. (USEPA, 1997). Mercury fever thermometers discarded in municipal trash annually contribute 18 tons of mercury and are the largest single source of mercury from households.

Mercury in a thermometer is not very biologically available. However, when mercury air emissions leave an incinerator, like dioxin, they may travel long distances before falling to the ground. When mercury happens to fall into a lake or river, microorganisms in the water convert it to methylmercury, which is much more bioavailable and much more dangerous.

This methylmercury builds up in the food chain, much like dioxin, but with one important exception: mercury accumulates in muscle tissue. So subsistence and recreational fishers can reduce their exposure to dioxin from fish by trimming the fat and by baking or grilling the fish instead of frying it. With mercury, this isn't possible, since the muscle is the portion of the fish that is eaten.

Mercury is a potent neurotoxin. Because it can cross the placenta and the blood–brain barrier, it is particularly dangerous to the developing fetus and young children (Committee on Environmental Health, 1998). The National Academy of Sciences (NAS) released a report concluding that the limits for mercury in food set by the EPA, which are more protective than those established by the Food and Drug Administration, are still not protective enough. The NAS study said that pregnant women who consume more than 3 oz. of ocean fish such as tuna, shark, swordfish, or king mackerel per day are putting their babies at risk for lower IQ and learning disabilities. This could affect at least 60,000 babies per year (Cone, 2000).

Forty states have fish consumption advisories because of mercury contamination. It is especially important for nurses working in obstetrics or pediatrics to make sure that parents are aware of the risks of eating fish from areas where there are advisories.

WHAT NURSES CAN DO TO LEARN MORE ABOUT MERCURY IN FOOD

1. Nurses should check with state departments of health and/or natural resources to find out whether the state has mercury-based fish advisories and if so, where. Subsistence fishers (people who eat fish for cultural, religious and economic reasons) are at greater risk than the rest of the population and are not always considered when agencies generate statistics or advisories.
2. Those working in obstetrics, pediatrics or family practice can work with education departments or state agencies to make copies of fish consumption advisory information available to patients. When possible, work with community groups or service agencies to find or create information that is accessible to patients—that is, in their native language and with graphics or photos that are culturally appropriate—and give them information on how to take some action.
3. Work with others in your facility to phase out the use of mercury-containing products so that the hospital or clinic is not contributing to mercury pollution of food and the environment.
4. Use fish consumption advisories to eat fish wisely, not to avoid fish. Fish remain an important source of protein, and often an inexpensive one. Choose fish that are not predator species. Find fishing areas that have been tested and found to be low in contamination.

BIBLIOGRAPHY

Center for Health, Environment and Justice. (1999). *America's choice: Children's health corporate profit* (Technical Support Document.) Falls Church, VA: Author.

Committee on Environmental Health. (1998). Mercury. *Handbook of Pediatric Environmental Health*, pp. 145–154.

Cone, M. (2000, July 12). Panel issues warning on mercury risk. *Los Angeles Times*.

Environmental Working Group. (1999). *How bout' them apples? Pesticides in children's food ten years after alar*. Washington, DC: Author.

Halverson, M. (2000a). *The price we pay for corporate hogs*. Minneapolis: Institute for Agriculture and Trade Policy. 33.

Halverson, M. (2000b). The Price We Pay for Corporate Hogs, 32. Minneapolis: Institute for Agriculture and Trade Policy, 2000. Citing PRNewswire. (1999, June 10). Smithfield Foods, Inc. Achieves Record Earnings for Third Consecutive Year in Fiscal 1999. Smithfield, VA: PRNewswire. and Nakashima, E., "Court Fines Smithfield $12.6 Million: Va. Firm is Assessed Largest Such Pollution Penalty in U.S. History," *Washington Post* (August 9, 1997): A1.

International Agency for Research on Cancer. (1997, February 14). IARC evaluates carcinogenic risk associated with dioxins (press release).

Levy, S. B. (1998, March). The challenge of antibiotic resistance. *Scientific American.*

Lewis, D. (1999, January 27). Editorial: Sludge M. *Journal of Commerce.*

Mackenzie, D. (1998, August 29). Waste not. *New Scientist.*

McBride, M. B. (1998). Growing food crops on sludge-amended soils: Problems with the U.S. Environmental Protection Agency method of estimating toxic metal transfer. *Environmental Toxicology and Chemistry, 17*(11), 2274–2281.

Raloff, J. Sickening food. *Science News,* 156:19.

Skrzycki, C., & Warrick, J. (2000, May 17). EPA links dioxin to cancer. *The Washington Post,* p. A01.

United States Environmental Protection Agency. (1997, December). *Mercury study report to Congress: Volume I: Executive summary.* United States Environmental Protection Agency, Office of Air Quality Planning & Standards and Office of Research and Development. (EPA-452/R-97-003).

CHAPTER 15

Environmental Tobacco Smoke and Smoking Cessation

Sophie Balk

This chapter provides information about the health effects of environmental tobacco smoke (ETS)—"second-hand smoke"—and then focuses on smoking cessation strategies for the clinician. Smoking cessation is the best means of preventing or ameliorating the negative health effects of ETS. The health effects of active smoking on the smoker are beyond the scope of this chapter and will not be discussed.

DEFINITION AND HEALTH EFFECTS

Environmental tobacco smoke consists of "mainstream" smoke exhaled by an active smoker, and "sidestream" smoke released from the smoldering end of a cigarette, pipe or cigar. ETS contains more than 3,800 different chemicals. ETS is qualitatively similar to mainstream smoke, but contains higher quantities of certain toxins such as ammonia, formaldehyde, and nitrosamines. It is the main source of particulate matter of less than 2.5 microns, a size that reaches the lower airways.

In 1998, more than 47.2 million U.S. adults, 24% of the population, were cigarette smokers (Centers for Disease Control and Prevention, 2000). Forty-three percent of children aged 2 months to 11 years lived in a home with a cigarette smoker (Pirkle, Flegal, Bernert, et al., 1996). Young children may spend a significant amount of their time indoors, in their own homes, relatives' homes, and child care settings, exposing them to ETS and making them passive smokers.

EFFECTS ON ADULTS

Adults may be exposed to ETS through a tobacco-using spouse or house-mate. ETS has been classified as a group A human carcinogen, indicating that there is sufficient scientific evidence supporting a causal relationship between exposure to ETS and the development of cancer. The U.S. Environmental Protection Agency has estimated that ETS is responsible for approximately 3,000 lung cancer deaths per year in nonsmokers in the United States. In addition, exposure to ETS has been linked with an increased risk of developing myocardial infarction, reduced pulmonary function, cough, headache, nasal congestion, and eye irritation.

EFFECTS ON CHILDREN

Children exposed to ETS through maternal smoking may show a number of negative health effects (American Academy of Pediatrics, 1999) including (1) *Lower respiratory tract infections:* These infants are 38% more likely to be hospitalized for pneumonia in the first year of life than children whose mothers do not smoke; when both parents smoke, the infants are twice as likely to be hospitalized than children whose parents do not smoke. (2) *Middle ear effusions:* Children of parents who smoke are more likely to develop middle ear effusion and otitis media. (3) *Asthma:* These children are more likely to develop asthma, and those with asthma may have more severe symptoms and more frequent exacerbations. (4) *Sudden infant death syndrome* (SIDS): A growing body of evidence links ETS exposure to an increased incidence of SIDS, independent of gestational age or birth weight.

Exposure to ETS before age 10 raises the risk of developing leukemia and lymphoma in adulthood.

SMOKING CESSATION

Smoking cessation efforts directed towards the smoker can benefit the smoker and are the most effective way to diminish a nonsmoker's exposure to ETS. It is now well-established that primary care clinicians can have a positive effect on smokers who wish to quit. At least 70% of smokers visit a physician each year, more than 50% visit a dentist, and many visit other clinicians. More than 70% of smokers wish to quit, and almost 50% of them try to quit each year. Although effective treatments are available, most smokers wishing to quit do not obtain the benefits of these treatments but try to quit on their own.

In 2000, the U.S. Public Health Service published *Treating Tobacco Use and Dependence: A Clinical Practice Guideline* (Fiore, Bailey, Cohen, et al., 2000), which provided recommendations for brief and intensive clinical interventions and for systems changes to promote treatment of tobacco dependence. The 2000 guideline updated the 1996 Agency for Health Care Policy and Research *Smoking Cessation: Clinical Practice Guideline* (Fiore, Bailey, Cohen, et al., 1996), which reflected the information gained from a review of 3,000 articles published between 1975 and 1994. For the 2,000 guideline, more than 6,000 research papers were reviewed, including 3,000 articles published between 1995 and 1999. This review provided the basis for more than 50 meta-analyses.

The updated guideline underscores the fact that tobacco dependence has come to be viewed as a true drug dependence comparable to dependence on opiates or cocaine. Because tobacco dependence is a chronic condition, changing the behavior of the tobacco user requires repeated clinical interventions. Even if a tobacco user wishes to quit permanently, there will generally be multiple cycles of relapse and remission. In order to successfully treat patients who are dependent on tobacco, clinicians must adopt approaches similar to those used to treat other chronic conditions such as hypertension, diabetes, and hyperlipidemia. Patients who are dependent on tobacco need simple advice, support, and pharmacotherapy. Clinicians must appreciate that tobacco use is a chronic addictive condition requiring repeated interventions, lest they become discouraged if the patient relapses.

The following is a list of key findings of the updated guideline.*

1. Tobacco dependence is a chronic condition that often requires repeated intervention.
2. Because effective tobacco dependence treatments are available, every patient who uses tobacco should be offered at least one of these treatments.
   a. Patients who are willing to try to quit tobacco use should be provided treatments identified as effective.
   b. Patients who are unwilling to quit tobacco use should be provided a brief intervention designed to increase their motivation to quit.
3. Clinicians and health care delivery systems must institutionalize the consistent identification, documentation, and treatment of every tobacco user seen in a health care setting.

---

* Adapted from Fiore 2000.

4. Brief tobacco dependence treatment is effective, and every patient who uses tobacco should be offered at least brief treatment.
5. There is a strong dose–response relation between the intensity of tobacco dependence counseling and its effectiveness.
6. Three types of counseling and behavioral therapies were found to be especially effective and should be used with all patients attempting tobacco cessation:
   a. Provision of practical counseling (problem-solving skills and training)
   b. Provision of social support as part of treatment (intratreatment social support)
   c. Help in securing social support outside of treatment (extratreatment social support)
7. Numerous effective pharmacotherapies for smoking cessation now exist. Except in the presence of contraindications, these should be used with all patients attempting to quit smoking.
8. Tobacco dependence treatments are both clinically effective and cost-effective relative to other medical and disease prevention interventions. Thus, insurance plans should ensure that they include, as a reimbursed benefit, the counseling and pharmacotherapies identified as effective and that clinicians are reimbursed for providing tobacco dependence treatment, just as they are reimbursed for the treatment of other chronic conditions.

Numerous pharmocotherapies and counseling strategies have been developed to help clinicians provide effective treatment and support. Long-term success rates can be increased from about 7% of smokers who try to quit on their own to 15–30% when smokers are offered treatment strategies suggested by the guideline. The most effective and cost-effective treatments are intensive counseling and pharmacotherapy, and there is a strong dose–response relationship between intensity of counseling and successful quitting. Even brief smoking cessation advice, when delivered by a physician during an office visit, is effective in increasing quitting rates. Brief interventions are most relevant to primary care settings where time constraints are common. Interventions have been shown to be cost-effective: smokers who quit use fewer health care resources. Many interventions are reimbursable, providing additional incentive for clinicians to counsel smokers to quit.

The updated guideline recommends that interventions, either brief or intensive, be used with all populations, including teenagers, pregnant women, and older smokers. Special consideration must be given when considering pharmacotherapy in certain populations, such as those patients with medical contraindications, those who are smoking fewer than 10 cigarettes per day, smokers who are pregnant or breastfeeding, and teen smokers.

The 2000 *Guideline* recommends that brief interventions be used for three categories of patients: current tobacco users who are willing to make a quit attempt, current users who are unwilling to make a quit attempt at this time, and former users who have recently quit. No attempt is made to intervene with adults who have never used tobacco or who have been abstinent for a long period of time.

THE "5 A's" APPROACH

The majority of tobacco users visit a primary care setting each year, and so the *Guideline* stresses the importance of identifying those patients who are willing to quit, using the "5 A's" approach: (1) *Ask:* Systematically identify tobacco users at every visit. Clinicians are urged to obtain a smoking history from patients to assess current and past smoking. (2) *Advise:* All users should be strongly urged to quit. (3) *Assess:* Clinicians should assess the patient's willingness to quit. If the patient is willing, the clinician should provide assistance, including specific referrals to local smoking cessation experts and other resources. (4) *Assist:* Clinicians should assist patients to set goals. These include setting a quit date; telling family, friends and co-workers about the quit date and enlisting their support for the cessation effort; anticipating challenges to quitting, particularly during the first few weeks when the relapse rate is highest; and removing all tobacco products from the environment before quitting. (5) *Arrange follow-up:* Follow-up contact should be made soon after the quit date, either during a health visit, or through a telephone call.

PHARMACOTHERAPY

Nicotine is an extremely addictive substance, acting on the hypothalamic center, which controls arousal, concentration, and stress reduction. Nicotine releases dopamine and norepinephrine, resulting in increased energy and euphoria, improved concentration, improved hand–eye coordination, and anorexia. A true drug dependence develops and physiologic withdrawal occurs after the patient stops using nicotine. Psychological dependence is also likely to occur, with cravings to start using tobacco again. Nicotine withdrawal symptoms are more likely if the patient smokes more than 10 cigarettes per day. "Nicotine withdrawal syndrome" is characterized by at least five of the following within 24 hours: (1) dysmorphic or depressed mood; (2) insomnia; (3) irritability, frustration or anger; (4) anxiety, restlessness, or impatience; (5) difficulty concentrating; (6) decreased heart rate; (7) increased appetite or weight gain.

Because of the addictive properties of nicotine, all patients willing to quit should also be offered pharmacotherapy unless there is a contraindication. Medications increase smoking cessation rates and reduce withdrawal symptoms. The first-line pharmacotherapies recommended are sustained-release bupropion hydrochloride, nicotine gum, nicotine inhaler, nicotine nasal spray, and the nicotine patch. The choice of a first-line medication is determined by the clinician's familiarity with the medication, the patient's previous experience with the medication, specific contraindications, and patient characteristics (such as history of depression or concern about weight gain). Second-line therapies, such as clonidine hydrochloride and nortriptyline hydrochloride, are suggested when patients are unable to use first-line therapies because of contraindications or when first-line therapies fail. A summary of recommended medications is listed as follows:

First-line medications

- *Nicotine replacement therapy (NRT):* Smokers should quit smoking entirely before beginning nicotine replacement and should not resume smoking during therapy.
- *Transdermal nicotine patch:* Several different transdermal patches are available, and all have lower doses used during tapering. Full-dose patches are recommended for most smokers for the first 1–3 months, followed by 1–2 tapering doses for 2–4 weeks each. The main side effect is local irritation. The patch is preferred by many clinicians because of ease of instruction in use and fewer compliance problems compared to nicotine gum.
- *Nicotine gum:* 2- and 4-mg gum is available over the counter. Users should not chew too rapidly, chewing for 20–30 minutes per piece. Instruction in use requires considerable education. Side effects are primarily local and include jaw fatigue, sore mouth and throat, upset stomach, and hiccups.
- *Nicotine nasal spray:* Patients administer one spray per nostril when they feel the urge to smoke. Because the resulting blood nicotine level is higher than that produced by the patch or gum, it may be more effec-

tive than other NRT delivery systems in highly addicted smokers. Side effects are irritation of the nose causing burning, sneezing, and watery eyes; tolerance to these effects usually develops in 1–2 days.

- *Nicotine vapor inhaler:* The inhaler is marketed in a cigarette-like plastic device and has a unique role because it fulfills the "hand-mouth" behavior of smoking. It can be used as frequently as desired. Nearly 80 puffs are required to achieve nicotine doses equivalent to a cigarette.
- *Bupropion:* Smokers are more likely than nonsmokers to have a history of major depression; nicotine may act as an antidepressant in some smokers. Bupropion, an antidepressant, is effective in some smokers. It is dosed at 150–300 mg per day for 7 days before quitting, then at 300 mg per day for the next 6–12 weeks. Bupropion can also be used in conjunction with a nicotine patch. In excessive doses, bupropion can cause seizures and should not be used in patients with a history of seizures or eating disorders.

Second-line medications

- *Clonidine*
- *Nortriptyline*

SMOKERS UNWILLING TO QUIT

Clinicians are urged to provide a motivational message to those smokers unwilling to quit. Success in effecting behavioral change is more likely if a clinician delivers the message in an empathetic and nonjudgmental manner. The "5 R's" approach is suggested by the *Guideline:* (1) *Relevance:* Smokers are encouraged to consider the personal importance of quitting, such as ameliorating the negative health effects of smoking on themselves or their children. (2) *Risks:* Smokers are asked to identify the negative effects of using tobacco. These include acute risks such as shortness of breath and exacerbation of asthma; chronic risks such as heart attacks, strokes, and lung cancer; and environmental risks such as increased risk of lung cancer and heart disease in spouses of smokers, and increased risk of sudden infant death syndrome, asthma, and ear infections in children of smokers. (3) *Rewards:* Smokers are asked to list potential benefits of stopping tobacco use. These include improved health of the smoker and his or her family, and setting a good example for children. (4) *Roadblocks:* Smokers are asked to identify possible barriers to quitting (such as fear of withdrawal symptoms or weight gain) and to note elements of treatment that could address barriers. 5. *Repetition:* Clinicians are encouraged to repeat the message at each health care visit; smokers should be reminded that most people make multiple attempts before successfully quitting.

RECENT QUITTERS: RELAPSE PREVENTION TREATMENT

The *Guideline* advises clinicians to continue to offer relapse prevention treatment to smokers who have recently quit. Tobacco addiction is a chronically relapsing condition; most relapses occur early in the process of quitting, although some occur months and years later. Brief relapse prevention advice should be part of every encounter with a patient who has recently quit. The patient should be congratulated about quitting and encouraged to remain abstinent. Discussion should include benefits of cessation and problems anticipated or encountered, such as depression, weight gain, or the influence of other tobacco users in the home.

Specific problems may need more intense follow-up and therapy during a dedicated follow-up encounter (either in person or by telephone) or through referral to a specialized clinic or program. Specific problems include. (1) *Lack of support:* The clinician can schedule an in-person or telephone follow-up to help the patient identify sources of support. This may include a referral to an appropriate agency that can offer support. (2) *Mood:* Depression or negative mood is common and may require medication or referral to a specialist. (3) *Prolonged or strong withdrawal symptoms:* For prolonged or severe symptoms, medication may be needed for a lengthy period. This may include adding or combining medications. (4) *Weight gain:* Reassurance is needed that although weight gain is common, it is usually self-limiting. The majority of smokers who quit gain 10 pounds or less. Clinicians can advise patients about the importance of a healthy diet and exercise and advise against drastic diets. Medications such as bupropion with or without nicotine replacement therapy and referral to a specialist may be needed. (5) *Feelings of deprivation, flagging motivation:* Clinicians can make patients aware that these feelings are common but that resuming smoking makes quitting more difficult. They can suggest other activities that may be rewarding.

Patients should be encouraged to identify situations in which they are likely to smoke. These may be situations of stress, or habitual situations such as drinking coffee in the morning, or relaxing with co-workers who smoke. The "4 D's" approach has been suggested to help patients overcome these situations: (1) *Do something else:* This could include going for a walk, or being prepared with a healthy snack to eat at coffee-break time instead of reaching for a cigarette. (2) *Drink water*; (3) *Deep breathe*; (4) *Delay:* This strategy helps patients until the craving for a cigarette passes.

Other strategies include staying away from smokers or leaving the room when others are smoking; asking friends and spouses to stop smoking too; and finding a supportive person who will provide encouragement.

Systems Interventions

The *Guideline* underscores that insurers such as managed care organizations can promote the implementation of systems and policies to encourage tobacco use assessment and treatment as an integral part of patient care. Changes in systems have increased the utilization of tobacco dependence treatment and reduced the prevalence of smoking among the enrollees of managed health care plans.

Office-wide interventions include: (1) *Office policy:* The office should have signs stating a no-smoking policy. Office staff should not smoke in the vicinity of the office. Literature that has pro-smoking messages should be removed from the waiting room. (2) *Systematic assessment of the patient's smoking:* Smoking status can be added as an item on the office intake form filled out by the patient. Office-wide systems, such as tobacco-use status stickers or adding tobacco use as a vital sign, are helpful in reminding clinicians to gather information. (3) *Involving staff in smoking cessation education:* Because cessation rates increase with the number of contacts a patient has with staff, the goal is to have all professionals, including receptionists, ask about smoking as part of the visit. Health educators can be a vital part of this effort. (4) *Providing patient education materials:* Materials are available free or at low cost from local affiliates of the American Cancer Society, American Heart Association, American Lung Association, and the National Cancer Institute's Cancer Information Service. Many agencies also provide self-help materials. (5) *Utilizing local resources:* Clinicians can compile a list of local agencies or programs to be given to motivated patients.

THE SPECIFIC ROLE OF CLINICIANS

Working with Pregnant Women

Many women who are pregnant stop smoking during the pregnancy. Pregnant women are often motivated to quit by information about the deleterious effects of smoking on the fetus, including increased risk of prematurity, low birth weight, and placental abruption. All pregnant women should be encouraged to quit smoking.

WORKING WITH CHILDREN AND THEIR MOTHERS

Offering smoking cessation to adults is not just the job of adult or women's health clinicians. Pediatricians and pediatric nurses are in a good position to provide counseling because parents frequently visit pediatricians, particularly in the child's first year of life or when the child has a medical problem. In fact, pediatricians may be the only doctors parents of young children visit.

As many as two-thirds of mothers who stop smoking during pregnancy may relapse within three months after the baby's birth. Smoking cessation counseling offered to parents is the most effective method of ensuring that children will not be exposed to ETS. Any of the strategies described in the *Guideline* can be used with parents, including offering advice, giving out literature, and providing information about medications. If a child's illness can be linked to parental smoking, clinicians may be able to use this instance as a "teachable moment" to reinforce the importance of not smoking. Parents can also be told that they have an important role modeling effect; children whose parents smoke are more likely to become smokers themselves. Pediatricians should familiarize themselves with the range of medications available and can make referrals to the parent's physician or to smoking cessation specialists for medication prescriptions.

WORKING WITH TEENAGERS

It is challenging to counsel teenagers who are smokers. Nine out of ten Americans who smoke began before they were 19 years old. Since 1991, adolescent tobacco use rates have increased while adult use has steadily decreased.

Clinicians can utilize the "5 A's" approach to *ask* teens about tobacco use (including smokeless tobacco). Honest responses are more likely if interviews are conducted in private, without a parent present and with a guarantee of confidentiality. Non-smokers should be praised for making a healthy choice. It is important for clinicians to *advise* smoking teens to quit. However, those who do smoke are often not receptive to ideas about their susceptibility to long-term negative health effects. With younger and less mature patients, it may be more effective to focus on short-term factors such as the expense of cigarettes; their effect on athletic performance; cosmetic effects such as bad breath, stained fingers and teeth; and the desirability for teens to resist peer pressure. Clinicians should *assess* the teen's readiness to quit. They should *assist* teen smokers in setting a quit date, provide self-help materials, encourage teens to think of situations in which they might be tempted to smoke, and help them develop strategies to avoid smoking. For patients who agree to setting a quit date, the clinician should *arrange follow-up* within one to two weeks to discuss smoking status, progress, and problems.

Clinicians should consider prescribing nicotine replacement therapy (NRT) for teenagers who want to quit smoking. Teens who smoke regularly may be as addicted to nicotine as are adults. There has been little research regarding NRT in teens, but it should nevertheless be considered for young smokers (Heymann, 1997) as the dangers of tobacco use almost certainly outweigh the risks associated with carefully monitored NRT. Like all other tobacco users, teens must avoid using tobacco products while on NRT because of the risk of nicotine toxicity.

CONCLUSION

The dangers of ETS are well known. Effective therapies for smoking cessation are available but are not always offered to patients who wish to quit. It is imperative that clinicians become familiar with smoking cessation strategies and make them available to all tobacco users.

BIBLIOGRAPHY

American Academy of Pediatrics' Committee on Environmental Health. (1999, October). Environmental tobacco smoke and smoking cessation. In R. A. Etzel & S. J. Balk (Eds.), *Handbook of pediatric environmental health* (pp.). Elk Grove Village IL: American Academy of Pediatrics.

Centers for Disease Control and Prevention. (2000). Strategies for reducing exposure to environmental tobacco smoke, increasing tobacco use cessation, and reducing initiation in communities and health care systems. *MMWR, 49*(RR12), 1.

Fiore, M. C., Bailey, W. C., Cohen S. J., et al. (1996). *Smoking cessation: Clinical practice guideline No. 18*. (AHCPR Publication No. 96-0692). Rockville MD: U.S. Department of Health and Human Services.

Fiore, M. C., Bailey, W. C., Cohen, S. J., et al. (2000). *Treating tobacco use and dependence. A clinical practice guideline*. (AHCPR Publication No. 00-0032). Rockville MD: U.S. Department of Health and Human Services.

Heymann, R. B. (1997). Tobacco: prevention and cessation strategies. *Adolescent Health Update, 9*, 1–8.

Pirkle, J. L., Flegal, K. M., Bernert, J. T., et al. (1996). Exposure of the U.S. population to environmental tobacco smoke: The Third National Health and Nutrition Examination Survey, 1988–1991. *Journal of the American Medical Association, 275*, 1233–1240.

CHAPTER 16

Hazardous and Municipal Waste Sites

Cherryll Ranger and Ralph O'Connor

H azardous waste is a multifaceted issue wrought with controversy in many areas including health impacts. This chapter presents in general terms the scope of the problem, common terminology, and the issues nurses will need to address to ensure safe environments through health promotion and prevention activities. Nurses will be required to use new approaches (1) for communication, (2) in prevention strategies, (3) to protect quality of life, (4) to create policies, and (5) to expand their collaboration networks. Nurses must balance science with elements of sensationalism and uncertainty. Trends and emerging issues are presented as nurses look to the future in addressing environmental health in their areas of practice. Recommendations for action are provided as points for exploration.

CHARACTERIZING HAZARDOUS AND MUNICIPAL WASTE

Hazardous waste and municipal waste have their own vocabulary such as *Superfund*. Superfund is a program established by Congress in 1980 in the wake of the Love Canal contamination in New York (Johnson, 1999). Superfund was created to clean up hazardous waste sites and chemical spills in the United States and it includes a revolving Superfund trust to help pay for the cleanups by taxing the chemical industry and then recovering cleanup costs from responsible parties. The monies collected are placed in the trust and are then administered by the U.S. Environmental Protection Agency (EPA). The legislation that created Superfund is the Comprehensive Environmental Response, Compensation, and Liability Act (CERCLA).

Note: Chapter is not under copyright—authors are federal employees.

Some hazardous waste sites are called National Priorities List (NPL) sites. NPL sites need extensive long-term cleanup under the Superfund program. EPA can place a site on the NPL by using criteria to rank sites according to the threat to the environment and to public health or if the Agency for Toxic Substances and Disease Registry (ATSDR), a federal public health agency, determines there is an imminent health risk and issues a health advisory for the site. Several states have separate programs for cleaning up their top priority sites.

Hazardous waste can be difficult to characterize. It can be referred to by specific toxin such as lead, arsenic, and trichloroethylene or by the class of toxins to which it belongs such as heavy metals, volatile organic compounds, polychlorinated biphenyls (PCBs), or pesticides. Sites may be classified according to their ownership such as private, local government, or federal government (e.g., Department of Energy or Department of Defense) sites. Hazardous wastes range from licensed landfills to illegal dumping areas (e.g., Times Beach in Missouri) to unintentional spills from transportation accidents or stationary facilities.

The more common types of waste sites are chemical waste landfills (e.g., the famous Love Canal), manufacturing or industrial facilities (e.g., Alabama Plating, Inc.) or mining sites (e.g., Libby, Montana; see Figure 16.1). In West Dallas, Texas, and Bunker Hill, Idaho, children were exposed to very high levels of lead in the air, in dust in their homes, and in the soil outside their homes, as a result of nearby smelters. Conventional weapons testing and firing has resulted in lead exposures at some military bases, and at Camp Lejeune military base in North Carolina, trichlorethylene (TCE) exposure occurred in the drinking water. Waste sites range from single family homes illegally treated with methyl parathion to contaminated aquifers to mining areas covering hundreds of square miles. There are 1,296 hazardous waste sites currently on the NPL and as of January 2001, 49 of the 50 U.S states had NPL sites, ranging from 1 in Nevada to 114 in New Jersey (U.S. Environmental Protection Agency, 2001). The trend for placement on the NPL is moving more toward removal actions that quickly clean up the worst contamination and away from long-term comprehensive remedial activities that require many years of cleanup. Many agencies become involved in hazardous waste remediation and risk assessment, on the local, state, and federal levels. Each agency may have a different method of assessment and different goals and missions. All of these can impact the decision making involved in cleanup.

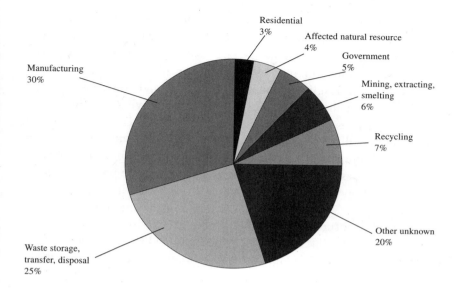

FIGURE 16.1 Types of site activities.

Additional legal definitions of hazardous substances and hazardous waste can be found in the CERCLA legislation language (42 U.S.C 9601 et seq.).

What then is municipal waste? Municipal waste is trash or garbage. It is generated from household waste and can contribute to toxic chemicals in the environment through improper disposal of items such as oil and paint, which end up in landfills and then leach into the ground water. When municipal waste is burned in incinerators there is often community concern about health effects from stack emissions. When it ferments in a landfill (a natural process), it produces methane gas that can be an explosion hazard in nearby basements and crawl spaces if not properly controlled.

THE HUMAN HEALTH PICTURE

For nurses, hazardous waste is not simply a matter of chemicals, laws, and terminology; it is a matter of health, both individual and collective. Among the 14 million people who live within 1 mile of a hazardous waste site, 11% are children under the age of 6, 12% are people aged 65 or older, and 24% are women of childbearing age (Agency for Toxic Substances and Disease Registry, 2000). This means that almost one half of the people living near hazardous waste sites are children, the elderly, or women of childbearing age, all of which are vulnerable to toxins because of biologic, developmental, and behavioral considerations. Other groups vulnerable to toxic chemical exposures are adolescents, migrant and transient workers, minority populations, the mentally ill, the chronically ill, the immuno-compromised, non-English speakers and the poor and homeless.

As discussed in chapter 6 on Toxicology, simply living or being near a toxic chemical does not cause negative health effects. Dose and duration of exposure determine health effects. Nurses can work with their communities and environmental health professionals to stop or prevent exposure by breaking at least one of the five links in an exposure pathway. Those links are as follows: (1) an environmental source of contamination at a waste site or spill, (2) the movement of contaminants and/or people to (3) a place where exposure occurs (called a point of exposure), (4) a route or means of exposure (oral, inhalation, or dermal), and (5) the people at risk (ATSDR, 1992). Even if people are exposed to toxic chemicals, certain biological conditions are required before disease occurs. This is best illustrated by Figures 16.2 and 16.3. Figure 16.3 also illustrates the actions that can occur at the different stages of disease development.

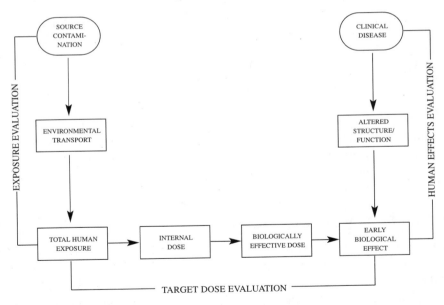

FIGURE 16.2 Continuum for Relating Environmental Contamination with Clinical Disease.

Adapted from National Research Council (1991).

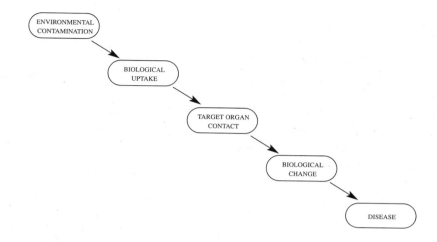

Key public health services needed to assess the relationship
between exposure to hazardous substances and disease

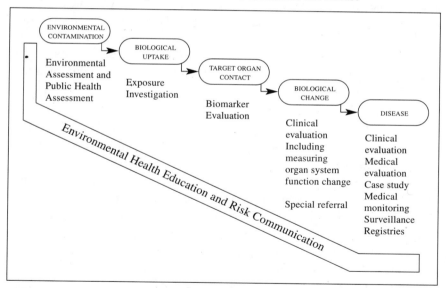

FIGURE 16.3 Model for the Relationship Between Exposure to Hazardous
Substances and Disease.

ROLE OF THE NURSE

Environmental health has come of age for nursing involvement. Nurses in all areas of practice have a role and responsibility to develop and maintain the appropriate skills to address environmental health concerns and issues in the populations they serve. The notion of holistic health is not complete without the inclusion of this vital concept in nursing practice. Nurses are making a difference by intervening all in areas of environmental health. One example is a Philadelphia nurse who noticed that a surprising number of her pediatric cancer patients were from Dover Township, New Jersey (New Jersey Department of Health and Senior Services, 1997). She communicated her concerns to the ATSDR regional office that triggered an investigation by the state health department into a possible childhood cancer cluster in the area. Surveillance alone did not answer the cancer cluster questions in this community but it led to several interventions. Other cluster investigation around hazardous waste sites have involve birth defects, autism, and multiple sclerosis. Causes of disease clusters are very difficult to determine unless the disease has a large number of cases in the cluster, is relatively rare, or is in an age group not usually affected by the disease. Aside from identifying patterns in health indicators and bringing them to the attention of the proper authorities, nurses can educate, advocate, assess, plan, intervene, and make referrals to stop health impacts of hazardous chemical exposures.

PREVENTION

All nurses need to become aware of opportunities to protect their clients and communities from the effects of toxic chemical exposures regardless of the age of the population, the nursing workplace setting, or the focus of their practice. Prevention in nursing practice is not a new idea, but its application to toxic chemicals is often uncharted territory for the uninitiated nurse. Prevention activities directed at breaking one or more links in the exposure pathway described earlier are the goals of nursing practice in the area of environmental health.

   Primary prevention occurs through nursing skill application in the areas of education, advocacy, and identification of potential exposure problems. It takes place before an actual exposure exists. Secondary forms of prevention occur once an exposure has occurred and the nurse is in a position to prevent further exposures. This usually happens when a screening for an exposure or a health effect. Tertiary prevention attempts to halt further disability when exposure-related illness is already present. Anticipation of possible existing conditions or exacerbation of current illnesses due to environmental triggers is a critical role of the nurse. Understanding and effectively communicating the pathophysiology of disease processes and the relationship of disease states and chemical exposures is becoming required of nurses everywhere.

As in other areas of nursing, the science and application of this science to hazardous waste problems is continually evolving. Thus, nurses need to actively listen for clients' environmental health concerns and apply the latest science in their decision making and action. Nurses can play a critical role as advocates by providing their patients with up-to-date, accurate, and timely science-based information.

PARADIGMS FOR PRACTICE

ASSESSMENT

Nurses are challenged to extend the traditional boundaries of their practices. In expanding their practice to include environmental health nurses must depend on their existing nursing skills and acquire new skills to protect clients from toxic substances. Nurses already have the ability to perform health assessments. This skill can be enhanced to include questions about individuals, families, and communities exposures. This health assessments guide environmental health intervention and planning.

SURVEILLANCE

Contributing to and ensuring complete reporting to birth, cancer, and chronic illness registries is one activity that can close data gaps in disease clusters investigation (Pew Environmental Health Commission, 2001). Nurses are often in a position to contribute skills and expertise for creating, strengthening, or improving such surveillance systems.

COLLABORATION

Intense collaboration within and across disciplines is a part of effective environmental health practice. Working with traditional disciplines such as medicine and ancillary health professions is familiar to most nurses, whereas working with geologists, toxicologists, environmental engineers, business people, and administrators may be a skill that needs to be developed.

COMMUNICATION

Effective communication about hazardous waste and health takes on different dimensions for the nurse. A tumult of emotions, perceptions, and attitudes have a great impact on the communication process when addressing toxic chemicals and exposure issues at hazardous waste sites. Not only are there outrage factors, as discussed in other chapters, but there is an the entire spectrum of levels of concern. Concern may be very low or nonexistent where real threats to health exist, or there may be extreme concern where no threat is identified. Perceptions and the reality of these perceptions for the people concerned about hazardous waste, demand respect. The nurse's ability to listen, avoid judgment, and provide support most significant contribution in chaotic communication scenarios. Credibility and trust are as important for nurses working with populations potentially exposed to toxins in hazardous waste sites as in any clinical situation.

Nurses need to develop and enhance skills in conflict resolution and negotiation in the often contentious, emotionally charged, and politically volatile situations involving hazardous waste sites. They should provide information about hazardous waste risks that are culturally appropriate, sensitive, and in understandable formats. They need to be prepared to respond to client questions about environmental exposures raised by the press (e.g., asbestos in crayons, phthalates in plastic, and lead in candle wicks).

QUALITY OF LIFE

For individuals and communities, the presence of hazardous waste, municipal waste, and toxic substances in their environment can have a significant impact on their quality of life (Tucker, 2000). Common recommendations to reduce exposure to toxic chemicals often result in disruption of activities of daily living such as dietary habits (e.g., fish consumption), drinking, bathing, and laundering. Other recommendations may interfere with leisure activities like swimming in lakes or rivers or gardening. Contamination of the local wild animals and birds threatens the traditional subsistence diet and culture of some Native American tribes. Economic hardships occur when environmental contamination prohibits or limits the sale of property, and temporary or permanent relocation burdens family resources and breaks the social fabric of communities. Just living with the uncertainty about possible health effects to family members from hazardous substances can cause emotional and psychologic turmoil and changes in coping patterns. Individual and community isolation is also a possibility. Nurses can ensure that clients affected by hazardous waste sites are provided the needed psychosocial support and can make appropriate referrals. Communities encountering hazardous waste are often simply responding normally to abnormal conditions.

POLICY

Nurses are charting new directions in standards of care in environmental health practice. These directions are based on recommendations for basic competencies that all nurses should develop as outlined in the Institute of Medicine report, *Nursing, Health, and the Environment* (1995). Policy development is an area for nursing leadership in clinics, hospitals, communities, and schools. The creation of local environmental coalitions for prevention and intervention similar to other health-related coalitions is breaking new ground for nursing involvement in improving public health through involvement in environmental health. In order to truly integrate environmental health into nursing practice, test questions about hazardous substances and health need to be addressed at all levels of nursing certification.

DILEMMAS IN PRACTICE

There is a paradox in environmental health: exposures to hazardous substances can cause harm in predictable, specific ways, but not everyone responds to a hazardous substance in a predictable way. It is generally agreed that environmental disease occurrence follows the model in Figure 16.2. However, because multiple factors can affect the physiologic process at each stage, the effects of exposure to a hazardous substance differ among individuals. These variables include smoking, lifestyle behaviors such as diet, or genetic susceptibility.

Many questions have led to uncertainties in the approach to identification and analysis of toxic exposures. For example, a client who lives near a hazardous waste site where several toxic chemicals have been found may in fact have only been exposed to two of those chemicals. How do those two chemicals affect the body as a mixture and what is the effect of one or more chemicals over time? Few data exist regarding synergistic effects of environmental contaminants on health. Other questions that have garnered interest are the effect of pharmaceutical chemicals and environmental exposure combinations and the potential for interference with a drug's action through synergy, potentiation, or diminishing of the therapeutic effect.

Government agencies often have conflicting positions on the levels of safety of chemicals (e.g. mercury), and scientific differences of opinion can cause confusion for the health care provider as well as the client or community member. Locating peer-reviewed, reliable information sources can help reduce controversy and misinformation. Some of these sources can be found in the resource section (Appendix) of this book.

DECISION MAKING

Uncertainties exist in addressing health issues for hazardous or toxic chemical exposures. The estimation of a safe dose for a chemical is one of these uncertainties. Because randomized clinical trials are not ethical for toxic chemical studies, observational epidemiologic studies or animal studies are used to estimate the risk associated with a specific hazord. In observational studies (e.g, case-control and cohort studies), exposure doses are often rough estimates and usually involve a mixture of chemicals. With animal studies, exposure conditions can be well controlled, but uncertainty exists when extrapolating the results from animals to people. The term *precautionary principle* is often applied in making decisions in the face of all these uncertainties. Although first coined in the 1970s and 1980s in reference to cost-effective action to guide cleanup actions for environmental degradation, it has also come to be used in environmental health science. Precautionary principle means that when there is a potential threat of serious damage to human health and insufficient scientific information exists, decisions to protect human health cannot be postponed. In effect, we need to make public health decisions even in the face of these uncertainties.

NEED FOR IMPROVED BIOLOGIC TESTING

Traditional medical methods generally rely on biologic testing to provide information on health status or to make a diagnosis. In environmental health, there are few scientifically accepted reliable biomarkers of exposure, effect, or susceptibility that are standardized for testing and analysis. We can reliably test for lead in blood, but standard laboratory tests for other substances such as vinyl chloride are not yet available. Unfortunately, unreliable tests such as hair and nail analysis are being sold to the public as indicators of exposure to toxic chemicals. Nurses need to determine which tests have been validated and have national reference ranges accepted by the scientific community so that their clients are not misled. There are many indications that until we further develop the ability to test for these chemical exposures reliably through biomarkers, our understanding and ability to intervene in environmental exposures will remain limited. This is an area that continues to lend itself to further research and development. Although much is known in environmental health science, at least an equal amount remains unknown. The amount, time, and period of exposures are often estimated or not known in detail. This leads to uncertainty in determining the exact health threat.

TRENDS FOR TODAY AND TOMORROW

Environmental health, like other health status indicators, is a reflection of our past, current, and future health policies and actions. Globalization of health issues has a major impact on environmental health along geographic borders, in allocation of resources, and in policy development. Demographics trends such as our aging population are leading to elderly workers experiencing increased cumulative occupational exposures, and the future may show an increase in manifestations of latent health effects from environmental exposures. Our poor and homeless are increasingly taking up shelter in abandoned and condemned hazardous waste sites, and this trend is likely to continue and to pose significant health and safety issues for this population.

The decoding of the human genome holds promise for the identification of genetic markers to assist in understanding variances in human susceptibility to chemical exposures (Sharp and Barrett, 2000). At the same time it opens the door to a variety of social, political, and privacy ramifications. There is increased attention and investigation into the relationship of diseases such as diabetes and chemical-specific exposures (i.e. nitrates, arsenic, and dioxin). Questions abound regarding endocrine disruptors and multiple chemical sensitivity. Future research is needed to addrress these issues. Emerging information on classes of chemicals such as polychlorinated naphthalenes (PCNs) is being developed; this information may change the direction of science and toxic chemical investigations.

Policy changes directed toward industry self regulation can have a positive or a negative impact on the future. Technology that addresses environmental health is rapidly advancing. Tools for remediation (e.g., the use of biofilm and information mapping systems such as GIS [geographic information systems]) are influencing the way we assess and intervene on health issues like cancer clusters and hazardous waste contamination, and the way we assess regional variances that indicate different exposure scenarios (e.g., rural and urban settings). Tele-health and -medicine have the potential to open doors to communication and services in medically underserved and isolated areas where environmental health investigations, environmental care, and consultation were previously difficult to access. Environmental litigation over the lack of appropriate, timely assessments and interventions by health care providers is bound to emerge as an issue for nurses in the future.

ACKMOWLEDGMENT

We would like to acknowledge the writing and editing assistance of Pamela Wigington.

BIBLIOGRAPHY

Agency for Toxic Substances and Disease Registry. (1992). *Public health assessment guidance manual.* Chelsea, Michigan: Lewis

Agency for Toxic Substances and Disease Registry. (2000). *Hazardous substances release/health effects database* (HazDat). Atlanta: U.S. Department of Health and Human Services.

Covello, V. (1999, January). *Health and environmental risk communication.* Presentation to ATSDR Partners Meeting, Atlanta, GA.

Institute of Medicine. (1995). *Nursing, health and the environment.* Washington, DC: National Academy Press.

Johnson, B. (1999). *Impact of hazardous waste on human health: Hazard, health effects, equity, and communications issues.* Washington, DC: Lewis.

New Jersey Department of Health and Human Services, Division of Environmental and Occupational Health Services. (1997). *Citizen's guide: childhood cancer incidence health consultation.* Trenton, N.J.

Pew Environmental Health Commission. (2001). *Transition report to the new administration: Strengthening our public health defense against environmental threats.* Available from http://pewenvirohealth.jhsph.edu/html/home/home.html.

Sharp, R. R., & Barrett, J. C. (2000). The environmental genome project: Ethical, legal, and social implications. *Environmental Health Perspectives, 108*(4), 279–281.

US Code 42 USC 9601 et seq.

U.S. Environmental Protection Agency. (2001). Auxiliary information: National priorities list proposed rule on January 11, 2001. *Intermittent Bulletin,* Internet volume 4, number 1. Available from http://www.epa.gov/superfund/sites/npl/info.htm

U.S. Environmental Protection Agency. (n.d.). Municipal and solid waste management. Available from http://www.epa.gov/epaoswer/non-hw/munccpl/facts.htm

CHAPTER 17

Pesticide Exposure

Patricia Butterfield and Phillip Butterfield

FROM THE PERSPECTIVE OF THE PUBLIC

There is probably no environmental health topic for which there is a greater level of citizen concern than exposure to pesticides. Public opinion ranges from those who object to any use of synthetic products in our nation's food supply to those who view the successes of American agricultural production as predicated on the use of pesticides and fertilizer on our crops. But public opinion can be easily swayed by misinformation and innuendo and the evidence addressing health risks from pesticide exposure is confusing at best. It is easy to understand how well-intentioned and well-informed people can disagree strongly about how pesticides should be used, evaluated, and regulated. Public views addressing pesticide use include the following.

- For some citizens, pesticides are composed of an indecipherable list of ingredients and a set of warnings. There is a lack of information to help people demystify technical information about pesticide labeling, formulations, and precautions. Pesticides are both needed and feared—a necessary evil that is reluctantly purchased when the dog brings fleas into the house or when the roses become covered with aphids.
- Farmers, gardeners, and ranchers are more likely to see pesticides as their first-line response in preventing and treating problems such as blights, insect infestations, and weed problems. In their line of work, they need pesticides to enssure that there is a crop that is worth harvesting at the end of the season. They see pesticides as an integral part of their efforts to produce high quality fruits and vegetables for the American consumer. Intensive farming practices require heavy applications of fertilizers and pesticides to produce high crop yields per acre. The technological advances in agriculture have been responsible for the

ability of our nation to feed vulnerable populations throughout the world during times of famine and floods.

- Still other citizens and health professionals view pesticides as a mainstay of public health protection against vector-borne disease in our country and elsewhere. Many health providers have lived in areas with high mortality from malaria and other vector-borne diseases and view pesticides as part of a risk–benefit ratio that needs to consider the benefits as well as the dangers of pesticide use.

- Many people whose lives have been impacted by diseases of unknown etiology wonder about the possible role of pesticides in the development of cancer, neurologic disease, and conditions of the immune system. How can something that, by its very nature is designed to kill animals or plants, have any beneficial role in an advanced society? It just makes sense that we would all be better off if we outlawed all pesticides and let the rules of nature reestablish themselves throughout the world.

Like many other complex health issues, the topic of pesticide use requires a sound understanding of the principles of pathophysiology, pharmacology, and epidemiology. A basic understanding of toxicology is essential to understanding concepts such as dose-response, individual susceptibility, and system-specific toxic effects. Finally, learning about the processes by which pesticides are tested, marketed, and regulated is critical to our understanding of pesticides continuing use.

CHAPTER OBJECTIVES

The primary goal of this chapter is to enable health providers to provide effective care for persons at risk for health problems due to pesticide exposure. Within this context, specific objectives address health providers' abilities to

1. Understand classes of pesticides and basic mechanisms of pesticide toxicity
2. Intervene effectively to treat acute pesticide poisoning
3. Conduct a client assessment to elicit sources of pesticide exposure
4. Provide education to prevent and minimize exposure to pesticides
5. Describe chronic health problems that have been associated with pesticide exposure

6. Understand the complexity of evidence from epidemiologic studies of long-term pesticide exposure
7. Understand the challenges of identifying health risks associated with exposure to multiple pesticide products
8. Describe policies addressing pesticide regulation and use
9. Use evidence addressing pesticides in potable water sources as a means to understanding the risk of pesticide exposure throughout the life span

Throughout the chapter, examples from studies addressing pesticides in drinking water will be used to demonstrate the complexity of human pesticide exposure and the controversies over the long-term consequences of exposure. In this way the reader can develop an understanding of the challenges of studying pesticide exposure in a manner that is consistent with cumulative lifetime exposure in humans. This information also makes it easier to understand why there is not conclusive scientific evidence addressing many of the hypothesized health effects from long-term pesticide exposure.

HISTORICAL OVERVIEW

A common misconception about pesticides is that such products were first used within the past few decades. In reality, plants and chemicals containing pesticidal properties have been used for centuries. Chinese farmers used sulfur as a fumigant as early as 1000 BC. In the 1700s, extracts from the tobacco plant were used to kill insects, and a primitive derivative of strychnine was used to kill rodents (Ecobichon, 1996). Arsenic-based compounds such as copper arsenite and lead arsenate became a mainstay in the battle against insect pests in the early 1900s. Pesticides made from synthetic chemicals were introduced in the 1930s, with major increases in agrochemical products following World War II (Ecobichon, 1996).

The 1962 release of Rachel Carson's *Silent Spring* focused attention on pesticides and their potential long-term consequences to a number of species. In her book, Ms. Carson emphasized the persistence of organochlorine insecticides in the environment. Since that time, many organochlorine compounds have been removed from the market and were replaced by organophosphate and carbamate pesticides, which have a shorter half-life. As of 1996, the global pesticide market was a $30 billion dollar per year industry, concentrated in ten multinational companies (Ciba-Geigy, DuPont, Monsanto, Zeneca, Bayer, DowElanco, Rhone-Poulenc, Hoechst, American

Cyanamid, and BASF); together these companies accounted for approximately two thirds of world food sales (World Health Organization, 1990). Over 60% of pesticides are used in the United States, western Europe, and Japan, where farming practices emphasize heavy applications of pesticides and fertilizers to increase crop yield (WHO, 1990).

TYPES OF PESTICIDES

The term *pesticide* refers to any physical, chemical, or biological agent that will kill an undesired plant or animal pest. By definition there can be no such product as a completely safe pesticide; otherwise the product will be ineffective in killing or controlling its intended target. Pesticide products are generally classified on the basis of the pattern of use (e.g., fumigant) and the organism killed (e.g., insecticide) (Ecobichon, 1996). In addition to the type of agent (e.g., herbicide), pesticides can be categorized by chemical class (e.g., triazines) and generic name (e.g., atrazine), as well as by a proprietary name (e.g., Atranex). In this way, the classification of pesticides resembles that of pharmaceuticals, where a general drug class (e.g., synthetic hormones) may also include more specific references to more specific trade names (e.g., Synthroid).

More than 600 chemicals are currently registered as pesticides in the U.S., with the majority of these products falling into the categories of insecticides, insect repellents, rodenticides, herbicides, and fumigants (American Academy of Pediatrics, 1999). Because new pesticides are being introduced into the market on an ongoing basis, the discussion of specific agents in this chapter is not meant to be comprehensive. In addition to new pesticides, changes in the formulation of existing pesticides on the market frequently occur. Material safety data sheets (MSDS), poison control centers, and product label information are easy ways to obtain timely information addressing a specific pesticide. Major classes of pesticides include the following.

INSECTICIDES

Insecticides are classified primarily by their mechanism of action. All chemical insecticides in current use are neurotoxins and act by destroying the nervous system of the target insect (Ecobichon, 1996). Major categories include organophosphates, organochlorines, carbamates, pyrethrum and pyrethroids, and other products.

Organophosphate insecticides poison insects by inhibiting the enzyme acetylcholinesterase at nerve endings. As a result, the excess of acetylcholine overstimulates the effector organ. The transmission of nerve impulses is predicated on the correct balance of acetylcholine and acetylcholinesterase within the nerve junction, and the loss of enzyme function leads to several types of problems within the central and peripheral nervous system (Environmental Protection Agency, 1999). In the cholinergic nerve junctions of smooth muscle and gland cells, excessive concentrations of acetylcholine cause muscle contraction and secretion. At skeletal nerve junctions, acetylcholine precipitates symptoms that are both excitatory (e.g., muscle twitching) and depressive (e.g., muscle weakness or paralysis) (EPA, 1999). In addition to use as an insecticide, organophosphorus compounds have a variety of industrial and residential uses, such as catalysts, flame retardants, and antistatic agents. Products in this family have also been developed as nerve gases, including the nerve gas sarin. In many parts of the world, organophosphate insecticides are a central part of efforts to reduce the occurrence of vector-borne diseases in humans and animals (Lotti, 2000). Products within this category include diazinon, malathion, and methyl parathion (generic names), and Dursban and Thimet (commercial names).

Organophosphate insecticides are absorbed through dermal, respiratory, and gastrointestinal routes (Lotti, 2000). Depending on the exposure dose and time frame of events, the patient may present with a variety of acute symptoms, including headache, fatigue, blurred vision, nausea, vomiting, diarrhea, abdominal cramping, and excessive sweating (Weeks, Levy, and Wagner, 1991). More severe cases of poisoning may present with shortness of breath, constricted pupils, and unconsciousness. The importance of health providers' initiating prompt treatment of acutely poisoned individuals cannot be overestimated.

Many organochlorine insecticides have been removed from commercial use by the Environmental Protection Agency; however, some of these products are still used in tick and flea products (EPA, 1999). In addition, some other organochlorines are applied to seeds to protect them from insect or fungal infestations. The mechanism of action of the organochlorines is similar to that of organophosphate insecticides, with exposure resulting in a hyperexcitable state in the central nervous system. Symptoms of acute poisoning include myoclonic jerking, seizures, paresthesias, tremor, and hyperreflexia. Fatalities occur primarily through metabolic acidosis, which occurs from seizures and impaired pulmonary gas exchange (EPA, 1999). Organochlorines are lipophilic compounds and are stored in fatty organs such as the breast and stomach. Because they stay in the body for an extended period of time, there are concerns about the long-term consequences of exposure as well as excretion of pesticide metabolites in breast milk. Most citizens are familiar with DDT, an organochlorine that was widely used in the 1960s but is no longer in use in the U.S. Other organochlorines include aldrin, dieldrin, heptachlor, and toxaphine (generic names); these products are marketed under a variety of commercial names.

Carbamate insecticides induce toxicity through a process similar, but not identical, to that of organophosphates. Both types of insecticides produce an accumulation of acetylcholine at the neural junction; however, carbamates cause a reversible carbamylation of acetylcholinesterase, whereas organophosphates induce a one-way process that is only reversed by the generation of new enyzme in affected tissues (EPA, 1999). Compared with organophosphate poisoning, poisoning with carbamate insecticides tends to be of shorter duration and less severe. However, life-threatening toxicity can occur, with patients presenting with seizures, coma, and cardiopulmonary depression. Dithiocarbamate compounds are also used as fungicides. Generally these products have a low level of toxicity that manifests primarily as a contact dermatitis, but descriptions of neurotoxic reactions, ranging from convulsions to Parkinson-like symptoms, have been noted in a few case reports. However, doses incurred in most cases of human poisoning with carbamate compounds have not resulted in permanent serious consequences to those affected (Ecobichon, 2000). Products within this category include carbaryl, aldicarb, and carbofuran (generic names), and Sevin and Temik (commercial names).

Pyrethrum is an extract of dried chrysanthemum flowers that has insecticidal properties, of which the active ingredients are known as pyrethrins. Synthetically derived products, called pyrethroids, are similar to pyrethrins. These products paralyze the nervous systems of insects; however, the effect is not always lethal. For that reason, pyrethrins are sometimes combined with other types of agents that extend the duration of pyrethrins (EPA, 1999). These products are commonly used for indoor pest control because they break down when exposed to light. Hence, they are not widely used in agricultural production. Because of their widespread use indoors, pyrethrin and pyrethroid products are frequently linked to cases of pesticide poisoning. Severe neurotoxicity rarely occurs in humans or other mammals (e.g., dogs and cats); more frequent symptoms of poisoning include tremor, excess salivation, and labored breathing (EPA, 1999).

Other types of insecticides include biologicals (e.g., bacteria), alkaloid agents (such as nicotine and sabadilla), and other products of plant origin, in addition to pyrethrin-based formulations (EPA, 1999). *Bacillus thuringien-*

sis, a bacterium that in its spore form contains properties pathogenic to some insects, has been used to control outbreaks of gypsy moths and other pests. Rotenone, which is derived from dried derris root, is also used as an insecticide, although its high toxicity to fish limits its application. Because potential health consequences from exposure vary widely according to agent, health providers need to consult specific toxicity information when considering the possibility of pesticide poisoning with any of these agents.

HERBICIDES

Herbicides are used to control weeds in lawns and gardens and are widely used in agricultural production. Compared with insecticides, herbicides are linked to fewer poisoning cases annually; however both intentional (i.e., suicide attempts) and unintentional poisonings do occur. Categories of herbicides include chlorophenoxy herbicides, nitrophenolic and nitrocresolic herbicides, dipyridyl compounds, and others.

Several hundred commercial products incorporate chlorophenoxy herbicides to control broadleaf weeds. In humans these products cause irritation to the skin, eyes, and gastrointestinal tract. They are absorbed through both the skin and the lungs; the half-life of most products is measured in hours rather than days or weeks. Severe cases of poisoning with chlorophenoxy herbicides have resulted in metabolic acidosis, as well as vomiting, anorexia, and mouth and throat ulcers (EPA, 1999). Damage to striated muscle can also occur, which can be expressed as muscle weakness and myoglobinuria. In experimental animals, reports of central (e.g., myotonia) and peripheral (uncoordination in the hind extremities) nervous system damage have also been reported. Products in this category include 2,4-dichlorophenoxyacetic acid (2,4-D) and 2,4,5-trichlorophenoxy acetic acid (2,4,5-T).

Nitrophenolic and nitrocresolic herbicides are used in fungal outbreaks as well as for their weed-killing properties. These products are highly toxic to both animals and humans. Although skin irritation is most commonly associated with dermal contact, fatal poisonings have occurred following skin contact (versus inhalation or ingestion) alone. Toxicity occurs through the stimulation of oxidative metabolism within cell mitochondria, with the hepatic, renal, and nervous systems primarily affected (EPA, 1999). Symptoms include tachycardia, headache, malaise, dehydration, and hyperthermia. Symptoms may be exacerbated when the outdoor temperature is high, due to the difficulty of dissipating heat from hyperthermic changes. Yellow stains on the skin and hair can be associated with nitrophenolic herbicide poisoning; this sign can give providers an important diagnostic clue. Products in this category include dinocap, dinitrophenol, and dinoseb; in the U.S., registration on a number of nitrophenolic herbicides has been cancelled.

Paraquat and diquat are dipyridal compounds that are widely used to control weeds. Commercial names for paraquat include Gramoxone, Dextrone, and Goldquat; commercial names for diquat include Aquacide and Ortho Diquat. The lungs are the primary organs affected in dipyridal herbicide poisoning; oxidative damage to the lungs occurs primarily through the generation of free radical compounds (EPA, 1999). Unfortunately, ingestion of paraquat has been a commonly used method of suicide; studies of suicide survivors have provided clinicians with much of the information regarding the consequences of this kind of poisoning.

There are a variety of other herbicide products in use, both domestically and abroad. Many products kill weeds selectively by impairing metabolic processes that are unique to plants. Health providers need to carefully assess exposure and identify potential agents whenever possible through interviews with family members and others.

OTHER TYPES OF PESTICIDES

It is important for providers to understand that, in addition to killing bugs and weeds, pesticides are used for a variety of other purposes. Wood preservatives, fungicides, fumigants, and rodenticides are also classified as pesticides, and, depending on the geographic setting and climate, may be widely used in close proximity to humans. In addition, insect repellants such as diethyltoluamide (DEET) are applied directly to the skin in a lotion, stick, or aerosol form (American Academy of Pediatrics, 1999). Health providers are well served by understanding products commonly used in their communities. Informal discussion with farmers, gardeners, pest control personnel, and lawn care personnel is an effective way to gather this type of information.

PESTICIDES IN DRINKING WATER

Surface waters (streams, rivers, lakes, and reservoirs) and ground waters are the source of nearly all water used for human consumption in the United States. Ground water serves as the source of drinking water for nearly 90% of rural residents and nearly three quarters of cities in the United States (Goodrich, Lykins, & Clark, 1991). In Europe it is estimated that 65% of the drinking water supply is derived from ground water sources (Holt, 2000). Water is the universal solvent and is capable of containing in solution a large variety of chemicals, natural organic and inorganic compounds, and microbial contaminants.

Extensive water quality monitoring during the 1980s and 1990s has demonstrated that pesticides can be found in most surface waters and groundwaters affected by agriculture or urban land uses (Gilliom, Barbash, Kolpin, and Larson, 1999). The introduction of pesticides into the aquatic ecosystem presents the potential for chronic effects due to long-term exposure, typically at very low concentrations and in mixtures with other pesticides or chemicals of public health concern. The topic of pesticides in drinking water is so extensive and broad that an entire book has been devoted to the subject (Gustafson, 1993).

REGULATION OF PESTICIDES IN DRINKING WATER

In 1974 the United States Congress enacted the Safe Drinking Water Act (SDWA) directing the Environmental Protection Agency (EPA) to establish regulations to control the level of pesticides and other contaminants found in drinking water. The SDWA has subsequently been amended in 1986 and 1996. The EPA has established a maximum contaminant level goal (MCLG) and a maximum contaminant level (MCL) for specific pesticide compounds that have been determined to be potentially harmful to human health. An MCLG is the maximum level of a compound or contaminant in drinking water at which there are no known or anticipated adverse health effects. MCLGs are nonenforceable health goals whereas MCLs are enforceable maximum permissible levels of a contaminant. The MCLG for a particular contaminant can be less than or equal to the MCL. Standards for pesticide concentrations in drinking water are contained within the National Primary Drinking Water Regulations (NPDWR, 2000) (USEPA, 2000) for organic contaminants. The EPA has also established Health Advisory Levels (HALs) for a large number of pesticides and chemical compounds (USEPA, 2000). Health advisories (milligrams per liter) are provided for a 1-day and 10-day exposure for a 10-kg child. In addition, the reference dose (RfD) and HALs for the drinking water equivalent level (DWEL), lifetime and 10^{-4} cancer risk level are provided for adults. The DWEL assumes a lifetime exposure from only the consumption of drinking water. Health Advisory concentrations can be referenced when no MCL has been established for a pesticide of concern.

The World Health Organization (WHO) Guidelines for Drinking Water Quality (GDWQ) (WHO, 1993; WHO, 1996; WHO, 1998) are health-based guidelines established in a manner similar to the approach used by the EPA (Younes and Galal-Gorchez, 2000). In contrast to the health-based approach taken by the EPA and the WHO, the European Union Drinking Water Directorate has established standards for pesticides in drinking water based on analytical limits of detection available at the time standards were originally established (Harrison, Watt, & Allister Vale, 2000). EC Council Directive 80/778/EEC (Council of the European Communities, 1980) sets a Maximum Admissable Concentration (MAC) of 0.1 micrograms per liter for each individual pesticide in drinking water, and a limit of 5 micrograms per liter for total pesticides. The most recent EC standards, Council Directive 98/83/EC (Council of the European Communities, 1998), have lowered standards for aldrin, dieldrin, heptachlor, and heptachlor epoxide to 0.030 micrograms per liter.

PESTICIDE PRODUCTS AND BYPRODUCTS IN THE ENVIRONMENT: EXAMPLES ADDRESSING WATER QUALITY

The occurrence of pesticides in surface waters and ground waters has been shown to be widespread in the United States, dependent upon geographical and seasonal uses of pesticides in both agricultural and urban settings. The National Water Quality Assessment (NAWQA) Program, conducted by the U.S. Geological Survey, has been one of the most extensive investigations of pesticides in U.S. waters (Gilliom et al., 1999). During the period 1992 to 1996, 20 study units were selected for the NAWQA to represent a wide variety of agricultural and urban settings where pesticides were utilized. Results of the initial NAWQA monitoring program indicated that pesticide concentrations were typically below maximum contaminant levels (MCLs) set for drinking water; however drinking water criteria did not exist for many of the 83 pesticides that were analyzed.

Many factors influence the movement and fate of pesticides to surface waters and groundwater in agricultural and urban settings. Some of the more important factors are (1) biogeochemical properties of pesticides; (2) geographic location of crop types, amount of land in particular crops, and the time when pesticides are applied; (3) soil type and its sorptive capacity for particular pesticides; (4) farming practices; and (5) variations in climate and seasonal patterns of precipitation and runoff (Pereira and Hostettler, 1993). Pesticide solubility in water, soil half-life, and the ability of soil to adsorb pesticides are important parameters when evaluating potential pollution from pesticides applied to crops or lawns, gardens and rights-of-way in urban areas. A pesticide that is soluble in water can be transported more easily to surface water and ground water where it can be present in concentrations greater than drinking water standards. The soil half-life of a pesticide indicates the time required for the pesticide concentration to be reduced by one half in soil. All other factors being equal, a pesticide with a long soil half-life is predicted to persist longer in soil than a pesticide that has a short half-life, making it more likely to be transported to surface water or ground water. However, not all factors are equal and multiple factors must be taken into account. How well a pesticide adsorbs to soil particles affects the retention of the pesticide in soil. Soil contains natural organic matter (such as humic and fulvic acids) that can adsorb pesticides, reducing their movement from unsaturated soil to groundwater. Pesticides in soil can undergo biodegradation by soil microorganisms, creating degradation products. While degradation decreases the concentration of the parent pesticide, little is known about the fate and transport of the degradation products.

Atrazine, deethylatrazine (DEA—a degradation product of atrazine), metolachlor, cyanazine and alachlor were the most frequently detected herbicides in agricultural areas during the initial NAWQA study. Atrazine, metolachlor, cyanazine and alachlor ranked first, second, fourth and fifth in national herbicide use for agriculture (Gilliom et al., 1999). In urban areas the herbicides most frequently detected were simazine, prometon, 2,4-D, diuron, and tebuthiuron. The herbicides 2,4-D and prometon rank first and fourteenth in their frequency of application in urban settings. The NAWQA study found insecticides more frequently in urban streams than in those from agricultural areas. The most frequently detected insecticides were diazinon, chlorpyrifos, carbaryl, and malathion and these insecticides ranked first, fourth, eighth, thirteenth and for their frequency of application in urban areas (Gilliom et al.).

Numerous studies, some associated with the NAWQA efforts, have reported the presence of pesticides in surface waters. A series of articles by Stamer (Stamer, 1996, Stamer and Wieczorek, 1996, Stamer and Zelt, 1994) described the frequency of detection and temporal changes in concentration for herbicides from three large river basins in Kansas and Nebraska. The river drainages were characterized by significant corn, sorghum, and soybean production. Atrazine, metolachlor, cyanazine, simazine, and alachlor were the most frequently detected herbicides in the surface waters sampled, with atrazine detected most often. The major pesticides detected had their greatest concentration during higher stream flows in the spring and early summer, implying that herbicides were being carried by surface runoff to receiving streams following their application and precipitation-runoff events. However, most pesticides continued to be detected during the fall and winter months. Individual sample concentrations of certain herbicides, such as atrazine, most often exceeded drinking water MCLs during the spring and summer runoff events. The insecticide diazinon was detected downstream of areas that have urban land uses where diazinon is commonly applied to lawns and gardens (Stamer and Wieczorek, 1996). It was noted that cities along the Platte River obtain water from wells located in the river alluvium, and pumping of the wells typically induces flow from the river to the well. Although the water pumped from the wells received conventional water treatment (chemical coagulation, sedimentation, and granular media filtration), these water treatment processes have limited capability to remove pesticides (Adams and Randtke, 1992; Miltner, Baker, and Speth, 1989).

The Mississippi River and its tributaries were shown to contain herbicides commonly used in the agricultural areas they drained (Pereira & Hostettler, 1993). The most common herbicides detected and in greatest concentrations were atrazine, cyanazine, metolachlor, alachlor, and simazine. Concentrations of pesticides followed a similar cycle as was seen in the studies in Nebraska and Kansas: Concentrations were highest following spring applications and precipitation and runoff events. Continued detection of herbicides in the Mississippi River during the fall and winter months when base flows are derived primarily from groundwater indicates pesticides are present in the groundwater. Atrazine was found in concentrations higher than most other detected herbicides in the lower Mississippi River, and its degradation product. (DEA) and deisopropylatrazine (DIA), were also found in significant concentrations. The year-round presence of atrazine and its degradation products indicates the persistence of atrazine in the ecosystem.

Studies of pesticides in the Great Lakes (Schottler and Eisenreich, 1994) resulted in the detection of atrazine and its degradation product DEA in 100% of 490 samples taken during the period 1990 to 1992 from Lakes Huron, Michigan, Erie, and Ontario. While the concentrations were quite low (< 110 nanograms per liter), the herbicides were detected deep in the lake, indicating long half-lives in the lakes. A study of two lakes in northeastern Nebraska (Spalding, Snow, Cassada, and Burbach, 1994) found atrazine concentrations above the drinking water MCLs; neither lake was used as a source of drinking water. Factors such as watershed slope, land use, rainfall, and soil drainage capacity influenced the amount of pesticides transported to the lakes by runoff or ground water.

Urban pesticide uses also contribute significantly to the presence of these compounds in both surface water and ground water. Kimbrough and Litke (1996) reported the results of a study that investigated the presence of pesticides in streams draining an agricultural area and an urban area of Colorado. For the two study areas the herbicide prometon was the most frequently detected, while DCPA and atrazine were found in the highest concentrations in the agricultural and urban drainages respectively. DCPA was used for weed control in onion fields and atrazine was used for application to road rights-of-way in the urban area. The insecticides carbaryl, chlorpyrifos, diazinon, and malathion were the most frequently detected in both areas, with carbaryl found at the highest concentrations. The results of most samples indicated the concentrations were below drinking water MCLs and HALs, with the highest concentrations associated with precipitation and runoff events for both areas. Atrazine and prometon persisted in the agricultural stream at nearly the same concentration during the months when runoff was not occurring (late summer, fall, and winter). The same trend was seen for simazine and prometon in the urban stream. The detection of these pesticides year-round indicated their persistence in the alluvial ground water systems associated with the two streams investigated.

Certain pesticides enter the atmosphere through volatilization from the soil or crop to which they are applied. The concentration of semivolatile organochlorine compounds in mountain snows of western Canada has been found to increase by a factor of 10 to 100 at high elevations of 770 to 3,100 meters (Blais et al., 1998). The presence of pesticides in snow results from transport in the atmosphere, precipitation, and a process termed "cold condensation." As moisture-laden air containing volatilized organochlorine compounds is forced upward by the mountains, the temperature drops and the compounds condense with snow, thus the term cold condensation. One implication of this phenomenon is the transport and deposition of pesticides to snow in mountains that eventually supplies water to lakes and streams used for drinking water by small and large cities in the Rocky Mountains of the U.S.

The results of the NAWQA clearly show that pesticides are present in groundwaters at low concentrations. Many studies have shown pesticides can enter and persist in groundwater (Bushway et al., 1992; Castaneda and Bhuiyan, 1996; Goodrich, Lykins, and Clarks, 1991; Goss, Barry, and

Rudolph, 1998; Wade, York, Morey, Padmore, and Rudo, 1998). Most studies of pesticides in groundwater have analyzed the parent compounds. Recent work has shown that pesticide degradation products can comprise 60 to 99% of the measured herbicide's concentration in ground water (Kolpin, Thurman, and Linhart, 1998). Failure to determine the concentration of degradation products can provide false information regarding the presence of pesticides in water, particularly because many of the degradation products can have similar toxicity effects as the parent compound (Kolpin et al., 1998). Pesticides with short soil half-lives, such as alachlor, had a higher ratio of degradation product detection frequencies to parent product detection frequencies. The herbicide atrazine, with a long soil half-life, was detected nearly as frequently as its degradation products.

ESTIMATES OF ACUTE PESTICIDE POISONING

Global and national estimates of cases of pesticide poisoning vary widely, primarily due to the underrecognition and underreporting of cases. Like many other conditions, signs and symptoms of acute pesticide poisoning are highly variable and range from a nonspecific rash to death from respiratory failure. Existing estimates include the following.

- Worldwide, as many as three million cases of acute pesticide poisoning occur annually, with the majority of these cases involving suicide attempts (WHO, 1990).
- In 1995, an estimated 79,000 U.S. children were involved in a household pesticide-related poisoning (EPA, 1999).
- 1,332 cases of definite, probable, or possible pesticide poisoning were reported to the California Pesticide Illness Surveillance Program in 1994 (O'Malley, 1997).
- Of 22,433 cases of pesticide poisoning cases reported nationwide in 1996, the five pesticide classes most commonly implicated included organophosphates (4,002 cases), pyrethrins and pyrethroids (3,950 cases), pine oil disinfectants (2,246 cases), hypochlorite disinfectants (2,109 cases), and insect repellants (2,086) (EPA, 1999).
- In developing nations, the incidence of pediatric pesticide poisoning is extremely difficult to assess. However, because children are typically involved in their family's work and participate in pesticide application, it is reasonable to assume that poisoning rates would be high (Khare et al., 1990).

ASSESSING AND EDUCATING TO REDUCE PESTICIDE-RELATED RISKS

Nurses can be involved in prevention, treatment, and educational interventions on behalf of individuals and groups at risk for pesticide exposure. Although the majority of nurses do not work in occupational or environmental clinics, most clinical settings provide ample opportunities to address pesticide-related health concerns. Assessing actual and potential exposures is the first step in risk reduction. Prior to addressing a client's concerns about a specific pesticide, it is important for the nurse to obtain accurate and timely information about the agent of concern. In considering opportunities for pesticide exposure, it is important for the health provider to consider current products and formulations as well as products that may no longer be sold, but still may be stored in people's homes, such as DDT. This information is best assessed as part of a clinical exposure history; within this context, questions addressing acute exposure include:

• What pesticide(s) was the person exposed to?
• What time did exposure occur?
• Describe the event and what was happening at the time of exposure.
• Were any other people affected?
• Did the pesticide product get in or on the person's eyes, mouth, skin, nose, hair, clothing, or boots?

In all situations, encourage the person or family member to identify the possible source of exposure. However, open bottles, spray packs, or other dispersal units should not be brought into the clinical setting. All pesticides bear a label containing the product name, manufacturer, EPA registration number, list of active ingredients, and precautionary statements (EPA, 1999). Obtaining this information is critical in all situations involving pesticide exposure.

For persons who are not acutely exposed to pesticides, there are fewer immediate needs and the exposure can focus on opportunities for risk reduction and prevention of exposure. Assessment questions for the nurse may include:

• What pesticides are used in the home and yard?
• Where are they stored and can children access them?
• What are the occupations of all family members?

- Do family members have hobbies that involve pesticide use?
- Is their lawn treated with commercial fertilizers and/or pesticides?
- Are pesticides ever used inside the home to kill fleas, ants, rats, mice, or cockroaches? How and where are these products sprayed, fogged, or placed on the floor?
- How are clothes that may have pesticides on them laundered and stored?
- Do people enter the home wearing clothes or boots that were used when spraying pesticides?
- Are there pets or livestock that are treated with pesticides?
- Are there any industrial facilities or farms/ranches where children could be inadvertently exposed to pesticides?
- Does the family's water source come from a private or municipal well? If water comes from a private well, how and how often is the water tested? What is the water tested for?

Risk reduction interventions focus on targeting areas where people could be inadvertently exposed. Many of the common sense interventions for poison-proofing a home will reduce opportunities for children's exposure to pesticides. In addition, talking with the family about practical steps to reduce the incidence of pesticides coming into the home, safe laundering practices, and adhering to any reentry times following in-home pesticide use will help reduce family exposure.

Because of citizens' concerns about health problems with a possible environmental etiology, pesticides are frequently limplicated as a cause of disease, before a proper health history is taken. Many citizens are worried about pesticide use and how it affects their daily lives. Rather than asking specific questions about toxicology, citizens and patients are more likely to frame their questions in a way that reflects concern about the potential of pesticides to cause specific health problems. Examples of questions that nurses may encounter (EPA 2000, p. 17) include:

- I received a report from my water utility that said the water contained 0.5ppb of dibromochloropropane. What is this chemical, what does it mean for my health, and what should I do?
- I just read in the newspaper that schools in my state are spraying their buildings with toxic pesticides. I'm worried because my child has asthma and sometimes feels worse at school. Could it be the pesticides?

- I have a 6-month-old child and the cat has fleas. Is it safe to have the exterminator flea-bomb the house? The exterminator says it's safe if we stay out for a few hours and open the windows afterwards.
- My husband and I are having trouble conceiving a child. We own a farm and he sprays pesticides. I want to know if the pesticides may be causing a problem.
- I get a headache and have difficulty concentrating at the office. I think it may be because the janitor sprays pesticides at night.
- I am a farm worker and was picking celery in the fields. Today I have a rash on my hands and arms. Is it from the chemicals?

SIGNS AND SYMPTOMS OF ACUTE ORGANOPHOSPHATE AND CARBAMATE INSECTICIDE POISONING

Because symptoms of acute pesticide poisoning are nonspecific in nature, many people fail to link their symptoms with exposure to pesticides. Furthermore, health providers often fail to associate a patient's illness with pesticide exposure and do not ask salient questions that would elicit more clues about the nature of the exposure (Weeks et al., 1991). Most often it is easier to identify a link between pesticide exposure and acute symptoms in patients who have occupations and hobbies where they encounter pesticides as a part of their daily lives. Because of the wide use of pesticides, health providers are well served by learning the constellation of symptoms that are associated with organophosphate and carbamate insecticides and asking focused questions of patients who present with these symptoms. In addition, knowing what pesticides are used locally, in both agricultural and residential settings, can help health providers focus their questions and diagnostic reasoning.

A combination of muscarinic (e.g., lacrimation, sweating, abdominal cramping), nicotinic (e.g., muscular weakness, hypertension, tachycardia), and central nervous system (e.g., tremor, convulsions, coma) signs/symptoms occur following organophosphate pesticide poisoning (Lotti, 2000). Clinical presentation varies according to dose and route of exposure, with symptoms generally occurring four to twelve hours post exposure (Schlenker, Albertson, and Saiki, 1992). However, given the diversity of specific organophosphate and carbamate insecticides, there can be considerable variation in presenting signs and symptoms following acute exposure.

O'Malley (1997) suggests using the mnemonic MUDDLES (miosis, urination, diarrhea, diaphoresis, lacrimation, excitation of the central nervous system, and salivation) to aid clinicians in remembering common signs and symptoms of pesticide poisoning. Because organophosphate insecticides are lipidphilic and have a high chemical reactivity, plasma levels of the compound may represent only a small proportion of the body burden. In addition redistribution of the compounds may occur when treatment is discontinued. Organophosphate insecticides are excreted in the urine, and the time course for excretion varies by dose and specific compound (Lotti, 2000). Common signs and symptoms by body system are listed in Table 17.1.

ACUTE ORGANOCHLORINE INSECTICIDE POISONING

Overall, organochlorine insecticides have low acute toxicity compared with organophosphates; however, these agents have a long-half life in the body and can sometimes be measured for months to years following exposure. One exception is Endrin, which is quickly metabolized and falls below detectable limits approximately 2 weeks following exposure (O'Malley, 1997). However, despite the lower toxicity of organochlorine compounds, fatal poisonings have occurred with ingestion of high doses. Early manifestations of organochlorine poisoning include paresthesias of the face and extremities, headache, dizziness, seizures, vomiting, incoordination, tremor, and confusion; as with the organophosophates, signs and symptoms vary by agent, dose, and route of exposure.

TABLE 17.1 Signs and Symptoms of Acute Organophosphate and Carbamate Insecticide Poisoning

Central nervous system	Musculo skeletal system	Gastrointestinal system	Respiratory system	Cardiovascular system
Salivation	Muscle twitching	Vomiting	Wheezing	Bradycardia
Headache	Weakness	Diarrhea	Rhinorrhea	Early tachycardia
Nausea	Sweating	Cramping	Pulmonary edema	Hypertension
Dizziness	Tremor		Respiratory paralysis	Sinus arrest
	Incoordination			
	Paralysis			

(Adapted from Ecobichon, 2000).

OTHER TYPES OF PESTICIDE POISONING

Pesticide poisoning can also occur from exposure to herbicides, fungicides, and rodenticides. Because there are significant differences in the mechanisms both within and between these classes of pesticides, it is critical that an emergency treatment plan is developed by a clinician with expertise in pesticide-related emergencies. In addition to active ingredients, poisoning can also occur from solvents that are used to suspend the pesticidal agents. Ingestion or inhalation of solvents such as toluene or xylene can have serious health consequences; on pesticide containers all nonpesticide compounds are labeled as inert ingredients. It is important to understand that the term inert refers to an agent's use as a pesticide, and not to its toxicologic potential (Agency for Toxic Substances and Disease Registry, 1993).

EMERGENCY TREATMENT

Although emergency management of affected persons varies by the type of pesticide, some general treatment guidelines can be implemented with all exposed persons. They include the following.

1. Continuously observe the patient until he or she is stable.
2. Maintain an open airway and provide respiratory support. Suction to remove secretions if necessary. Intubate if there is evidence of respiratory depression or severe neurologic impairment. Administer oxygen if necessary; however it is critical to note that oxygen is contraindicated in cases of paraquat and diquat poisoning. It is important to seek detailed information prior to administering oxygen to patients with suspected poisoning (EPA, 1999).
3. Decontaminate the eyes, skin, and hair to eliminate residual pesticides. To reduce continued exposure, decontamination procedures should proceed concurrently with resuscitative and antidote treatments (EPA, 1999). Clothing should be removed and bagged and then the patient should be given a complete bath and shampoo while lying recumbent. In cases involving possible eye contact, flushing with copious amount of water or normal saline should proceed for 10–15 minutes (Ecobichon, 2000; EPA, 1999).
4. The gastrointestinal tract should be decontaminated by gastric lavage, administration of activated charcoal, or syrup of ipecac. Induction of vomiting and administration of activated charcoal is indicated in the treatment of most pesticide poisonings; however, emergency procedures

vary by specific agent. Advice from the poison center and emergency personnel should be based on the specific product(s) ingested (Weeks et al., 1991).

5. Obtain laboratory specimens to assess biologic indicators of pesticide exposure. In general, detection of organophosphate and carbamates in the blood can only be obtained soon after exposure. Metabolites of carbamates and organophosphates can often be detected in urine up to 2 days post exposure (ATSDR, 1993).

6. Administer antidotes to reverse the effects of specific pesticides. High doses of atropine sulfate are frequently administered to patients with organophosphate or carbamate insecticide poisoning. The goal of atropine therapy is to antagonize the effects of excessive acetylcholine in the peripheral neuroeffector junctions (muscarinic effects). In addition, pralidoxime (2-PAM) can be ordered in severe cases of organophosphate poisoning; however, this cholinesterase reactivator is of limited value in the treatment of carbamate poisonings (EPA, 1999). Because the pharmaceutical regime varies considerably by pesticide class and dose, it is necessary to obtain detailed treatment parameters from emergency department physicians.

In addition to decontamination and treatment of the patient, it is important to protect all emergency responders and health providers from secondary contamination from exposed persons. All contaminated clothing should be removed and disposed of, and the patient should be decontaminated with large amounts of soap and water.

GUIDELINES FOR ASSESSMENT AND CONTROL OF PESTICIDES IN DRINKING WATER

The large number of available pesticides and the complex regulations regarding their use and permissible concentrations in drinking water compound the difficulties for environmental health professionals who deal with pesticide issues. Because pesticides rarely exist in drinking water at concentrations greater than their MCLs or HALs it is difficult to assess whether chronic exposure to those compounds will have any adverse health consequences. Knowing the source of water for an individual or population is the first step in assessing possible chronic exposure, and understanding the potential for pesticides in drinking water is the next step. In cases where pesticides are suspected in drinking water, but their actual presence is not known, actual testing of the water may be necessary. If pesticides are present in drinking water at levels of concern, the person may be forced to develop a new source of water or install treatment for removal of pesticides.

In agricultural areas, knowledge of the crops grown within the drainage area for a particular water supply can be very helpful in determining the most commonly used pesticides. Comparison of those pesticides with information on pesticides most commonly found in water can help identify compounds of concern. Local, state, and county agricultural extension agents can provide information about the most common pesticides used in a particular area. Other helpful information pertains to the time of application for particular pesticides. As noted above, pesticide concentrations in surface waters are typically greatest following application periods and precipitation-runoff events. Temporal variations of pesticides in ground water are less well defined. Groundwater impacted by urban and suburban areas is more likely to contain insecticides than are those impacted by agriculture.

Pesticide use in urban areas will also lead to their presence in water. While most persons living in urban areas receive water from a centralized provider, some persons living down gradient from the urban area and using groundwater as a water source may be exposed to those pesticides used within the urban area. Common pesticides in urban areas will be herbicides and insecticides used on lawns, gardens, and road rights-of-way.

Knowledge of the source of water for an individual or population will provide valuable insight to the potential for long-term pesticide exposure from drinking water. Approximately 55,000 community water supply systems supply 90% of the drinking water in the United States. Ninety-three percent of those systems serve populations of fewer than 10,000 customers. Persons whose water source is a community water system now have access to that system's water quality monitoring data through the Consumer Confidence Report (CCR). Starting in October of 1999, each community water system was required by the CCR Rule (EPA, 1998) to publish and distribute a CCR on an annual basis. CCRs are typically distributed by enclosing a copy in water bills, publishing in newspapers with local circulation, and posting on the Internet by larger utilities. The CCR must provide the basic information shown in Table 17.2.

Public water supply systems are required to monitor quarterly for the presence of pesticides. If the annual mean concentration of pesticides is found to be below the MCLs, less frequent monitoring is generally approved by the regulatory agencies (USEPA, 2000). For example, if results of quarterly samples indicate a pesticide's concentration is below the analytical detection limit, then the regulatory agency can approve sampling once per

TABLE 17.2 Basic Information Found in Consumer Confidence Reports

- Source of drinking water
- Susceptibility of source water to contamination
- How to obtain a copy of the system's source water assessment
- Level of contaminants found in drinking water, range of levels and MCLs for contaminants
- Likely source of contaminants
- Potential health effects of any contaminant found in excess of MCL
- Compliance with drinking water-related rules
- Educational statements for susceptible populations on how to avoid a contaminant, such as *Cryptosporidium*
- Source(s) of additional information on the system's water quality

year. If the water system uses ground water and has not detected a pesticide for three consecutive years of annual sampling, then the water system can request to sample for that pesticide only once every 6 years. If the CCR does not supply the desired information about pesticides, additional water quality information can be obtained by contacting the water service provider using the information provided in the CCR.

Public water supplies are required to meet all applicable standards for contaminants in drinking water. If a contaminant exceeds its respective MCL the water utility must notify its customers and implement a program to meet the MCL for the contaminant in question. Generally some form of treatment must be provided to remove the contaminant or a new water supply source must be developed.

Almost 90% of people living in rural areas rely on ground water as their source of drinking water (Goodrich et al., 1991). Because monitoring water for pesticides is expensive, very few individual well owners have their water tested for pesticides. Few pesticide data are likely to exist unless local, state, or federal agencies have monitored ground water in the area of interest. Most state agencies responsible for drinking water maintain laboratories capable of performing pesticide analyses in water. The testing procedures are expensive and require sophisticated equipment and trained laboratory personnel. However, these state agencies can provide information on how to properly collect a water sample from a private well and can interpret the results of the tests performed (make a comparison with MCLs or HALs).

The EPA lists granular activated carbon (GAC) as the best available treatment process for removal of pesticides in drinking water, with the exception of glyphosate (i.e., Roundup), for which oxidation is the recommended treatment process. GAC consists of granular charcoal or soft coal that has been heat-treated to improve its adsorption characteristics. Centralized treatment is not an option for people who must rely on private wells for their water supply. Point-of-entry (POE) treatment units for individual homes are manufactured by many companies and are typically sold by home water-conditioning companies. In the case of pesticides, contacting the water with GAC is the usual treatment process. GAC for POE treatment is typically placed in a cylindrical canister and water is allowed to flow through the granular media at a controlled rate to allow contact between the contaminants in the water and porous surfaces of the GAC. Contaminants are sorbed to the surfaces of the GAC, removing the contaminant from the water. GAC contact units can provide an environment where microorganisms in the water can grow and multiply. Therefore most POE systems will provide a disinfection unit, such as an ultraviolet light device, to reduce the bacterial concentrations in the GAC-treated water. These disinfection units are particularly important where susceptible persons such as young children, the elderly, or immunocompromised individuals will consume the water.

GAC has a limited capacity to adsorb organic compounds such as pesticides. Once the GAC's adsorption capacity is exhausted it must be replaced with fresh GAC. Continued operation of exhausted GAC used to remove pesticides can result in pesticide concentrations greater than in the source water (Goodrich et al., 1991). Ultraviolet light disinfection units require periodic cleaning and UV-light bulb replacement. POE devices can provide reliable treatment when properly installed, operated, and maintained. Because most homeowners do not have the technical background to monitor the operation and performance of POE treatment devices, their use and effectiveness have been seriously questioned (Goodrich et al., 1991). The long-term maintenance contracts offered to homeowners by POE providers are recommended to enssure proper treatment.

HUMAN BIOMARKERS OF PESTICIDE EXPOSURE

In some cases that involve ingesting large doses of pesticide in a suicide attempt, it may be possible to obtain direct blood levels of pesticide, depending on the agent and time elapsed since exposure. Serum levels of the herbicide paraquat have been obtained following suicide attempts and have been found to be effective in determining patient prognosis (Erickson, Brown, Wigder, & Gillespie, 1997). However, except in rare cases, it is typically difficult to obtain measures of organophosphate and carbamate compounds in the blood of exposed persons. Urine metabolites of organophosphates and carbamate insecticides may be detected up to 48 hours post exposure (ATSDR, 1993).

Blood measurement of cholinesterase activity has been found to be useful in monitoring organophosphate and carbamate pesticide exposure, either following a single exposure or over time. Cholinesterase enzymes can be measured either in red blood cells (RBCs) or in plasma, and serve as surrogate indicators of neuroreceptor site activity (ATSDR, 1993). Cholinesterase depression in plasma can be detected within a few hours of significant exposure to organophosphate insecticides, with depressed levels persisting for several days to weeks. Depression of RBC cholinesterase activity may not be noted until several days post exposure, and may persist up to one to three months post exposure (EPA, 1999). Finger stick tests to assess RBC cholinesterase are commercially available; such tests have greatly enhanced opportunities to evaluate high risk groups such as farmers and farmworkers (McConnell, Cedillo, Keifer, & Palamo, 1992). Ciesielski, Loomis, Mims, and Auer (1994) compared RBC cholinesterase in 244 North Carolina farmworkers and non-farm workers; farmw orkers (mean 30.18 U/g hemoglobin) had significantly lower enzyme levels than non-farmworkers (mean 32.20 U/g hemoglobin. p = 0.01). Twenty-four farmworkers and zero non-farm workers had very low levels of cholinesterase. However, it is important to note that there are a number of different analytic methods used to determine cholinesterase levels in humans. Health providers should become familiar with the specific method used by their clinic or lab and how lab results should be interpreted.

The greatest challenge in interpreting cholinesterase levels is that baseline levels (i.e., preexposure) are typically not available; this issue is complicated by the fact that normal values vary widely among humans. Inhibition of 25 to 50% of an individual's baseline level is generally regarded as evidence of pesticide toxicity. It is important to keep in mind that this level of enzyme depression may not be associated with clinical signs or symptoms of acute poisoning (ATSDR, 1993).

HYPOTHESIZED ASSOCIATIONS BETWEEN PESTICIDE EXPOSURE AND CHRONIC HEALTH PROBLEMS

Pesticide exposure has been associated with a number of chronic health problems such as cancer, neurologic impairments, pulmonary disease, and reproductive disorders (National Research Council, 1993). In addition, there is increasing evidence that in some individuals, pesticide exposure may have a deleterious effect on the immune and endocrine systems. There is a high degree of controversy addressing chronic consequences of pesticide exposure, despite extensive research in both animals and humans. Some of the greatest concerns are for the health of children, who are biologically more susceptible than adults to most chemical exposures (National Research Council).

In the area of neurologic function, there is sufficient evidence to conclude that some organophosphate insecticides can induce a syndrome called organophosphate-induced delayed polyneuropathy, otherwise known as OPIDP. This condition is manifested primarily by paresthesia, weakness, and paralysis of the extremities, which can persist for weeks to years (EPA, 1999). Initial symptoms occur one to four weeks following exposure and include leg cramps, followed by numbness in the legs and occasionally in the forearms. The symptoms occur as a result of damage to the afferent fibers in the central and peripheral nervous system. Well-documented cases of OPIDP are rare but provide evidence of long-term neurologic consequences from organophosphate exposure. OPIOP has been induced in animal experiments, with the key pathologic hallmark consisting of axonal degeneration of the distal portion of sensory and motor neurons (Lotti, 2000). Compounds associated with the development of OPIDN include Trichlorphon, Merphos, triorthocresyl phosphate (OPIOP), and triortho-tolyl phosphate (TOTP) (ATSDR, 1993).

In addition to OPIDP, some findings from neurobehavioral studies of organophosphate-exposed individuals have provided evidence in support of long-term neuropsychiatric problems following insecticide exposure. Overall, studies with positive findings note significant differences between exposed and nonexposed persons in regard to memory, mood, and concentration (EPA, 1999). In their review of studies addressing pesticide exposure and children, the National Research Council (1993) concluded that "the evidence of chronic effects, particularly neurobehavioral effects of organophosphate and carbamate exposure, is less well established, but is strongly suggestive" (pp. 63–64).

Some scientists think that evidence from both human and animal studies demonstrates the potential for pesticide exposure to induce problems with immune functioning. Proposed mechanisms of toxicity include links between pesticide and reduced T cell populations, reduced lymphocyte responses, diminished cell-killing activity, and altered levels of circulating antibodies. The World Resources Institute (1996) notes that while links between immune dysfunction and pesticide exposure are not conclusive, the weight of evidence demonstrates a need for concern. Immune system alterations associated with pesticide exposure may manifest as hypersensitivity, immunosuppression, altered host resistance against infections of neoplastic agents, or the proliferation of immune components such as lymphoma or leukemia (NRC, 1993). A recent area of concern is the possibility that pesticides that contain estrogen-like compounds may act to disrupt endocrine function in humans; this concern has focused primarily on children as they approach puberty. There is evidence that high estrogen levels (which could potentially occur through exposure to some pesticides) during puberty can decrease the achievement of optimum height in adulthood (NRC).

A high degree of concern involves the potential for exposure to pesticides to play a role in the development of cancers. Carcinogenesis is a complex multistage process in which exogenous chemicals may play a number of roles in initiating cell mutations such as transitions or small deletions, or complex genetic alterations such as gene amplification or irreversible changes in gene expression (Pitot and Dragan, 1996). The most controversial area addresses the potential for some phenoxy herbicides to induce cancer in humans. The basis for this argument extends from human and animal evidence implicating TCDD (i.e., Agent Orange) and other polyhalogenated dioxins in the development of several types of cancer. Of concern is that phenoxy herbicides are often contaminated with dioxin compounds (Pitot and Dragan). While some pesticides may exert a direct effect on tumor development, it is plausible that other agents may act primarily by altering immune function (WRI, 1996). Because of the diversity of pesticides, there can be no sound rationale for making blanket statements implicating all pesticides as a cause of cancer in humans; however there is evidence supporting the carcinogenic potential of several specific agents. Studies of agents with long half-lives and those with evidence of carcinogenicity in animals are continuing to be conducted within the scientific community.

Blair and Zahm have examined cancer rates in both farmers and farm workers and have concluded that cancer patterns differ among these groups, compared with the general population. Overall, mortality rates for farmers are favorable, and cancers of the lung, bladder, and esophagus are generally low among this group. Part of these differences may be attributed to the lower prevalence of smoking in farmers versus nonfarmers and the physically demanding nature of agricultural work. Elevated rates of multiple myeloma, non-Hodgkin's lymphoma, melanoma, prostate cancer, and malignant brain tumors have been noted in previous studies of farmers, although the evidence is not consistent across studies (Blair and Zahm, 1995). Because of the overlap between tumors that are elevated in farmers and those associated with immunodeficiencies, there is continuing concern about the potential for long-term exposure to pesticide to induce immunologic changes that culminate in tumor development. However, data addressing cancer links in farmers are far from conclusive and fail to provide evidence on behalf of a link between specific pesticides and cancer incidence. It is important to keep in mind that farming involves multiple exposure to pesticides, fertilizers, gasoline, diesel, solvents, dusts, and sunlight, as well as biologic agents such as fungi and viruses; further research is needed to elucidate the nature of association between cancer occurrence and pesticide exposure (Blair and Zahm).

Compared with farmers, fewer epidemiologic studies have focused on health risks to migrant and seasonal farm worker, because of the challenges (e.g., migration, language barriers) in studying this group. Like farmers, farm workers comprise a heterogeneous group of persons, who differ in regard to race, ethnicity, occupational work tasks, residency patterns, and opportunities for formal education. Depending on the site and crop, farm workers may participate in a number of agricultural-related work tasks; however, pesticide exposure is prevalent among this group. In a survey of farm workers employed in Northern Mexico, Chaín-Castro, Barrón-Aragón, and Haro-Garcia (1998) found the highest rates of poisoning in workers who mixed pesticides, followed by those who were both mixers and sprayers, and those who worked exclusively as sprayers. Of 200 workers sampled, only one could identify a single pesticide by name; 30% did not wear any personal protective equipment when working with pesticides (Chaín-Castro et al.). Zahm and Blair (1993) have systematically assessed previous studies of cancer occurrence involving farm workers. Like farmers, there is some evidence that farm workers have elevated rates of multiple myeloma as well as cancers of the stomach, prostate, and testis. In addition, there is some evidence that supports the hypothesis that farm workers may have increased cancer rates for tumors of the oral cavity and pharynx, lung, liver, and cervix. The methodologic challenges of studying cancer occurrence in farm workers are well documented and research in this area continues.

PESTICIDE DEGRADATES AND MIXTURES IN DRINKING WATER AND THEIR IMPLICATION IN CHRONIC EXPOSURE

It has been estimated that in the past toxicologists devoted 95% of their efforts to studying the effects of single compounds (Groten, 2000). An awareness and interest in the toxicology and potential risks of combined compounds have spurred new research and approaches to protecting public health (Feron, Groten, and van Bladeren, 1998; Groten, 2000). The combined effects of a mixture of chemicals existing at levels below the no-observed-adverse-effect level (NOAEL) may still pose possible long-term health problems. An example would be assessing the potential carcinogenicity of a mixture of disinfection byproducts and pesticides, all at levels below standards set for the individual compounds in drinking water. Approaches such as using the NOAEL of the "most risky chemical in the mixture" or using the common "dose addition" concept may not be suitable for the many complex mixtures found in drinking water. Recent animal studies (Porter, Jaeger, and Carlson, 1999) have found that a mixture of aldicarb, atrazine, and nitrate at the MCLs for drinking water can affect the endocrine and immune systems as well as influence neurologic behavior. The effects detected using mixtures were not as significant when single compounds were tested. This recent study points out the importance of assessing the effects of mixtures versus the traditional approach of assessing one agent at a time.

Further complicating the issue of mixtures in drinking water is the fact that pesticide mixtures do not only contain the parent compounds, but also contain the degradation products of the parent compounds. As demonstrated in the study by Kolpin et al. (1998) the concentration in ground water of the degradates for herbicides with short soil half-lives can be much greater than the concentration of the parent compound, ranging from 60 to 99% of the measured herbicide concentration. Other studies have clearly demonstrated that chlorination of drinking water (the most widely practiced treatment technique for water disinfection) leads to creation of numerous chemical degradation products, many of which have similar toxic effects as the parent compound (Aizawa, Magara, Takagi, and Soona, 1994; Miles, 1991). It is becoming more apparent to all concerned with the safety of drinking water that mixtures of chemicals and their degradation products, from environmental degradation and/or treatment processes, must be taken into account in assessing the risks to public health.

RISK ASSESSMENT FOR PESTICIDES IN WATER

The basic four elements used by the EPA for human health risk assessment include (1) hazard identification (toxicology), (2) dose–response assessment, (3) exposure assessment, and 4. risk characterization. Chronic toxicity testing includes both chronic effects (non-cancer) and carcinogenicity (cancer). Included in chronic testing are developmental and reproductive testing, mutagenicity testing, and hormone disruption testing. When data do not exist on the effects of long-term exposure of healthy humans to pesticides, development of maximum contaminant level goals (MCLGs) for pesticides in drinking water often requires chronic (long-term) testing of the pesticide's toxic effects on test animals (Gustafson, 1993). The pesticide of concern is placed in the food of test animals at various dose levels and fed over a long period of time. Toxic effects such as liver and kidney damage are monitored over the course of the study and results are typically given in terms of milligrams of pesticide per kilogram of body weight per day (mg/kg bw/day). An NOAEL for the pesticide would be the dose at which no significant adverse health effects were observed. When an NOAEL cannot be demonstrated experimentally, the lowest-observed-adverse-effect level (LOAEL) is used. Unless specific dose–response information is available for humans, the NOAEL is extrapolated to humans by applying a factor of safety with the final result being a reference dose (RfD) expressed as mg/kg/day. Factors of safety include both an uncertainty factor (UF) and a modifying factor (MF), the former taking into account the type of studies used to determine the NOAEL and exposures to vulnerable populations such as children, and the latter based on professional judgment. The total factor of safety can range from 10 for the case where sufficient human dose–response data is available to values of 1000 or greater. The RfD is calculated using the following equation:

$$RfD = NOAEL / (UF \times MF)$$

To establish an MCL for drinking water, all exposure routes, such as food products, air inhalation, cosmetics, and so on, are taken into account during the exposure assessment. A typical assumption is that 10 to 20%

of a person's exposure results from drinking water, (Gustafson, 1993; Younes and Galal-Gorchez, 2000); therefore the MCLG would be set based on 10 to 20% of the RfD, taking into account body weight (60 kg for an adult) and typical water consumption per day (2 liters for adults) (Gustafson, 1993). The actual process used to set MCLs once the RfD has been estimated generally involves a complex risk assessment approach. MCLs are set as close as possible to MCLGs but must take into account the limitations of analytical techniques. Setting an MCL below the best available detection limits for a pesticide would be of no practical use. Establishment of an MCL can also take into account the best available treatment techniques for a particular contaminant to account for the realities of water treatment technologies.

A similar approach to that described above is used by the EPA to assess risks associated with chronic exposure to pesticides having known or possible carcinogenic or mutagenic effects. The hazard identification step uses both human studies, if available, and long-term animal studies to assess the carcinogenicity of a chemical. Table 17.3 (USEPA Office of Research and Development, 1992) lists the five categories used by the EPA for describing carcinogenic effects of a chemical. If a pesticide is shown to have carcinogenic effects (Group A or B) the MCLG is set to zero (Gustafson, 1993). Again, the MCL for the pesticide takes into account best available analytical and treatment capabilities. Because many of the studies used to assess carcinogenic effects of pesticides use test animals fed relatively high doses of a pesticide, typically in the parts per million range, the validity of the approach has been questioned by many scientists (Lave, Ennever, Rosenkranz, & Omenn, 1988).

TABLE 17.3 Carcinogenic Effects

Group	Category
A	Human carcinogen
B	Probable human carcinogen
	• B1: indicates limited human evidence
	• B2: indicates sufficient evidence in animals and inadequate or no evidence in humans
C	Possible human carcinogen
D	Not classifiable as to human carcinogenicity
E	Evidence of noncarcinogenicity for humans

SUMMARY

Although the acute effects of pesticide poisoning are well documented, incomplete science characterizes studies that address the potential for chronic adverse health effects from pesticides. Because the majority of studies have focused on single agents, the nature and magnitude of risk associated with mixtures and multiple agents, is, for the most part, unknown. A key role for nursing can be in the area of risk reduction through minimizing exposures. Clear advice from nurses can go far in helping families select products wisely, use and store them in a judicious manner, and wear appropriate personal protective gear when using pesticides. Reading product labels and following instructions for product mixing and dilution can help significantly in preventing spills and mishaps in the home setting. Because of metabolic and exposure differences between children and adults, minimizing children's exposure should be emphasized in all settings. Because of profound differences in pesticide use in different areas of the country, nurses are well advised to become familiar with local agricultural practices, industries using pesticides, and any contamination sites from historical pesticide use. Because of the complexity of technical information addressing pesticide use and exposure, enlisting advice from other professionals in agriculture, engineering, and medicine can help extend the expertise of the nurse. Finally, community involvement in activities to monitor and encourage safe use practices will go far in preventing tomorrow's cases of acute and chronic disease. Public health advocacy by nurses can be a force that promotes the development and use of safer pesticides for the future.

ACKNOWLEDGMENT

The authors would like to thank Sania Amr, M.S., M.D., Assistant Professor, Department of Epidemiology and Preventive Medicine, University of Maryland School of Medicine, for her review of this chapter.

BIBLIOGRAPHY

Adams, C. D., & Randtke, S. J. (1992). Removal of atrazine from drinking water by ozonation. *American Water Works Association Journal, 84*(9), 91–102.

Agency for Toxic Substances and Disease Registry. (1993). *Cholinesterase-inhibiting pesticide toxicity* (Report 22). Atlanta, GA: Department of Health and Human Services.

Aizawa, T., Magara, Y., Takagi, H., & Souna, F. (1994). Chlorination by-products of pesticides in drinking water. *Water Supply, 12*(1–2), SS11-6–SS11-9.

American Academy of Pediatrics. (1999). *Handbook of pediatric environmental health*. Elk Grove Village, IL: Author.

Blair, A., & Zahm, S. H. (1995). Epidemiologic studies of cancer among agricultural population. In H. H. McDuffie, J. A. Dosman, K. M. Semchuk, S. A. Olenchock, & A. Senthilselvan (Eds.), *Agricultural health and safety: Workplace, environment, sustainability* (pp. 111–117). Boca Raton, FL: CRC Press.

Blais, J. M., Schindler, D. W., Muir, D. C. G., Kimpes, L. E., Donald, D. B., & Rosenberg, B. (1998). Accumulation of persistent organochlorine compounds in mountains of western Canada. *Nature, 395*, 585–588.

Bushway, R. J., Hurst, H. L., Perkins, L. B., Tian, L., Guiberteau Cabanillas, C., Young, B. E. S., Ferguson, B. S., & Jennings, H. S. (1992). Atrazine, alachlor, and carbofuran contamination of well water in central Maine. *Bulletin of Environmental Contamination and Toxicology, 49*, 1–9.

Castaneda, A. R., & Bhuiyan, S. I. (1996). Groundwater contamination by ricefield pesticides and some influencing factors. *Journal of Environmental Science and Health, A31*(1), 83–99.

Chaín-Castro, T. D., Barrón-Aragón, R., & Haro-Garcia, L. (1998). Pesticide poisoning in Mexican seasonal farm workers. *International Journal of Occupational and Environmental Health, 4*, 202–203.

Ciesielski, S., Loomis, D. P., Mims, S. R., & Auer, A. (1994). Pesticide exposures, cholinesterase depression, and symptoms among North Carolina migrant farmworkers. *American Journal of Public Health, 84*(3), 446–451.

Council of the European Communities. (1980). *EC directive relating to the quality of water intended for human consumption, 80/778/EC*. Luxembourg: Office for Official Publications of the European Communities.

Council of the European Communities. (1998). *EC directive relating to the quality of water intended for human consumption, 98/83/EC*. Luxembourg: Office for Official Publications of the European Communities.

Ecobichon, D. J. (1996). Toxic effects of pesticides. In C. D. Klaassen (Ed.), *Casarett and Doull's toxicology: The basic science of poisons* (pp. 643–689). New York: McGraw-Hill.

Ecobichon, D. J. (2000). Carbamates. In P. S. Spencer, H. H. Schaumburg, & A. C. Ludolph (Eds.), *Experimental and clinical neurotoxicology.* (pp. 289–298). New York: Oxford University Press.

Environmental Protection Agency. (2000). *Pesticides and national strategies for health care providers (draft implementation plan)*. Washington, DC: Author.

Environmental Protection Agency, Office of Prevention, Pesticides and Toxic Substances. (1999). *Recognition and management of pesticide poisonings* (5th. ed.). Washington, DC: Author.

Erickson, T., Brown, K. M., Wigder, H., & Gillespie, M. (1997). A case of paraquat poisoning and subsequent fatality presenting to an emergency department. *Journal of Emergency Medicine, 15*(5), 649–652.

Feron, V. J., Groten, J. P., & van Bladeren, P. J. (1998). Exposure of humans to complex chemical mixtures: hazard identification and risk assessment. *Archives of Toxicology, 363*, 377.

Gilliom, R. J., Barbash, J. E., Kolpin, D. W., & Larson, S. J. (1999). Testing water quality for pesticide pollution. *Environmental Science and Technology, 33*(7), 164A–169A.

Goodrich, J. A., Lykins, B. W., Jr., & Clark, R. M. (1991). Drinking water from agriculturally contaminated groundwater. *Journal of Environmental Quality, 20*, 707–717.

Goss, M. J., Barry, D. A. J., & Rudolph, D. L. (1998). Contamination in Ontario farmstead domestic wells and its association with agriculture: 1. Results from drinking water wells. *Journal of Environmental Quality, 32*, 267–293.

Groten, J. P. (2000). Mixtures and interactions. *Food and Chemical Toxicology, 38*(Suppl. I), S65–S71.

Gustafson, D. I. (1993). *Pesticides in drinking water*. New York: Van Nostrand Reinhold.

Harrison, W. N., Watt, B. E., & Allister Vale, J. (2000). Pesticides in drinking water: What should be the standard? *Journal of Toxicology: Clinical Toxicology, 38*(2), 145.

Holt, M. S. (2000). Sources of chemical contaminants and routes into the freshwater environment. *Food and Chemical Toxicology, 38*(Suppl. I), S21–S27.

Khare, M., Bhide, M., Ranade, A., Jaykay, A., Panicker, L., & Patnekar, P. N. (1990). Poisoning in children—analysis of 250 cases. *Journal of Postgraduate Medicine, 36*, 203–206.

Kimbrough, R. A., & Litke, D. W. (1996). Pesticides in streams draining agricultural and urban areas in Colorado. *Environmental Science and Technology, 30*(3), 908–916.

Kolpin, D. W., Thurman, E. M., & Linhart, S. M. (1998). The environmental occurrence of herbicides: The importance of degradates in ground water. *Archives of Environmental Contamination and Toxicology, 35*, 385–390.

Lave, L. B., Ennever, F. K., Rosenkranz, H. S., & Omenn, G. S. (1988). Information value of the rodent bioassay. *Nature, 336*, 631–633.

Lotti, M. (2000). Organophosphorus compounds. In P. S. Spencer, H. H. Schaumburg, & A. C. Ludolph (Eds.), *Experimental and clinical neurotoxicology* (pp. 897–925). New York: Oxford University Press.

McConnell, R., Cedillo, L., Keifer, M., & Palomo, M. R. (1992). Monitoring organophosphate insecticide-exposed workers for cholinesterase depression: New technology for office or field use. *Journal of Occupational Medicine, January*, 34–37.

Miles, C. J. (1991). Degradation of aldicarb, aldicarb sulfoxide and aldicarb sulfone in chlorinated water. *Environmental Science and Technology, 25*(10), 1774–1779.

Miltner, R. J., Baker, D. B., & Speth, T. F. (1989). Treatment of seasonal pesticides in surface waters. *American Water Works Association Journal, 81*(1), 43–52.

National Research Council. (1993). *Pesticides in the diets of infants and children.* Washington, DC: National Academy Press.

O'Malley, M. (1997). Clinical evaluation of pesticide exposure and poisonings. *Lancet, 349,* 1161–1166.

Pereira, W. E., & Hostettler, F. D. (1993). Nonpoint source contamination of the Mississippi River and its tributaries by herbicides. *Environmental Science and Technology, 27*(8), 1542–1552.

Pitot, H. C., & Dragan, Y. P. (1996). Chemical carcinogenesis. In C. D. Klaassen (Ed.), *Casarett and Doull's toxicology: The basic science of poisons.* (pp. 201–267). New York: McGraw-Hill.

Porter, W. P., Jaeger, J. W., & Carlson, I. H. (1999). Endocrine, immune, and behavioral effects of aldicarb (carbamate), atrazine (triazine) and nitrate (fertilizer) mixtures at groundwater concentration. *Toxicology and Industrial Health, 15*(1–2), 133–150.

Schlenker, M. B., Alberson, T. E., & Saiki, C. L. (1992). Pesticides. In W. N. Rom (Ed.), *Environmental and occupational medicine* (pp. 887–902). Boston: Little, Brown.

Schottler, S. P., & Eisenreich, S. J. (1994). Herbicides in the Great Lakes. *Environmental Science and Technology, 28*(12), 2228–2232.

Spalding, R. F., Snow, D. D., Cassada, D. A., & Burbach, M. E. (1994). Study of pesticide occurrence in two closely spaced lakes in northeastern Nebraska. *Journal of Environmental Quality, 23,* 571–578.

Stamer, J. K. (1996). Water supply implications of herbicide sampling. *American Water Works Association Journal, 88*(2), 76–85.

Stamer, J. K., & Wieczorek, M. E. (1996). Pesticide distributions in surface water. *American Water Works Association Journal, 88*(11), 79–87.

Stamer, J. K., & Zelt, R. B. (1994). Organonitrogen herbicides in the lower Kansas River basin. *American Water Works Association Journal, 86*(1), 93–104.

United States Environmental Protection Agency. (1998). Consumer confidence reports. Final rule. *Federal Register, 63*(160), 44512–44536.

United States Environmental Protection Agency. (2000). *Drinking water standards and health advisories.* (EPA 822-B-00-001). Washington, DC: U.S. Environmental Protection Agency, Office of Water.

National Primary Drinking Water Regulations. (2000). Code of Federal Regulations, 40 CFR Ch. 1, Part 141, pp. 334–561.

United States Environmental Protection Agency. Office of Research and Development, National Center for Environmental Assessment IRIS. (1992). EPA's approach for assessing the risks associated with chronic exposures to carcinogens: (Background document 2). http://www.epa.gov/ngispgm3/iris/carcino.htm.

Wade, H. F., York, A. C., Morey, E., Padmore, J. M., & Rudo, K. M. (1998). The impact of pesticide use on groundwater in North Carolina. *Journal of Environmental Quality, 27,* 1018–1026.

Weeks, J. L., Levy, B. S., & Wagner, G. R. (1991). *Preventing occupational disease and injury.* Washington, DC: American Public Health Association.

World Health Organization. (1990). *Public health impact of pesticides used in agriculture*. Geneva: Author.

WHO. (1993). *Guidelines for drinking water quality: Vol. 1—Recommendations* (2nd ed.). Geneva: Author.

WHO. (1996). *Guidelines for drinking water quality: Vol. 2—Health criteria and other supporting information* (2nd ed.). Geneva: Author.

WHO. (1998). *Guidelines for drinking water quality: Addendum to Vol. 2—Health criteria and other supporting information* (2nd ed.). Geneva: Author.

World Resources Institute. (1996). *Pesticides and the immune system: The public health risks*. Washington, DC: Author.

Younes, M., & Galal-Gorchez, H. (2000). Pesticides in drinking water—a case study. *Food and Chemical Toxicology, 38*(Suppl. I), S87–S90

Zahm, S. H., & Blair, A. (1993). Cancer among migrant and seasonal farmworkers: An epidemiologic review and research agenda. *American Journal of Industrial Medicine, 24*, 753–766.

PART III

Environmental Health Risks in Specific Populations and Settings

CHAPTER 18

Environmental Hazards in the Home

Barbara Sattler

W e like to think that our homes are a safe haven. However, in recent years we have been discovering that certain products, designs, and even the siting of our homes can create health risks. When families moved into a new development in Waynesville, North Carolina called "Barber Orchard," they were ecstatic about their new surroundings—the fresh air, mountain views, and clean water. When one of the new residents had his well water tested their dream homes took on a different character. The water was reflective of the years of pesticide use on the former orchard on which their homes were sited: it contained DDT, DDE, and benzene hydrochlorides (Manual, 2000). The soil was contaminated with lead and arsenic, also the result of pesticide applications. The Environmental Protection Agency (EPA) sent in an emergency response team, removed topsoil, and advised residents to install carbon filters on their water systems.

Sometimes we unintentionally bring pollution into our homes. In the homes of middle-income families with small children, vacuum dust was found to have pesticide concentrations 10 to 100 times greater than those found in the surface soils surrounding the houses (Lewis, Fortmann, and Camann, 1994). In the agricultural area of Washington State, 47 of 48 farm homes had chlorpyrifos (a pesticide) measured in the house dust. The litany of human health risks associated with chlorpyrifos is substantial (including headaches, dizziness, muscle twitching, vomiting, and blurred vision), hence its EPA ban in 2000 for many applications.

Several building materials have evolved into bad actors in terms of their health risks. Lead-based paint, found in over 50 million American homes, is a prime example. Asbestos, which had a number of uses in home building, is associated with chronic lung conditions, including lung cancer. Formaldehyde is a chemical found in many of the pressed wood materials in modern homes. It is an irritant and a carcinogen. This chapter focuses on just a few of the environmental health risks associated with housing.

Indoor pollution sources that release gases or particles into the air are the primary cause of air quality problems in homes. Studies from the United States and Europe show that people in industrialized nations spend more than 90% of their time indoors. For infants, the elderly, persons with chronic diseases, and most urban residents of any age, the proportion is probably higher. Well-documented triggers of allergies and asthma include pet dander, molds, dust mites, cockroaches, and environmental tobacco smoke. The EPA's Office of Indoor Air (http://www.epa.gov/iaq) and the American Lung Association (http://www.lungusa.org) have excellent resources on these issues.

MOLDS

Molds are microscopic fungi that comprise 25% of the earth's biomass. They can grow on virtually any organic substance: wood, paper, carpet, foods, and insulation. When moldy material becomes damaged or disturbed, spores (reproductive bodies similar to seeds) can be released into the air. Exposure can occur if people inhale the spores, directly handle moldy materials, or accidentally ingest them. Mold sometimes produces toxic chemicals called mycotoxins that may cause illness in sensitive people. It is impossible to eliminate all mold and mold spores in the indoor environment. However, mold growth can be controlled indoors by controlling moisture. All types of mold have the potential to cause adverse health effects. They produce allergens that can trigger allergic reactions or asthma attacks. The most common symptoms of overexposure are cough, congestion, runny nose, eye irritation, and aggravation of asthma, as well as more serious problems such as fevers and breathing problems. Mold prevention and remediation can help to avoid such health risks.

MOLD PREVENTION AND REMEDIATION TIPS

Prevention

1. Fix leaky plumbing and leaks in the home as soon as possible.
2. Prevent moisture from condensation by increasing surface temperature or reducing the moisture level in air (humidity). To increase surface

temperature, insulate or increase air circulation. To reduce the moisture level in air, repair leaks, increase ventilation (if outside air is cold and dry), or dehumidify (if outdoor air is warm and humid).

3. Keep heating, ventilation, and air conditioning (HVAC) drip pans clean, flowing properly, and unobstructed.
4. Vent moisture-generating appliances, such as dryers, to the outside where possible.
5. Maintain low indoor humidity, below 60% relative humidity (RH), ideally 30–50%, if possible.
6. Clean and dry wet or damp spots within 48 hours. Provide drainage and slope the ground away from the foundation.
7. Wash mold from hard surfaces and dry completely.
   (Available on-line at http://www.epa.gov/iaq/molds/prevention.html)

Remediation

1. Always use gloves and eye protection when cleaning up mold. For extensive mold cleanup personal protective equipment (PPE) should be used. An explanation of PPE use can be found at   http://www.epa.gov/iaq/molds/i-e-r_ppe.html.
2. A variety of mold cleanup methods are available for remediating damage to building materials and furnishings. The specific method or group of methods used will depend on the type of material affected. For an explanation of remediation methods, go to http://www.epa.gov/iaq/molds/i-e-r_cm.html.
3. Absorbent materials, such as ceiling tiles and carpet, may have to be replaced if they are contaminated with mold.
4. Dust mites are microscopic animals that are found in every home. They survive by consuming dead skin cells and can be powerful triggers for asthma and allergies. Dust mites live in mattresses, pillows, carpets, fabric-covered furniture, bedcovers, clothes, and stuffed toys. There are a few simple steps that can be taken to minimize reactions to dust mites.
   a. Wash sheets and blankets once a week in hot water.
   b. Choose washable stuffed toys, wash them often in hot water, and dry thoroughly. Keep stuffed toys off beds.
   c. Cover mattresses and pillows in dust-proof (allergen-impermeable) zippered covers.
   d. Maintain low indoor humidity.

RADON

Radon is a naturally occurring radioactive gas that is found in soil and may seep into buildings from the surrounding soil. The EPA ranks indoor radon among the most serious environmental health problems facing us today. After smoking, it is the second leading cause of lung cancer in the United States, causing an estimated 14,000 lung cancer deaths a year (available online http://www.epa.gov/iaq/radon/pubs/citguide.html). The combination of exposure to radon and smoking significantly increases the risk of cancer. Approximately 1 out of every 15 homes in the U.S. is estimated to have elevated radon levels. You cannot see, taste, or smell radon. However, radon's decaying radioactive particles can be trapped in the lungs where they damage lung tissue and may lead to lung cancer. The risk of developing lung cancer from radon exposure depends on the amount of radon in the home (dose), the amount of time spent in the home (duration), and whether the individual is a smoker or has ever smoked (host factor).

Radon enters buildings by the following means:

1. Cracks in concrete slabs
2. Spaces behind brick veneer walls that rest on uncapped hollow-brick foundation
3. Pores and cracks in concrete blocks
4. Floor-wall joints
5. Exposed soil, as in a sump
6. Weeping (drain) tile, if drained to open sump
7. Mortar joints
8. Loose-fitting pipe penetrations
9. Open tops of block walls
10. Building materials such as some rock
11. Water (from some wells)

Testing is the only way to know if a home has an elevated radon level. The EPA and the Surgeon General recommend testing all homes below the third floor for radon. There are many kinds of low-cost do-it-yourself radon test kits that homeowners can purchase in hardware stores and other retail outlets. State radon offices also provide a list of trained contractors who conduct the tests. Nurses should test their homes and encourage neighbors and patients to test theirs.

CARBON MONOXIDE

Carbon monoxide (CO) is another colorless, odorless, tasteless poisonous gas. It is the leading cause of poisoning deaths in the U.S., with more than 3,800 people known to die annually from CO poisoning (accidental and intentional). It is produced by the incomplete combustion of carbon materials. Any flame or combustion device such as a stove or furnace is likely to emit carbon monoxide.

Carbon monoxide combines with hemoglobin to form carboxyhemoglobin, rendering the red blood cells incapable of carrying oxygen, which in turn results in tissue anoxia. The health threat from exposure to CO is especially serious for unborn babies, infants, and people with anemia or a history of heart or respiratory disease. At moderate levels, carbon monoxide can cause severe headaches, dizziness, confusion, and nausea. If these levels persist for a long time, death can occur. Low levels can cause shortness of breath, mild nausea, and mild headaches, and may have longer-term effects on health. These flu-like symptoms are often mistaken for the flu or other illnesses, an error that may result in delayed or misdiagnosed treatment.

To prevent and address low-level, chronic CO exposures, utilizing CO monitors, maintaining appliances, and recognizing symptoms of possible poisoning are essential.

Important Tips

1. Never burn charcoal inside a home, garage, vehicle, or tent.
2. Never use portable fuel-burning camping equipment inside a home, garage, vehicle, or tent.
3. Never leave a car running in an attached garage, even with the garage door open.
4. Never service fuel-burning appliances without proper knowledge, skills, and tools. Always refer to the owner's manual when performing minor adjustments or servicing fuel-burning appliances.
5. Never use gas appliances such as ranges, ovens, or clothes dryers for heating your home.
6. Never operate unvented fuel-burning appliances in any room with closed doors or windows or in any room where people are sleeping.
7. Do not use gasoline-powered tools and engines indoors. If use is unavoidable, ensure that adequate ventilation is available and whenever possible, place the engine unit to exhaust outdoors.

(Available on-line from the Consumer Product Safety Commission: http://cpsc.gov/cpscpub/pubs/cospot.html#prevention).

If the CO detector alarm goes off, check to see if any members of the household are experiencing symptoms of poisoning. If they are, get them out of the house immediately and seek medical attention. If no one is feeling symptoms, ventilate the building with fresh air; turn off all potential sources of CO—oil or gas furnace, gas water heater, gas range and oven, gas dryer, gas or kerosene space heater, and any vehicle or small engine. Have a qualified technician inspect fuel-burning appliances and chimneys to make sure they are operating correctly and that there is nothing blocking the fumes from being vented out of the house. (Source: www.epa.gov/iaq/pubs/coftsht.html).

ASBESTOS

Asbestos is a mineral used in a variety of building materials Unlike most minerals, which turn into dust particles when crushed, asbestos breaks up into fine fibers that are too small to be seen by the human eye. It becomes a health threat when these fibers become airborne. Asbestos fibers are persistent in the air because they are small and extremely light. Once inhaled, they easily penetrate body tissues. Asbestos fibers remain in the lung and are highly resistant to elimination, so that each new exposure increases the likelihood of developing an asbestos-related disease. There is no safe threshold level for exposure to airborne asbestos. Constant exposure can result in lung damage known as asbestosis or white lung, a chronic obstructive pulmonary disease. Exposure can also cause a rare type of cancer called mesothelioma. Asbestos is commonly used as insulation wrapping for pipes. When the insulation becomes dried, damaged, and airborne, it is referred to as "friable." In homes and buildings where insulation wrap is used, the wrap should be tested by professionals to determine whether it is asbestos. If it is, it should be removed or encapsulated by licensed professionals so there is no risk of fiber exposures.

VOLATILE ORGANIC COMPOUNDS

A volatile organic compound (VOC) is a chemical that vaporizes or "off-gasses" at normal room temperatures. Formaldehyde, a colorless chemical compound with a strong odor, is one example of a VOC. Formaldehyde is found in many of the pressed or particle board products that are commonly used in modern furniture and home buildings. It can cause irritation to nose, eyes, and throat, as well as coughing, skin rashes, fatigue, and allergic reactions. If extensive exposure to formaldehyde occurs, it can cause damage to the liver, kidneys, and central nervous system and it is a carcinogen.

Other VOCs include acetone, butyl and isopropyl (emitted from cleaners and tobacco smoke), aromatic hydrocarbons (from adhesives, sealants, caulking, gasoline, paint, pesticides, solvents, resilient flooring, and tobacco smoke), chlorinated hydrocarbons (from wood preservatives and solvents) phenols (from furnishings and tobacco smoke), and styrene (from carpeting). Each of these has its own constellation of adverse health effects. Certain products are now labeled as to the relative amounts of formaldehyde and VOC off-gassing. Purchasing low VOC products can reduce the indoor air level of these gases.

LEAD

Though there are many products in which lead can be found, the primary source in homes is lead-based paint. Exposure to lead creates a whole host of health risks. Lead is a powerful neurotoxin. It affects both the central and peripheral nervous systems. It is also toxic to the kidneys, gums, hemopoeitic system, reproduction (both male and female), and causes hypertension. Discussions in this chapter will be limited to the nursing role associated with lead-based paint.

NURSES' ROLE IN LEAD POISONING PREVENTION

Primary prevention efforts involve identifying and eliminating lead hazards before children are poisoned. Until this can be achieved, screening and follow-up of lead-poisoned children is essential. Tests for blood lead levels are recommended for children at ages 1 and 2, and more frequently for children if they are at higher risk. Any home built before 1978 should be tested for lead exposure. Nurses and homeowners can test for lead dust or the presence of lead in the paint.

Education efforts can include the provision of information to parents regarding federal regulations, which require that property sellers and landlords provide families with information about lead poisoning and about any known lead-based paint or lead hazards in a dwelling before its sale or lease. The only way to prevent lead poisoning is to remove the source of exposure. However, the process of removal often creates more exposure. If lead-based paint is in good condition (not chipped, flaking, or in areas of high friction), it is safer and easier to simply cover the area with non-lead-based paint. The outermost paint surface should be lead free. If there is lead-based paint underneath the intact paint, and the top surface is lead free, there will not be an exposure unless the surface begins to deteriorate or if renovations or other activities are implemented that compromise the integrity of the paint.

Nurses should educate parents and local health care providers about lead poisoning and the importance of screening homes and children. Excellent materials exist from the EPA, the Alliance to End Childhood Lead Poisoning, and the National Safety Council. A helpful publication entitled "Lead in Your Home: A Parents' Reference Guide" can be accessed from the brochure and training section of the EPA website (http://www. epa.gov/lead).

SCREENING HOMES FOR LEAD EXPOSURES

Nurses can perform dust sampling and/or train family and community members to sample for lead-based paint dust. There are also professional inspectors who can help homeowners make a lead assessment. The requisite "tools" for dust sampling are a tape measure, a baby wipe, and a ziplock plastic bag. Dust wipe sampling for lead should be done where children spend the most time (bedroom, kitchen, playroom, etc.), at the most used entrance door, where there are areas of failing paint, and in areas where renovation is underway or planned. Spots in the room to sample are the inside windowsill, the window trough, and the floor in front of the most used entrance. Materials needed are baby or hand wipes (use thin wipes that pull through a hole in the top of the container and avoid wipes with aloe, scent, or alcohol), a container (sealed plastic freezer bag, 35-mm film container, or centrifuge tube), a permanent marking pen, disposable gloves, a ruler or tape measure, a mailing envelope, and a form to identify and record samples.

How to take a sample

Throw out the first baby wipe, as it may be dry or dirty. Measure a 12-inch by 12-inch area. Using a moderate amount of pressure, wipe the 12-inch square in one direction, side to side, in a zigzag motion. Try to wipe the entire surface with a minimum of overlap. Fold the wipe, dirty side in, and wipe the same square in the same way in the opposite direction (top to bottom). Place the wipe in a sealed plastic bag and label it. For the windowsill and trough follow the same procedure as above, but instead of a 12-inch square, wipe the entire sill. Measure the length and width and label the bag with the information. Take a separate dust sample for the floor in front of the most used door.

Composite Samples

Composite samples combine samples from several sites and provide an average exposure level. Composite sampling can help to rule out lead-safe houses and indicate the need for further evaluation in homes where elevated lead levels are found. The advantage is that composite sampling is less expensive. The disadvantage is that the composite will only give an average. Put up to four wipes from different floor areas in one container. Do not put windowsill and floor wipes in same container. Send the samples to a lab that is recognized by the National Lead Laboratory Accreditation Plan. A list of these labs can be obtained by calling 1-800-424-5323. Make sure the a lab will take composite tests and will accept samples in a sealed plastic bag. Some labs will only accept centrifuge tubes. Use a lab that charges $10 or less per individual or composite sample (Livingston, 1997).

SUMMARY

In our homes, there are a number of environmentally related health threats that can be avoided by good assessment activities and the removal of the threats. All homes should be tested for the presence of radon. In homes where fuel powers the heating system, furnaces should be inspected annually. Carbon monoxide detectors should be considered for homes where gas fuels the furnace or stoves. Homes built before 1978 (when lead-based paint was banned from indoor use) should be tested for lead-based paint. Nurses, as role models for their families and communities, should be the first to know whether such environmental health threats exist in their own homes and then include such assessments when they do home visits or prepare new mothers or recovering patients for their return home from hospital stays. The website for the Childrens Health and Environment Coalition has a wonderful "virtual" interactive home, with excellent information on environmental health issues associated with our homes. See: www.chec.org —look for the health-e-home.

So many of the environmental health threats in homes can endanger children and their ability to learn. Working with day care settings and schools to incorporate environmental health education can help to improve the community's knowledge about preventable environmental diseases.

Nurses are uniquely qualified members of the community to initiate educational and awareness programs in schools, as well as incorporating them into home visiting activities, when teaching new mothers, and when sending patients home.

REFERENCES

Lewis, R. G., Fortmann, R. C., & Camann, D. D. (1994). Evaluation of methods for the monitoring of the potential exposure of small children to pesticides in the residential environment. *Archives of Environmental Contaminant Toxicology, 26*, 37–46.

Livingston D. (1997). Maintaining a lead safe home (Rev. ed.). Baltimore, MD: Community Resources, Inc.

Manual, J. S., (2000). Land use: A toxic house in the country. *Environmental Health Perspectives, 8*(3), 115.

CHAPTER 19

Children's Environmental Health

Barbara Sattler

Much like canaries in coal mines, children may unwittingly serve as environmental health sentinels for our society, as they are becoming the first to manifest adverse responses to environmental exposures.

Children's Environmental Health Network

More than 70,000 chemicals are used commonly today. Little is known about the impact of these substances on humans, but particularly troubling is that almost nothing is known about the effects on children or the effects of in utero exposure. Children have not been routinely included in the risk assessment process by which our environmental protection standards are set. When human exposure data is developed or projected, it is based on adult males.

Traditionally a disease associated with aging, cancer is even more devastating when it strikes children. The good news about childhood cancer is the increasing success in treatment. However, the very bad news is that childhood cancer rates appear to be increasing at a rate of 10% each year (Schmidt, 1998). Leukemia and tumors of the central nervous system combined account for approximately 50%. The list of possible causes of children's cancer includes genetic abnormalities, ultraviolet and ionizing radiation, electromagnetic fields, viral infections, certain medications, food additives, tobacco, alcohol, and industrial and agricultural chemicals (Schmidt). Clearly, the environment is playing an important role.

Children are exposed to environmental health threats in their first environment—the womb—and in their homes, day care and school settings, and in the community. There are a variety of characteristics that make children more susceptible to the impacts of hazardous environmental exposures.

Sandra Steingraber's beautifully written book, having faith, chronicals the environmental health risks to children from pre-conception through early infancy.

CHILDREN'S SPECIAL VULNERABILITIES

Children are not just little adults. They are different organisms in many ways, particularly with regard to their exposures and responses to the environment. Their status as developing organisms, their heightened biological sensitivity, their diet, and their unique exploratory nature enhance their vulnerability to many toxic threats in their environments.

To review, toxicology is the study of the negative effect of a physical stressor (chemical, biological, or radioactive) on a biological system—a cell, tissue, organ, organ system, or organism. The key variables in determining the relationship between an exposure to a stressor and a health effect are (1) the "dose" of the exposure, (2) the duration of the exposure, (3) the toxicity or strength of the toxin, and (4) a variety of host factors (such as age, sex, weight, health status, other exposures). Environmental toxins can enter the human body via ingestion, inhalation, and dermal exposure. People may ingest toxic chemicals in their drinking water as well as in foods and other beverages. Air pollution toxins, both indoor and outdoor, are absorbed in the lungs, and some toxic exposures, such as solvents and some pesticides, can be absorbed through the skin.

In the same way that the desired effects of pharmacological agents are dose dependent and also depend on the characteristics of the person receiving the medication, the effects elicited by toxic chemicals in our environment are dose dependent and dependent on the characteristics of the host. This concept is extremely important when discussing children's special vulnerabilities to environmental exposures because there are a number of variables that influence the dose of toxic chemicals to which children are exposed and their response to the chemicals.

Metabolic and physiological processes of children differ dramatically from those of adults. Children's skin, respiratory, and gastrointestinal absorption of toxic materials is greater than adults'. They cannot metabolize, detoxify, and excrete certain toxins as well as adults, and are thus more vulnerable to adverse health effects (Snodgrass, 1992). Infants and young children breathe more rapidly than adults. This increase in respiratory rate translates to a proportionately greater exposure to air pollutants. While infants' lungs are developing they are particularly susceptible to environmental toxicants. Children are short and, as such, their breathing zones are lower than adults', causing them to have closer contact to the chemical and biological agents that accumulate on floors and carpeting.

Infants and young children drink more fluids per body weight than adults do, thus increasing the dose of contaminants found in their drinking water, milk (hormones and antibiotics), and juices (particularly pesticides). If an adult were to drink a proportionate amount of water to the amount an infant drinks, he would have to drink about 50 glasses of water a day. Children also eat more per body weight and they eat different proportions of food. How many adults could eat the same amount of raisins pound for pound as the average 2-year-old? Children eat much more fruit and drink much more fruit juice than adults do, once again causing heightened exposure to doses of pesticide residues. In proportion to body weight, the average infant consumes 15–17 times more apple juice than the national average (National Research Council, 1993).

Children also drink proportionately more milk than adults and they drink both human and cow's milk. When averaged over the first year, cow milk products comprise 36% and 58% of the diets of nursing and non-nursing infants, respectively, while in adults these products amount to only about 29% (NRC, 1993). Several major toxic pollutants are lipophilic and therefore accumulate in milk fats (including human breast milk, which is approximately 3% fat). Both cow's and human milk have been found to have PCBs and dioxins (Rogan et al., 1986).

Children play on the floor, the grass, and the playground, placing them at increased risk for exposure to toxic chemicals that fall to earth, including lead-based paint dust, cleaning product residues, and horticultural/agricultural chemicals (fertilizers, herbicides, pesticides). The hand-to-mouth exploration of the infant and young child that helps them learn about their world also places them at much higher risks of exposures. This is particularly true in the case of lead-based paint dust when it is present in houses. When this hand-to-mouth behavior is observed and every encounter is viewed as another "dose," the point is brought to high relief. See Table 19.1 for a chart of hand-to-mouth contacts by children 2–6 years old (Reed, Jimenez, Freeman, & Lioy, 1999). Children's circulation is more rapid than adults', causing increased exposure to the individual organs of the body by circulating toxic chemicals.

Children's bodies also operate differently. They are more able to absorb calcium and other nutrients, an important mechanism for growing bodies.

Table 19.1 Range and Frequency of Mouthing Behaviors (contacts/hour)

Behavior	Mean	Minimum	Maximum
Hand-to-Clothing	66.6	22.8	129.2
Hand-to-Dirt	11.4	0.0	146.3
Hand-to-Hand	21.1	6.3	116.4
Hand-to-Mouth	9.5	0.4	25.7
Hand-to-Object	122.9	56.2	312.0
Object-to-Mouth	16.3	0.0	86.2
Hand-to-Other Itema	82.9	8.3	243.6
Hand-to-Smooth Surface	83.7	13.6	190.4
Hand-to-Textured Surface	22.1	0.2	68.7

adapted from Reed et al., 1999
aIncluding paper, grass, and pets

But this accelerated process also enhances the uptake of unwanted chemicals such as lead and other heavy metals. Newborns have lower pH in their gastric fluids that may increase the absorption of environmental pollutants and infectious agents (Bucuvalas & Balisitreri, 1997). Some of the protective mechanisms that are well developed in adults, like the blood-brain barrier, are immature in young children, thereby making them more vulnerable to the effects of toxic chemicals. Their immature immune system places them at higher risk of infection from pathogens in water or on foods.

The nervous system is the most vulnerable during embryonic, fetal, and early infant development. In the absence of a blood-brain barrier during these developmental stages, toxic exposures have unhampered access to the developing central nervous system (Rodier, 1995). Children's metabolism may affect their responses to toxic chemicals. In the same way that prescription drugs such as Ritalin will have a distinctly different response in an adult versus a child, environmental toxicants can also cause different responses. The half-life of caffeine is more than 10 times longer in newborns than in adults (Pelkonen, 1980). The kidneys of newborns and very young children are less effective at filtering out undesirable, toxic chemicals, resulting in their continued circulation and accumulation. Developmental differences in the body's ability to excrete toxic chemicals may affect the overall exposure to these chemicals. Kidney function does not reach adult capacity until about 16 months of age (Plunkett, Turnbull, & Rodricks, 1992)

Even before conception, maternal exposures (as well as paternal exposures) can play a role in compromising fetal and child development. For example, the fetus may be affected by the lifelong accumulation of lead in the mother's body that may have been stored in the bone and is mobilized into the bloodstream during pregnancy. Thirty percent of the maternal skeleton becomes available to the fetus to supply calcium needs. The freed lead that circulates in the maternal circulatory system passes freely through the placenta and into fetal circulation where it can do damage to the extremely vulnerable and immature central nervous system.

Persistent organic pollutants like dioxins are stored in the fatty tissues and have a very long half-life. They accumulate in the food chain and in breast milk. In utero and infant exposures to dioxin may account for as much as 10% of the lifelong exposure. The most spectacular rate of multiplicative growth (growth from cellular division) occurs before birth. Rapid cell growth makes fetal tissue particularly susceptible to the damage caused by environmental exposures. The more cell division occurs, the more opportunity for toxic chemicals to cause cells to make inaccurate copies of DNA, which in turn can lead to mutations and cancers. Neuronal cell division is complete by 6 months of age; however migration, differentiation, and myelination continue through adolescence. The lung tissue also continues postnatal cell division and cell differentiation. Babies exposed to environmental tobacco smoke have higher risk for smaller lung volumes, general developmental delays, and reductions in somatic growth.

The placenta does not provide a guaranteed protection for the fetus. As nurses, we know that some drugs pass through the placenta and others do not. The same is true for toxic chemicals. The following categories of compounds may cross the placenta.

1. Compounds of small molecular weight, such as carbon monoxide
2. Lipophilic compounds, such as ethanol
3. Compounds using an active transport mechanism, such as lead, which displaces calcium and is transported across the placenta

Mercury is another toxic substance that crosses the placenta barrier. For a 10-year period starting in 1956, residents of Minamata, Japan, consumed fish contaminated with methyl mercury discharged from a local industry. An increase in cerebral palsy was initially noted, as well as mental retardation, diffuse brain atrophy, and visual field deficits. Mothers were usually significantly less affected than their children. Umbilical cord sampling showed elevated levels of mercury in affected children.

Paternal exposure can also play a role in children's health. The short life span of sperm limits its exposure to toxic chemicals, yet the rapid differentiation of sperm increases its susceptibility to harm when exposure occurs. The most recent exploration of the relationship between paternal exposure and birth outcomes have included studies of veterans with their attendant exposures to Agent Orange in association with spina bifida in their offspring. Sperm abnormalities are associated with male cigarette smoking, which may induce mutagenesis and an increased risk of cancer in the man's offspring (Children's Environmental Health Network, 2001).

Although children are most vulnerable when they are very small, throughout childhood their susceptibilities may change. Adolescence is a case in point. Initiation of drinking and smoking, experimentation with recreational drugs, introduction of oral contraception, anabolic steroids, and other performance-enhancing drugs may have direct harmful effects but may also influence environmental toxicant metabolism (Golub, 2000). Recommendations for research that will help to create more appropriate environmental protection for adolescents include the following.

- Identify adolescence as a distinct developmental period in children's health research. Determine priorities for data needs in the area of adolescent toxicology.
- Identify end point methodologies that are appropriate for inclusion in animal toxicology studies conducted in the adolescent period.
- Establish in vivo and in vitro models for determining hazards unique to adolescence.
- Identify exposure periods in test species for the study of toxicology in adolescence. Establish guidelines for consistently including or excluding postweaning sexually immature animals in standard toxicology study designs.
- Consider adolescent development when establishing workplace exposure standards.

- Bracket the adolescent period when collecting age-dependent exposure data in survey studies.
- Examine the potential contribution of immunotoxicants and neurotoxicants to the high incidence of infection and injury in adolescents.

This excellent list of recommendations by Golub could and should be replicated for each of the major developmental stages of childhood development to ensure that stage-appropriate research continues to identify special vulnerabilities.

Clinicians should be alert to the unique physiology and behaviors of children and how they interface with their environment. Consideration of parents' take-home toxins from their occupational exposures should be noted. Incorporating environmental exposure factors into patients' histories is crucial, and then including these factors in the differential diagnosis will be key.

PROTECTING AND ADVOCATING FOR CHILDREN

Environmental standards that are "health based" almost never consider the effects on children or the unborn. Even the animal models are almost always adult animals. In those instances where research has been introduced using fetal, young, and adolescent animals, differences in toxicity are noted, indicating a critical need to explore toxicity in animal models across the life span. Health-based standards are typically set on the basis of preventing adverse health effects in white, adult (otherwise healthy) men who weigh 70 kilograms (about 160 pounds). Clearly, with such a model, the protection of our most vulnerable populations is jeopardized.

Passage of the Food Quality Protection Act in 1996, was the most recent indication that Congress was changing the course for children's environmental protection, as the Act demanded that children's diet, behavior, and vulnerabilities be taken into account when establishing safe standards for pesticide residues on food (see Table 19.2 for the major elements of the Food Quality Protection Act). Much debate and regular threats of repeal are indications of the power of the pesticide manufacturing and agricultural industries to influence the process by which children health is protected.

In the past two decades, there has been a major shift in awareness about children's environmental health that is very slowly influencing policy making. At the Environmental Protection Agency, a Child Health Protection Office was established to infuse an awareness of children's health within

Table 19.2 Food Quality Protection Act of 1996: New provisions related to protection of infants and children

---

Health-based standard: A new standard of a reasonably certainty of no harm" that prohibits taking into account economic considerations when children are at risk.

Additional margin of safety: Requires that the EPA use an additional 10-fold margin of safety when there are adequate data to assess prenatal and postnatal development risks.

Account for children's diet: Requires the use of age-appropriate estimates of dietary consumption in establishing allowable levels of pesticides on food to account for children's unique dietary patterns.

Account for all exposures: In establishing acceptable levels of a pesticide on food, the EPA must account for exposures that may occur through other routes, such as drinking water and residential application of the pesticide.

Cumulative impact: The EPA must consider the cumulative impacts of all pesticides that may share a common mechanism of action.

Tolerance reassessments: All existing pesticide food standards must be reassessed over a 10-year period to ensure that they meet the new standard to protect children.

Endocrine disruption testing: The EPA must screen and test all pesticides and pesticide ingredients for estrogen effects and other endocrine disruptor activity.

Registration renewal: Establishes a 15-year renewal process for all pesticides to ensure that they have up-to-date science evaluations over time.

---

the agency. This small office has maintained a strong and steady insistence that children should be considered when the EPA makes its policies and recommendations. The EPA's web site has an excellent children's section that links within the agency and to outside resources (www.epa.gov/children). Among the changes that have been influenced by the Office have been a significant increase in children's environmental health research and the reassessment of environmental standards to include concerns for children.

The Children's Environmental Health Network (CEHN) is a national advocacy organization that has had a powerful impact on national policy. This organization, with its impressive Scientific Board, has been able to present sound scientific rationales for the development of strong policies to protect children. It has also been very involved in training and education. Its "Training Manual on Pediatric Environmental Health: Putting it into Practice" (1999) is an excellent primer for health professionals on children's environmental health. This manual can be downloaded from CEHN's web site (www.cehn.org). Also found on the web site is a national resource guide that includes a large number of private and public organizations that relate to children's environmental health. The Children's Environmental Health Network continues to actively promote rigorous scientific discourse through national and international conferences.

Another national organization is the Children's Health Environmental Coalition which provides excellent materials for parents and communities on practical steps to take, as well as organized advocacy. Its web site (www.checnet.org) provides wonderful resources that nurses can use for community-based and patient environmental health education. Additionally, the group is producing a set of high quality videos in Spanish and English that could be used in clinics, closed-circuit TV within hospitals, and other settings.

Healthy children become healthy adults. Our investment in the health of our children should be an absolute priority. In the development of policies and practices, the health of our children should be paramount. Nurses are in many positions in which they can protect and promote children's environmental health. As informed parents, as professionals in clinical settings, in schools, and in communities, we have a unique presence to influence the environmental conditions in which are children live, play, and learn.

BIBLIOGRAPHY

Bearer, C. F. (1995). How are children different from adults? *Environmental Health Perspectives, 103*(Suppl. 6), 7–12.

Bucuvalas, J. D., & Balisitreri, W. F. (1997). The neonatal gastro intestinal tract. In A. A. Fanaroff, R. J. Marin (Eds.) *Neonatal-perinatal medicine. Diseases of the fetus and infant* (3rd ed., pp. 1288–1344). New York: Mosby.

Children's Environmental Health Network. (1999). *Training manual on pediatric environmental health: Putting it into practice.*

Golub, M. S. (2000). Adolescent health and the environment. *Environmental Health Perspectives, 108*(4), 355–362.

National Research Council. (1993). *Pesticides in the diets of infants and children.* Washington, DC: National Academy Press.

Pelkonen, O. (1980). Biotransformation of xenobiotics in the fetus. *Pharmacology and Therapeutics, 10,* 261.

Plunkett, L., Turnbull, D., & Rodricks, J. (1992). Differences between adults and children affecting exposure assessment. In P. S. Guzelian, D. J. Henry, & S. S. Olin (Eds.), *Similarities and differences between children and adults: Implication for risk assessment* (pp. 79–94). Washington, DC: International Life Sciences Institute Press.

Reed, K. J., Jimenez, M., Freemen, N. C., & Lioy, P. J. (1999). Quantification of children's hand and mouthing activities through a videotaping metholdology. *Journal of Exposure Analysis and Environmental Epidemiology, 9*(5), 513–520.

Rodier, P. M. (1995). Developing brain as a target of toxicity. *Environmental Health Perspectives, 103*(Suppl. 6), 73–76.

Rogan, W. F., Gladen, B. C., McKinney, J. D., Carreras, N., Hardy, P., Thullen, J., Tinglestad, J., & Tully, M. (1986). Polychlorinated biphenyls (PCSs) and dichlorodiphenyl dichlorethene (DDE) in human milk: Effect of maternal factors and previous lactation. *American Journal of Public Health, 76,* 172–177.

Schmidt, C. W. (1998). Childhood cancer: A growing problem. *Environmental Health Perspectives, 106,* 18–23.

Snodgrass, W. R. (1992). Physiological and biochemical differences between children and adults as determinants of toxic response to environmental pollutants. In P. S. Guzeliam, C. J. Henry, & S. S. Olin (Eds.). *Similarities and differences between children and adults: Implications for risk assessment* (pp. 35–42). Washington, DC: International Life Sciences Institute Press.

CHAPTER 20

Environmental Health Risks in the Work Setting: Recognizing Sentinel Events

Kathleen McPhaul

Sentinel occupational health events are preventable work-related or work-exacerbated disability, disease or death (Mullan and Murthy, 1991; Rutstein et al., 1983). A sentinel health event serves as a warning signal that preventive measures have failed. (Rutstein et al.). The occupational medicine literature is populated with papers describing sentinel occupational health conditions including solvent overexposures (Centers for Disease Control, 1989b), building-associated hypersensitivity pneumonitis (Weltermann et al., 1998), asthma associated with metal-working fluids (Rosenman, Reilly, and Kalinowski, 1997), pesticide poisoning, (Olson, Sax, Gunderson, and Sioris, 1991), and many others (CDC, 1984; Hoffman, Wood, and Kreiss, 1993; Lax et al., 1996; Rutstein et al., 1983), A list of 64 sentinel occupational diseases was developed as a model for a national surveillance system (Mullan and Murthy, 1991). Occupational health nurses have also incorporated the concept of sentinel occupational health events into their practices (Connon, Freund, and Ehlers, 1993; Randolph and Migliozzi, 1993) as evidenced in the literature (Cohen and Kaufman, 2000). The Occupational Health Nurses in Agriculture Communities Program (OHNAC) engages nurses to actively seek cases of occupational disease and injury in farming communities. Such targeted identification of cases leads to pragmatic public health interventions. For example, a nurse-initiated investigation of a sentinel scalping injury from a hay baler uncovered three earlier injuries from the same model machine and resulted in a published product alert broadcast to every cooperative extension agent in the country. (Connon et al., 1993).

Increasingly the reporting of occupational and environmental disease is considered the responsibility of health providers, especially physicians and nurses (Butterfield, 1990; Herbert, London, Nagin, and Beckett, 2000; Institute of Medicine, 1995; NEETF et al., 2000). Nurses who assess or diagnose and act upon sentinel occupational health events realize the goal of "thinking upstream" and "promot[ing] health through population-based interventions. (Butterfield, 1990, p. 2) This chapter provides a framework for nurses in all specialties to incorporate the concept of sentinel occupational health events into their practice. But how do nurses identify sentinel occupational events and what do they do once they have? Consider the following example of adult occupational lead poisoning. In the author's experience this fairly common illness of construction workers is generally not diagnosed on the initial healthcare visit, an omission that often leads to deteriorating health, unnecessary testing and treatment, and delays in protecting other workers at the site. In order for nursing practice to effectively utilize the concept of sentinel occupational health events (SHEO), the nurse must be able to recognize a preventable occupational illness or injury and to communicate with the public health agency responsible for taking action.

LEAD POISONING AS A MODEL OF A SENTINEL OCCUPA-TIONAL HEALTH EVENT

R. G. was working as an ironworker renovating a historic office building in the nation's capital. The job was behind schedule, and therefore the construction crew was working twelve-hour days, seven days a week. This schedule was particularly demanding, so when R. G. developed fatigue and irritability he attributed it to his long hours and long daily commute. When he developed stomach pains he went to see a physician in his off hours so he wouldn't miss much work. He didn't consider his using a power grinder to remove old paint from the ornate cornices of the historic building as contributing to his illness and no one asked him about his work. After several evening appointments at his local urgent care his stomach pains worsened. In agony he presented to his local emergency room and was prepped for an emergency appendectomy. At the last minute, a blood lead level was drawn on the recommendation of the gastroenterologist. Needless the say, the surgery was cancelled when his blood lead came back in the high 80's (normal range for an adult is less than 25 mcg/dl). The numerous missed opportunities for nurses and other clinicians to ask about this gentleman's occupation illustrate the profound consequences that can accompany a missed diagnosis. R. G. had a 3-year-old son whose blood lead increased due to lead dust contaminating the home when R. G. returned from work. His son's blood lead was only checked after his father's diagnosis of lead poisoning was confirmed (Keogh and Gordon, 1994).

An elevated blood lead level (greater than 25 mcg/dl) in an adult is a sentinel occupational health event. A discovery of occupational lead poisoning in one adult is the basis to take action to limit exposure to coworkers. Some states mandate laboratory reporting of elevated blood leads to the Adult Blood Lead Epidemiology Surveillance (ABLES) registry usually within the State Health Department (Freund et al., 1990). Fortunately, R. G. lived in a state requiring mandatory reporting of elevated blood leads to the ABLE's Registry. R. G.'s elevated blood lead was reported and the State Department of the Environment Heavy Metals Registry staff determined the reasons for the elevated blood lead, ensured appropriate medical follow-up, and made a referral to the Occupational Safety and Health Administration (OSHA). An adult diagnosis of lead poisoning is a signal that OSHA protective requirements are either not in place or have failed. Most U.S. workers are covered by the federal OSHA law requiring employers to protect against overexposures to lead. Depending on the state, either the ABLES registry or the health care provider can initiate a referral to OSHA. It is the responsibility of OSHA or a similar state agency to determine if human health is at risk at a work site. (See Table 20.1 for participating ABLES states.)

Nurses can play a key role in obtaining an occupational/environmental history during patient encounters. This history can be brief if a workplace exposure seems unlikely, or more detailed if exposures are reported (see chapter 23 on environmental history taking). If a connection is suspected between the workplace and the symptoms, a more in-depth investigation or referral is warranted. It is essential, however, that nurses utilize the sentinel health event or public health approach and ensure that the outbreak does not spread to other workers. Later in this chapter, several sentinel surveillance systems are reviewed. Nurses who work in states with sentinel occupational disease reporting systems may have access to preventive occupational health resources (see Table 20.1). Common medical conditions for which there can be an occupational etiology are also identified (see

TABLE 20.1 Selected Sentinel Occupational Health Surveillance Systems by Participating State

State	SENSOR	ABLES Lead	AOEC Clinic	Death Certificate I/O Coding	OHNAC
Alabama		X	X		
Arizona		X	X		
California	X	X	X		X
Colorado	X		X	X	
Connecticut		X	X		
Georgia			X	X	X
Hawaii				X	
Idaho				X	
Illinois	X		X		
Iowa		X	X		X
Kansas				X	
Kentucky			X	X	X
Louisiana			X		
Maine		X		X	X
Maryland		X	X		
Massachusetts	X	X	X		
Michigan	X		X	X	
Minnesota		X	X		
Nebraska		X			
Nevada				X	
N. Hampshire		X		X	
New Jersey	X	X	X	X	
New Mexico		X	X	X	
New York		X	X		
North Carolina		X	X	X	X
North Dakota					X

TABLE 20.1 *(continued)*

Ohio	X	X	X	X	X
Oklahoma		X			
Oregon	X	X			
Pennsylvania		X	X		
Rhode Island		X		X	
South Carolina		X		X	
Tennessee			X		
Texas	X	X	X		
Utah		X	X	X	
Vermont		X		X	
Virginia			X		
Washington		X	X		
West Virginia			X	X	
Wisconsin	X	X		X	
Wyoming		X			
District of Columbia			X		

Suggested key or legend for the acronyms:
SENSOR—Sentinel Event Notification for Occupational Risk
ABLES—Adult Blood Lead Epidemiologic Surveillance
AOEC—Association of Occupational and Environmental Clinics
OHNAC—Occupational Health Nurse in Agricultural Communities

Tables 20.2 and 20.3). It is important to know which occupational exposures may have medical testing required by federal OSHA law (see Table 20.4). These powerful laws can assist the health care provider and worker to determine when a worker can return to work safely.

Figure 20.1 graphically illustrates a paradigm for two possible pathways after occurrence of a sentinel occupational health event.

PREVALENCE OF WORK-RELATED DISEASE

How much work-related disease and injury exists? How often can a nurse expect to encounter occupational disease or injury? There is a broad spectrum of nurse generalists, nurse specialists, and nurse practitioners who

TABLE 20.2 Occupational Diseases and Injuries Most Likely to be Encountered by Nursing Specialty

Nursing Specialty	Sentinel Occupational Health Event
Emergency room nurses	Carbon monoxide (CO) poisoning; acute asthma attacks; lead poisoning; trauma from falls, accidents and violence; chemical overexposures
Obstetrical nurses/midwives	Infertility, miscarriages, birth defects from chemical overexposures or physical work factors
Cardiovascular nurses	Occupational stress-induced coronary disease/hypertension and toxic exposures
Pediatric nurses	Chemical exposures in children from "take home" exposures from parents' work (i.e., lead poisoning), adolescent chemical exposures in the workforce
Hospital employee health nurses	Needlestick injuries (with and without conversion to HIV, hepatitis B and C), back injuries, latex allergy, injuries from patient and visitor assault, allergies/asthma, chemical overexposure, radiation exposure
Infectious disease nurses	Tuberculosis, hepatitis B and C, legionnaires' disease
Community health nurses	Take home exposures, poor indoor and outdoor air quality, pesticide poisonings
Primary care adult/family nurse practitioners	Any and all occupational conditions, hearing loss, asthma, musculoskeletal conditions, occupational cancers, fibrotic lung disease, asthma, repetitive strain injuries
Nursing administrators/managers	Needlestick injuries (with and without conversion to HIV, hepatitis B and C), back injuries, latex allergy, injuries from patient and visitor assault, allergies/asthma, chemical overexposure, radiation exposure among their staff
Critical care/trauma nurses	Industrial and agricultural poisonings; construction, agricultural and industrial accidents; severe injuries from workplace violence; transportation accidents
Geriatric nurses	Fibrotic lung diseases, occupational cancers, occupational hearing loss
Oncology nurses	Occupational lung cancer (asbestos), leukemia (benzene) bladder cancer (beta-naphalene), soft tissue sarcoma (dioxin), angiosarcoma of the liver (vinyl choride), skin cancer

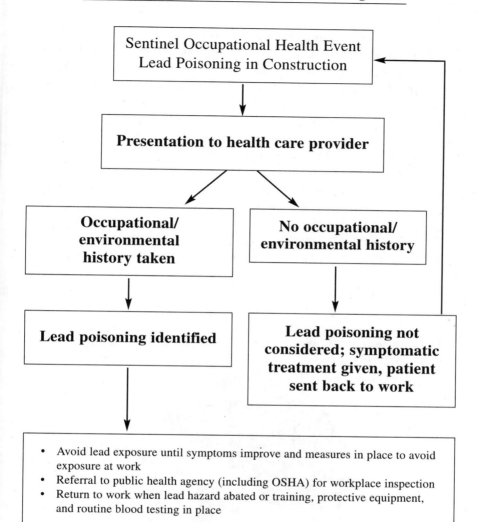

FIGURE 20.1 Adult lead poisoning as a model of sentinel occupational health event paradigm.

can realistically expect to encounter occupational sentinel health events in their practices. For example, nurses who care for any working adult in an ambulatory care clinic, during an acute hospitalization, or in the home setting, community, or workplace might encounter a sentinel occupational health event. Furthermore, retired persons are susceptible to occupational illnesses with long latency periods such as fibrotic lung (i.e. asbestosis), occupational cancers, noise-induced hearing loss, and musculoskeletal disorders long after they have retired from their jobs. Both permanently and temporarily disabled persons should be queried about their past occupational exposures and their plans for future work. It is possible that the disability arose from employment conditions. Nurses caring for men and women of child-bearing age, pregnant women, and infertile couples should pay particular attention to the occupational history because the reproductive system is unusually vulnerable. Finally, pediatric and neonatal nurses should be vigilant to the occupational exposures of the parents of their patients, and the occupational exposures of their older adolescent patients.

In 1998 the Annual Occupational Survey reported 144.8 million persons working in the United States (BLS, 1999). The BLS reports a total of 5.9 million injuries and illnesses in 1998 (non-governmental private industry workplaces). This is a rate of 6.7 cases per 100 full-time workers (BLS). Figures 20.2 and 20.3 reflect the relative proportion of types of occupational illnesses and injuries according to the Healthy People 2000 Progress Charts (Department of Health and Human Services, 2000).

In addition to the high number of *reported* occupational illness and

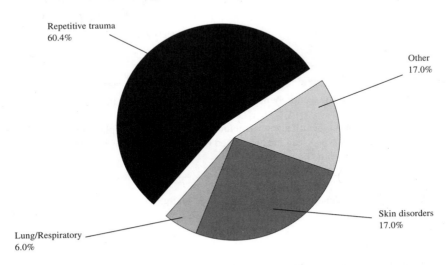

FIGURE 20.2 Chart from healthy people 2000 progress report—occupational illness.

From: Centers for Disease Control
National Center for Health Statistics
Occupational Safety and Health Progress Review
Healthy People 2000 Occupational Safety and Health Progress Review, November 17, 1999
(http://www.cdc.gov/nchs/about/otheract/hp2000/safety/safetycharts.htm).

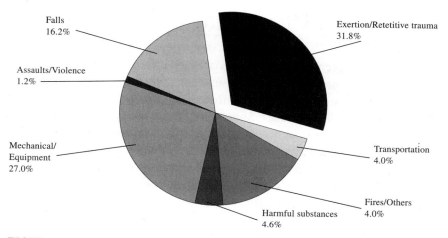

FIGURE 20.3 Chart from healthy people 2000 progress report—occupational illness.

From Healthy *People 2000 Occupational Safety and Health Progress Review*, November, 1999
(http://www.cdc.gov/nchs/about/otheract/hp2000/safety/safety.htm).

injury, occupational health researchers and practitioners acknowledge that
the reported numbers are only the tip of the iceberg (CDC, 1989a, 1990;
Jajosky et al., 1999; Levy and Wegman, 2000) The vast number of occu-
pation-related health conditions, especially illnesses are unrecognized and,
hence, unreported. The workplace is an environment where adults spend
substantial time, and, unfortunately, the workplace environment is the
source of significant environmental exposures with serious adverse health
effects (IOM, 1995).

THE IMPORTANCE OF THE OCCUPATIONAL/ENVIRONMEN-
TAL HISTORY

The link between work and disease is established by the occupational/envi-
ronmental history. Rather than create a complex algorithm for when and
how to take an occupational/environmental history it is recommended to
always inquire about a patient's work. Eliciting the work history will then
become as routine as asking about smoking, life style, medication, and
chronic health conditions. In addition to discovering possible links between
work and disease, the nurse can begin to formulate the impact of the client's
current health condition on his or her ability to work. Such thinking will
facilitate discharge planning processes for hospitalized working adults.
Details on taking an occupational history are outlined in chapter 23.

SELECTED SENTINEL OCCUPATIONAL HEALTH EVENT SURVEILLANCE MODELS

There is no comprehensive occupational disease or injury surveillance system in place in the United States. Some states however, do participate in active occupational surveillance utilizing "sentinel" providers to report specific occupational diseases. Some states also have passive occupational disease surveillance systems. Several systems are described in this section. For a comprehensive review of existing occupational surveillance systems the reader is referred to a series of articles devoted to occupational surveillance (Muldoon et al., 1987) or the most recent National Institute for Occupational Safety and Health *Worker Health Chart Book* (NIOSH, 2000). It is evident that by relying on fragmented state-based occupational disease and injury reporting systems it will never be possible to obtain an accurate picture of the true incidence and prevalence of occupational and environmental disease in the U.S. Therefore, it is incumbent upon, the health care providers, to identify local public health systems and resources to advocate for our patients.

Sentinel Event Notification Systems for Occupational Risks (SENSOR)

The Centers for Disease Control (CDC) National Institute for Occupational Safety and Health (NIOSH) has responsibility for occupational illness and injury research. NIOSH, in partnership with several states developed the Sentinel Event Notification Systems for Occupational Risks, known as SENSOR (Baker, 1989). It is a state-based and condition-specific surveillance and preventive intervention system. Currently SENSOR programs are in place for work-related asthma, silicosis, carpal tunnel syndrome, lead poisoning, noise-induced hearing loss, and pesticide poisoning. (CDC, 1989a, 1990; Jajosky et al., 1999) States participating in the SENSOR system generally have resources for following up reported sentinel cases and ensuring that protective measures are in place to prevent reoccurrences of the sentinel occupational health event (see Table 20.1 for participating states). These active surveillance systems have been shown to result in far more case reporting than passive reporting systems. For example, the SENSOR program in Texas noted only two reports in its first year before developing a system of sentinel case providers and actively following up with each one to ensure accurate reporting (Schnitzer and Shannon, 1999).

THE ADULT BLOOD LEAD EPIDEMIOLOGY AND SURVEILLANCE PROGRAM (ABLES)

The ABLES program is a surveillance system for identifying and preventing cases of elevated blood lead levels among U.S. adults. The public health objective of the ABLES program (Objective 20.7 "Reduce the number of persons who have elevated bloodlead concentrations from work exposures" in DHHS's *Healthy People 2010*) is, "Eliminate exposures which result in workers having blood lead concentrations greater than 25 micrograms per deciliter (mcg/dL) of whole blood." (p. B20–19).

State ABLES programs collect blood lead level data from local health departments, private health care providers, and from private and state reporting laboratories. State ABLES programs also analyze and report their data; conduct follow-ups with physicians, workers and employers; target on-site inspections of work sites; provide referrals to cooperating agencies; identify new exposures and failures in prevention; and target educational and other interventions (see Table 20.1 for participating states). It is worth noting that the ABLES program does not rely solely on health care provider reporting of adult lead poisoning, but rather requires the laboratories to report elevated blood lead levels. In the event that an emergency room visit or a workplace medical testing program identifies an elevated blood lead, the public health system will automatically be notified.

ASSOCIATION OF OCCUPATIONAL AND ENVIRONMENTAL CLINICS (AOEC) COMPUTERIZED DATABASE

The AOEC is committed to improving the practice of occupational and environmental health through information sharing, professional support, and collaborative research. The AOEC strives to aid in identifying, reporting, and preventing occupational and environmental health hazards and their effects. The AOEC has developed a confidential computer database of occupational and environmental diseases reported by AOEC member clinics. This database has centralized, deidentified episodes of disease induced by environmental or occupational circumstances reported by the AOEC member clinics. This resource is available to health care providers for analysis and comparison. AOEC clinics, especially the reporting clinics, recognize each occupational and environmental disease as a sentinel event. Regional AOEC clinics educate health care providers, assisting in workplace investigations, and conduct occupational disease and injury research (Welch, 1989).

Death Certificate Industry and Occupation Coding

NIOSH collaborates with the National Center for Health Statistics and the Bureau of Census to obtain data on the prevalence of occupational fatalities. The sentinel occupational health event concept has been successfully applied to several states' death certificate reporting systems (Lalich and Schuster, 1987). Death certificate cause of disease reporting has its limitations, however, by coding death certificates with both occupation and industry, the identification of trends, particularly in diseases with long latency periods, can be followed. Coal workers' pneumoconiosis and mesothelioma were the two most common occupational diseases in the analysis reported by Lalich and Schuster.

Occupational Health Nurses in Agriculture Communities Program (OHNAC)

The OHNAC program described earlier in this chapter is an example of active surveillance. The program utilizes trained nurses to work with agricultural communities to identify and report cases of occupational disease and injury in agricultural settings. The program has even experimented with obtaining occupational injury and illness reports from non-health care providers including the farmers themselves. Nurses play an important role in the education and outreach activities as well as the workplace hazard identification and control (Connon et al., 1993; see Table 20.1 for participating states).

Other Sentinel Occupational Health Event Surveillance Models

A successful partnership between a large union and a primary health care network has resulted in an effective sentinel occupational health clinic in New York. This model system demonstrates an effective collaboration among the workers, the primary care medical group, and the occupational health team. When an occupational health disease is diagnosed it is treated as a sentinel health event. An occupational health specialist functions as case manager, coordinating care and preventive follow-up activities (Herbert et al., 1997).

Some states use their Workers Compensation data system as a surveillance program for occupational injuries and diseases. The Safety and Health Assessment and Research for Prevention (SHARP) program in Washington conducts sentinel surveillance of occupational dermatologic conditions

(Cohen and Kaufman, 2000). Workers Compensation is a federally mandated system administered in each state. It is a logical database to monitor for sentinel occupational health events because each accepted claim has been determined to be work related or work exacerbated. This method of surveillance can be limited by the time interval between filing and acceptance of a claim. Nonetheless only a handful of states currently routinely monitor this source of occupational injury and illness data.

Poison control centers are not sentinel health surveillance systems; however, some investigators have analyzed poison control data for occupational overexposures (Olson, Sax, Gunderson, and Sioris, 1991; Woolf and Flynn, 2000). Adolescent chemical exposures were analyzed in this fashion bringing to light the unacceptably high number of chemical exposures in typical adolescent workplaces such as fast food restaurants and automotive shops (Woolf and Flynn). Pesticide poisoning has also been investigated through regional poison control data analysis (Olson et al.).

As indicated above, many nurses and physicians in the AOEC member clinics treat each occupational illness and injury as a sentinel health event. Furthermore, the occupational health professionals in these clinics are available for consultation, training, and referrals. The AOEC coordinates a database of occupational and environmental diseases reported from the member clinics. It also provides training and education to medical and nursing students and practicing physicians and nurses, often in collaboration with government agencies and local authorities. This organization, its clinics, and its web page, are extremely useful resources and should be considered by any nurses in need of consultation on an occupational health problem (AOEC, 2001; Welch, 1989).

SENTINEL OCCUPATIONAL HEALTH EVENTS COVERED BY OSHA REGULATIONS

Some sentinel occupational health events enjoy specific regulation by OSHA. The regulations, known as OSHA Standards, empower health care providers to request an inspection of a patient's workplace. A written health care provider referral should result in an inspection, which can improve health and safety conditions, not only for your patient but for his or her coworkers as well. For example, there is a specific OSHA Standard for Lead in the Workplace (OSHA CFR 1910.1025). An adult with an elevated blood lead should be queried about the conditions of the workplace. Did the worker know there was lead in the workplace? Was there a specific training program about the health effects of lead? Does the employer have blood lead levels drawn on a regular basis? Does the worker wear protective gear, such as a respirator, while working? In most cases of lead in the workplace, these are OSHA requirements and must be in place to ensure that workers do not get overexposed to lead.

Other examples of occupational hazards with special protections under OSHA are exposure to blood-borne pathogens, tuberculosis and formaldehyde. These hazards are very common in health care workplaces. Health care employers are now required to provide engineered sharps or safer needle devices in health care workplaces. Recently an OSHA Ergonomics Standard was promulgated and rescinded. The special protective requirements of this standard would have been activated by a single sentinel musculoskeletal injury resulting from a repetitive or other ergonomic exposure. Preventive ergonomics programs would be developed in response to the sentinel case identification.

RECOMMENDED NURSING ACTION FOR SENTINEL OCCUPATIONAL HEALTH EVENTS

In summary, sentinel occupational health events indicate that preventive workplace measures were either not in place or not effective. Preventive workplace measures can include engineering controls to reduce chemical, biological, or mechanical exposure; administrative controls to reduce the amount of time a worker is in contact with a hazard; education and training to raise awareness of hazards and their effects; personal protective equipment such as respiratory protection or goggles to prevent contact with exposure; and medical surveillance to watch for early medical signs of an exposure. It is not practical to memorize an exhaustive list of sentinel occupational health conditions. It is, however, practical and recommended that nurses always ask about occupational conditions and environmental exposures during health histories. A range of occupational health conditions, all of which are preventable and can be treated as sentinel occupational health events are listed by nursing specialty to illustrate the diversity of nurses who may encounter occupational conditions (Table 20.2). Occupational sentinel surveillance systems and occupational specialty clinics are in place in a patchwork of states. Nurses should make every effort to determine what resources are available in their states for reporting and following up workplace health hazards (Table 20.2). OSHA has regulated several of the most hazardous chemicals and workplace hazards. These regulations provide a powerful tool for working with employers to ensure that workplace conditions are safe for returning injured or ill workers (Tables 20.3 and 20.4). This chapter supports the Institute of Medicine's recommendations for nursing practice to incorporate taking a thorough occupational history and advocating for worker patients by utilizing the available public health resources (IOM, 1995).

TABLE 20.3 Selected Sentinel Occupational Illnesses and Injuries

Condition	Selected Occupations and Exposure Notes*	OSHA Standard
Asthma	Health care workers, metal-fluid workers, janitors, some manufacturing settings, wet buildings,	
Back pain/strain	Repetitive motions, awkward postures, heavy lifting (health care workers)	
Cancers/neoplasms	Asbestos workers, PVC	X
Carpal tunnel syndrome	Garment workers, butchers, grocery checkers, electronics assembly workers, typists, musicians, packers, housekeepers/cooks, carpenters	X
Contact and allergic dermatitis, dermatologic/skin disorders	Cutting oils, poison ivy, solvents, latex	
Fibrotic lung diseases (asbestosis, silicosis, coal worker's pneumoconiosis)	Shipyard workers, coal miners, concrete workers, construction workers	X
Hearing loss	High noise manufacturing and construction environments	X
Hepatitis A, B, C	Needlesticks, splashes	X
Human immunovirus (HIV)	Needlesticks, splashes	X
Infertility	Chemical exposures	
Lead poisoning	Construction workers, cable strippers, battery plant workers, secondary lead smelters	X

(continued)

TABLE 20.3 *(continued)*

Legionnaire's disease	Health care workers, problem buildings, water sources	
Mercury poisoning	thermometers, gauges	
Rabies	Animal workers, foresters	
Stress-related conditions	Firefighters, office workers, health care workers, many others	
Tenosynovitis	Repetitive motions	
Traumatic injury from violence	Retail workers, taxi drivers, mental health workers, other health care workers, public safety personnel, case workers, home health nurses	**
Tuberculosis	Health care workers, prison guards	X

* Nurses should not feel limited by this list of occupations. There are many occupations that have not been formally studied in terms of their link between work and disease.
** OSHA has guidelines but no specific standard at this time.

TABLE 20.4 Workplace Exposures for Which There Are Specific Medical Testing Requirements and the Corresponding OSHA standard. (http://www.osha.gov/)

Chemical	*OSHA Standard*
Acrylonitrile	CFR 1910.1045
Arsenic	CFR 1910.1018
Asbestos	CFR 1910.1001 CFR 1926.1101 (Construction) CFR 1915.1001 (Shipyard)
Benzene	CFR 1910.1028
Bloodborne pathogens	CFR 1910.1030
1,3-Butadiene	CFR 1910.1051
Cadmium	CFR 1910.1027
Carcinogens	CFR 1910.1003–1015.1016 1910.1003, 13 Carcinogens (4-Nitrobiphenyl, etc.) 1910.1004, alpha-Naphthylamine 1910.1006, Methyl Chloromethyl Ether 1910.1007, 3,3'-Dichlorobenzidine (and its salts) 1910.1008, bis-Chloromethyl Ether 1910.1009, beta-Naphthylamine

TABLE 20.4 *(continued)*

Coke oven emissions	CFR 1910.1029
Compressed air	CFR. 1926.803
Cotton dust	CFR 1910.1043
1,2,-Dibromo, 3-Chloropropane	CFR 1910.1044
Ethylene oxide	CFR 1910.1047
Formaldehyde	CFR 1910.1048
Hazardous waste Operations/emergency response	CFR 1910.120
Laboratories	CFR 1910.1450 Hazardous Chemical Exposures
Lead	CFR 1910.1025 CFR 1926.62 Lead in Construction
4,4,Methylenedianiline (MDA)	CFR 1910.1050 CFR 1926.60 Construction
Methylene chloride	CFR 1910.1052
Noise/hearing conservation	CFR 1910.95 CFR 1926.52
Respiratory protection	CFR 1910.134 CFR 1926.103
Silica, crystalline	Docket: 79-3185-P (1983)
Tuberculosis	
Vinyl chloride	CFR 1910.1017 CFR 1926.1117 Construction

ACKNOWLEDGMENT

This chapter is dedicated to the memory of James P. Keogh, M.D. (1950–1999) an occupational medicine physician, colleague, friend, and mentor who was a tireless worker advocate. It was the author's privilege to practice nursing in Jim Keogh's clinic, an AOEC clinic where sentinel occupational health events prompted community worksite visits, union and employer outreach, and medical and nursing education. I would also like to acknowledge Dr. Jane Lipscomb and Dr. Barbara Sattler for their support and assistance on this project.

BIBLIOGRAPHY

Association of Occupational and Environmental Clinics. (2001, February 22). *Association of Occupational and Environmental Clinics website*. Available (http://www.aoec.org).

Baker, E. (1989). Sentinel event notification system for occupational risks (SENSOR): The concept. *American Journal of Public Health, 79*(Suppl.), 18–20.

Bureau of Labor Statistics. (1999). *Workplace injuries and illnesses in 1998* (Web Technical Report). U.S. Department of Labor. Available: http://stats.bls.gov/osh-home.htm

Butterfield, P. (1990). Thinking upstream: Nurturing a conceptual understanding of the societal context of health behavior. *Advances in Nursing Science, 12*(2), 1–8.

Centers for Disease Control. (1984). Dermatitis among hospital workers—Oregon. *Morbidity and Mortality Weekly Report, 33*(48), 681–682.

CDC. (1989a). Current trends in occupational disease surveillance: Carpal tunnel syndrome. *Morbidity and Mortality Weekly Report, 38*(28), 485–489.

CDC. (1989b). Epidemiologic notes and reports of acute occupational fatalities in a foundry—Indianna, 1974–1986. *Morbidity and Mortality Weekly Report, 38*(17), 293–297.

CDC. (1990). Occupational disease surveillance: Occupational asthma. *Morbidity and Mortality Weekly Report, 39*(7), 119–123.

Cohen, M., & Kaufman, J. (2000). Latex sensitivity in Washington State acute care hospitals. *AAOHN Journal, 48*(6), 297–303.

Connon, C., Freund, E., & Ehlers, J. (1993). The occupational health nurses in agricultural communities program. *AAOHN Journal, 41*(9), 422–428.

Department of Health and Human Services. (2000). Healthy People 2000 Final Review 382 pp (PHS) 2001-0256. *Healthy People 2000 Progress Charts*. Department of Health and Human Services. Available: http://www.cdc.gov /nchs/about/otheract/hp2000/safety/safetycharts.htm.

Freund, E., Seligman, P., Chorba, T., Safford, S., Drackman, J., & Hull, H. (1990). Mandatory reporting of occupational diseases by clinicians. *Morbidity and Mortality Weekly Report, 39*(RR-9), 19–23.

Herbert, R., London, M., Nagin, D., & Beckett, W. (2000). The diagnosis and treatment of occupational diseases: Integrating clinical practice with prevention. *American Journal of Industrial Medicine, 37*, 1–5.

Herbert, R., Plattus, B., Kellogg, L., Luo, J., Marcus, M., Mascolo, A., & Landrigan, P. (1997). The Union Health Center: A working model of clinical care linked to preventive occupational health services. *American Journal of Industrial Medicine, 31*, 263–273.

Hoffman, R., Wood, R., & Kreiss, K. (1993). Building-related asthma in Denver office workers. *American Journal of Public Health, 83*(1), 89–93.

Institute of Medicine. (1995). *Nursing, health, and the environment*. Washington, DC: National Academy Press.

Jajosky, R. A. R., Harrison, R., Reinisch, F., Flattery, J., Chan, J., Tumpowsky, C., Davis, L., Reilly, M. J., Rosenman, K. D., Kalinowski, D., Stanbury, M., Schill, D., & Wood, J. (1999, June 25). Surveillance of work-related asthma in selected U.S. states using surveillance guidelines for state health departments—California, Massachusettes, Michigan, and New Jersey, 1993–1995. *Morbidity and Mortality Weekly Report, 48*(SS03), 1–20.

Keogh, J., & Gordon, J. (1994). *The doctor never asked me.* Baltimore, MD: University of Maryland School of Medicine Occupational Health Project.

Lalich, N., & Schuster, L. (1987). An application of the sentinel health event (occupational) concept to death certificates. *American Journal of Public Health, 77*(10), 1310–1314.

Lax, M., Keogh, J., Jeffery, N., Henneberger, P., Klitzman, S., Simon, D., & Joyce, J. (1996). Lead poisoning in telephone cable strippers: A new setting for an old problem. *American Journal of Industrial Medicine, 30*, 351–354.

Levy, B., & Wegman, D. (2000). Occupational health—An overview. In B. Levy & D. Wegman (Eds.), *Occupational health recognizing and preventing work-related disease and injury* (4th ed.). Philadelphia: Lippincott Williams & Wilkins.

Muldoon, J., Wintermeyer, L., Eure, J., Fuortes, L., Merchant, J., Van Lier, S., & Richards, R. (1987). Occupational disease surveillance sources, 1985. *American Journal of Public Health, 77*(8), 1006–1008.

Mullan, R. J., & Murthy, L. (1991). Occupational sentinel health events: An up-dated list for physician recognition and public health surveillance. *American Journal of Industrial Medicine, 19*, 775–799.

National Environmental Education Training Foundation (NEETF), Environmental Protection Agency (EPA), U.S. Department of Agriculture (USDA), Department of Health and Human Services (DHHS), Department of Labor (DOL), & Foundation, N. E. E. T. (2000). *Pesticides and national strategies for health care providers—Draft implementation plan* Washington, DC: Environmental Protection Agency.

NIOSH. (2000). *Worker health chart book.* U.S. Department of Health and Human Services, Public Health Service, Centers for Disease Control, NIOSH Pub. No. 2000-17.

Olson, D., Sax, L., Gunderson, P., & Sioris, L. (1991). Pesticide poisoning surveillance through regional poison control centers. *American Journal of Public Health, 81*(6), 750–753.

Randolph, S., & Migliozzi, A. (1993). The role of the agricultural health nurse. *AAOHN Journal, 41*(9), 429–433.

Rosenman, K. D., Reilly, M. J., & Kalinowski, D. (1997). Work-related asthma and respiratory symptoms among workers exposed to metal-working fluids. *American Journal of Industrial Medicine, 32*, 325–331.

Rutstein, D. D., Mullan, R. J., Frazier, T., Halperin, W., Melius, J. M., & Sestito, J. (1983). Sentinel health events (occupational): A basis for physician recognition and public health surveillance. *American Journal of Public Health, 73*, 1054–1062.

Schnitzer, P., & Shannon, J. (1999). Development of a surveillance program for occupational pesticide poisoning: Lessons learned and future directions. *Public Health Reports, 114*(May/June), 242–248.

Welch, L. (1989). The role of occupational health clinics in surveillance of occupational disease. *American Journal of Public Health, 79*(Suppl.), 58–60.

Weltermann, B., Hodgson, M., Storey, E., DeGraff, A., Bracker, A., Groseclose, S., Cole, S., Cartter, M., & Phillips, D. (1998). Hypersenstivity pneumonitis: A sentinel event investigation in a wet building. *American Journal of Industrial Medicine, 34*, 499–505.

Woolf, A., & Flynn, E. (2000). Workplace toxic exposures involving adolescents aged 14–19 years: One poison center's experience. *Archives Pediatrics Adolescent Medicine, 154*(March), 234–239.

CHAPTER 21

Environmental Health Risks in Schools

Erin Balka, Marian Condon, Tonya McKee, and Barbara Sattler

There have been two gentle shifts in our environmental concerns. The first has been from a strictly ecological focus, where concerns centered on man's negative effects on the natural world to interest and concern about the risks posed to human health by our environment. Even more focused is our interest in children's health. The second shift has been to be more attentive to the environmental risks associated with the "built" environment: our homes, office buildings, and schools. This shift has helped to raise awareness about indoor air quality, the existence of and manner by which we control pests (including insects, molds, fungus/mildew, and rodents), and the health risks associated with the products that we use to construct buildings and that we bring into our homes, schools, and offices.

Increasingly, concerns are being raised about school buildings, the built environment that one sixth of the U.S. population can be found in, Monday through Friday, during the school year. Our concerns are further heightened because the majority of people found in school buildings are children, who have distinct vulnerabilities to environmental health risks. This chapter reviews basic concepts about the built environment and provides information and directions for nurses to assist them in their efforts to advocate for healthy and safe indoor air quality.

While the quality of outdoor air can pose health problems, indoor air can be even more troublesome. According to the EPA, indoor levels of pollutants may be 2 to 5 times higher than outdoor air. Furthermore, children are six times more vulnerable to indoor air contaminants than adults are due to faster respiration rates and lower body weights (CEHN, 2000). Poor indoor air quality (IAQ) can aggravate existing health conditions such as asthma and allergies, as well as induce symptoms in sensitive populations such as persons experiencing chemical sensitivity.

Nurses are unique in that they are often the only health care providers in the school setting. School nurses are aware of the health status of the students and those with particular vulnerabilities. This knowledge and awareness places school nurses in a special position to make a link between health effects experienced by the school population and the environmental conditions within the school. This chapter provides information about environmental health risks in schools and how to advocate for the health of all those in the school community.

Perhaps the most sensitive of school building inhabitants are asthmatic children. Asthma is a growing problem, according to the American Lung Association (ALA), which estimates that 17 million Americans suffer from asthma, with 5.3 million of these under the age of 18. The ALA also reports that (1) the prevalence rate for pediatric asthma rose from 40.1 to 74.9 per thousand persons between 1982 and 1995, (2) asthma is the number one ranking cause of hospitalizations among children under the age of 15, and (3) children with asthma average 7.6 days absence over a 12-month period, compared with 2.5 days for children without asthma. Minority groups are affected disproportionately, with death rates for blacks higher than for whites.

A survey of 600 school nurses in California and Colorado obtained information about the impact that asthma and allergies had on their students (Shering Plough, 1999). According to these nurse respondents, asthma and allergies caused 52.6% of asthmatics and 22.8% of children with allergies to miss school; adverse academic performance in 33.3% of asthmatics and 21% of those with allergies; disruptive classroom and other behavioral problems in 8.6% of asthmatics and 7.4% of allergic children; and symptoms of drowsiness or hyperactivity from taking medications

Poor indoor air quality can generate a constellation of symptoms known as Sick Building Syndrome (SBS), which manifests as an array of multisystem symptoms that usually go away when the individual leaves the building environment that is causing the condition. The symptoms are vague and generalized and may include eye irritation, dry throat, sinus congestion, dizziness, headache, fatigue, difficulty in wearing contact lenses, chest tightness, sneezing, nausea, dizziness, and dermatitis. Problems that may cause SBS include damaged roofs that create moisture problems that, in turn, promote mold growth, malfunctioning ventilation systems, and chemical emissions from a wide array of sources in the school building.

In September of 1992, school children and faculty were exposed to highly toxic volatile organic compounds (VOCs) during a renovation project at the Jefferson Middle School in Jamestown, New York. New carpeting was installed throughout the school using two adhesives: contact cement containing dichloromethane, and a glue containing mineral spirits. A week later, administrators began to receive complaints from students and staff. Symptoms such as headaches, dizziness, muscle fatigue, eye irritation, sinus problems, and difficulty breathing were reported. A teacher collapsed at school and was later diagnosed with peripheral nerve damage. Six other staff members also became ill and could not return to work. In late October of 1992, the school was closed due to severe indoor air quality problems and insufficient air supply. The school reopened at the end of October, but closed again in early November due to continuing health complaints ("Guide To School Renovation and Construction: What You Need to Know to Protect Child and Adult Environmental Health." Healthy Schools Network, 2000.).

While renovation and new construction are welcome, these projects can damage the health of children and school staff by creating the potential for a rise in environmental risks such as exposure to noise, dust, mold, asbestos and lead. New products brought into the school often emit toxic gases (Healthy Schools Network, (4). When schools undergo renovations, a variety of health complaints may occur including headache, dizziness, sinusitis, irritated eyes, itchy skin, allergies, shortness of breath, hoarseness, dry nose and throat, and upper respiratory infections. These complaints can be associated with a number of chemicals introduced during the renovations, possibly mixing with chemicals already present in the school, and/or an inadequate ventilation system.

Construction materials and new products can also be sources of pollutants. Many of these products contain volatile constituents, such as resins, solvents, and binders that emit volatile organic compounds (VOCs) for a period of time. VOCs can cause irritation to the nose, eyes, and throat, as well as coughing, skin rashes, fatigue, and allergic reactions. Extensive exposure to VOCs can cause damage to the liver, kidneys, and central nervous system.

INDICATIONS OF LEARNING AND DEVELOPMENTAL TRENDS

A growing number of children are being diagnosed with learning and behavioral disabilities.

- "It is estimated that nearly 12 million children (17%) in the United States under age 18 suffer from one or more developmental disabilities (defined as deafness, blindness, epilepsy, stuttering or other speech defects, cerebral palsy, delay in growth and development, emotional or behavioral problems, learning disabilities)."
- "Attention deficit hyperactivity disorder (ADHD), according to conservative estimates, affects 3 to 6% of all school children, though recent evidence suggests the prevalence may be as high as 17%."
- "The number of children in special education programs classified with learning disabilities increased 191% from 1977–1994."
- "The incidence of autism may be as high as 2 per 1000 children. One study of autism prevalence between 1966 and 1997 showed a doubling of rates over that time" (Schettler, Stein, Reich, and Valenti, 2000).

There are many variables that can contribute to learning and behavioral disorders; however, among them is an association with poor indoor air quality and verbal, perceptual, motor, and behavioral disorders in children.

Developmental disorders add additional stress to the resources of communities, families, and schools. Afflicted children risk early school dropout, teen parenting, drug abuse, crime, institutionalization, and suicide (Schettler et al., 2000). Although these disabilities are clearly the result of complex interactions among genetic, environmental, and social factors that have significant impacts on children during vulnerable periods of development, chemical exposures may contribute significantly to the epidemic of developmental disabilities. Experimental prenatal exposures in animals to dioxin, mercury, and lead have all resulted in increased risk of neurobehavioral problems. Human epidemiological studies have shown the association between learning problems, language skill development, and greater propensity to violent behavior when children are exposed to lead. (Sattler et al., 2000)

THE STATE OF U.S. SCHOOLS

In a recent federal report to Congress entitled "Condition of America's Schools " the Government Accounting Office found that "while laws com-pel children to attend school, some school buildings may be unsafe or even harmful to children's health" (GAO, 1995)   School buildings are aging, and overcrowding puts pressure on small classrooms not designed for today's growing student population. Storage room decreases as students begin to occupy areas not designated as classrooms.   Nearly 60% of schools surveyed by the GAO self-reported at least one unsatisfactory environmental condition.   Many of these conditions are associated with health risks for the school occupants.

Putting off renovations can have a domino effect that leads to further damage and higher repair costs; for example, roofing that is not maintained develops leaks and causes damage to interior walls. Moisture problems are the primary cause of paint failure.   In older schools, damaged lead-based paint may be a concern.   However, it is not always the older buildings that are in poor condition; modern buildings built after 1970 were often constructed cheaply and quickly.   These buildings were designed to have life spans of only 20 or 30 years.   They have now exceeded their predicted life spans and are often experiencing system failures.

In addition, the energy crisis of the 1970s is believed to have increased exposures to indoor pollutants.   Buildings were made to be tighter and better insulated in order to conserve energy and fuel costs.   Computerized controls were introduced in order to reduce energy use after hours, resulting in fewer air exchanges in the building in the evening when the cleaning activities typically occur. Just as uncontrolled industrial processes can foul the air outside, many of industry's products, important as many of them are, can contribute to air pollution in our homes, office buildings, and schools. This pollution can be trapped indoors. In the past, our need to save energy resulted in weatherizing our buildings. This process included adding storm windows, and weather stripping and sealing cracks. We have not always thought about the effect this can have on indoor air quality. As a result, researchers have found air pollution can be greater inside than outside (American Lung Association, 1993).

POLICY

Currently, there are no standards for indoor air established specifically for children in schools.   Human exposure guidelines for a number of indoor air pollutants have been established in regulations or recommended by various governmental agencies and professional organizations.   The Occupational Safety and Health Act has Permissible Exposure Limits (PELS) for nearly 500 hazardous chemicals.   However, these limits are for chemicals found in industrial settings and are based on research sometimes dating back to the 1950s and 1960s that has never been updated. The American Society of Heating, Refrigeration and Air-Conditioning Engineers (ASHRAE), identifies acceptable ventilation rates and indoor temperature conditions. However, these voluntary, nongovernmental standards may not be sufficient for the diverse conditions and populations found in schools.

The heating, ventilation, and air conditioning (HVAC) system maintains positive pressure, influencing the transfer of moisture from outside to inside the building. Outdoor contaminants such as pesticides, exhaust emissions, or fumes from rotting debris can be drawn into air intake grilles. If air movement is impeded and areas start to experience high humidity or moisture problems, microbial contaminants such as mold and mildew, along with viruses, begin to thrive. This may affect children with underlying diseases such as asthma or bronchitis.

> During August of 1998, and well into student orientation for the school year, a new polyurethane resin gym floor was installed in the Milton Terrace Primary School in Ballston Spa, New York. Volatile organic chemicals, including toluene, thylbenzene, xylenes, methyl ethyl ketone, and methyl isobutyl ketone were being poured during kindergarten orientation. As much as 30,000 pounds of chemicals were used. Children and staff complained of bad odors and a range of health problems. After teachers and parents joined together to protest at a school board meeting, the gym was closed. Health experts say that while the "off-gassing" decreases over time, it will never reach zero, and could take years to reach undetectable levels. The district has decided to remove and replace the gym floor.
> ("Guide To School Renovation and Construction: What You Need to Know to Protect Child and Adult Environmental Health." Healthy Schools Network, Inc. 2000.)

The selection of environmentally preferable cleaning and maintenance agents can have a significant effect on human health. Cleaning and maintenance products that add to the pollution load are not necessary; further, they contribute to a school's overall risk management problem. The use of less toxic products in schools helps to protect the children in our schools and decreases the manufacture and ultimate disposal of more than products.

Children are exposed to toxic chemicals in school cleaning and maintenance products in a variety of ways:

- When products are freshly applied or inappropriately applied in the presence of children
- If products are mixed improperly (some common cleaning products, when mixed together can give off deadly gas, such as ammonia and chlorine products)
- When products are used without diluting them according to directions
- If toxic products are stored in an unventilated hall closet
- When products leave a heavy residue

If janitorial workers are not sufficiently trained about the products they use, problems can arise. Language and literacy issues may hinder effective reading of labels with regard to sufficient diluting of industrial strength cleaners and/or other misunderstandings about directions that are necessary for the safe and healthy use of products. Improper dilution and unsafe work practices have been known to cause health problems for the janitorial staff when breathing the undiluted toxic chemicals. Organic solvents, used in some cleaning and maintenance agents, are a major concern for poisoning. Exposure to solvents can affect the central nervous system. It can result in disorientation, euphoria, giddiness, and confusion, progressing to unconsciousness, paralysis, convulsion, and death from respiratory or cardiac arrest.

Chemicals used in arts and crafts supplies and biological and chemical agents used for laboratory sciences may be toxic. Paints, glues, and other art, science, and vocational supplies may contain chemicals that can be toxic to children. Industrial arts courses can expose children to metal dusts, fumes, and wood dust. Chemicals such as acetic acid, aminophenol, ammonia, hydrochloric acid, and so on, are found in photo labs and may be a problem if there is not sufficient ventilation and safety equipment. Kiln firing can release clay dust, which can contain silica (known to cause fibrosis), toxic gases such as carbon monoxide, and heavy metals from the glazes. Home economics and theater exposures may include fabric dyes, oven cleaners, cosmetics, hairsprays, and fog and smoke effects generated from machines using glycols and mineral oil. Copy machines produce ozone, which has been linked to lung problems and should be run only in well-ventilated rooms.

Environmental hazards in our nation's schools are an increasing concern. Pervasive substances such as mercury, lead, PCBs, and pesticides are toxic to the developing child's brain. Rubber cement, permanent felt tip markers, pottery glazes, enamels, spray fixatives, and other potentially hazardous materials are sold for use in schools despite the fact that there are often animal and human studies demonstrating their toxicity. Involvement in product selection for use in our schools is of critical importance.

SCHOOL-WIDE ACTION STEPS FOR SCHOOLS

These are some affirmative steps to make your school safer and healthier.

1. Find out who is in charge of the school environment and who makes purchasing decisions for your school or district.
2. Contact the Environmental Protection Agency. Indoor Air Quality / Tools for Schools Program.
3. Contact the state or local health department, department of environmental quality, or department of education to determine their ability to provide technical assistance.
4. Contact the Healthy Schools Network, Inc. Their publications include guides on air quality, lead, pesticides, nontoxic custodial products, health and safety committees, and many other relevant topics.

CREATING AN ENVIRONMENTALLY HEALTHY AND SAFE "HEALTH SUITE"

All school nurses are busy people, so tackling the environmental health status of the whole school may seem like a daunting task. Perhaps starting with your own area, the nurse's office or health suite will feel like a more manageable place to start. There are some really simple things to start with, what some might call the low-hanging fruit.

Do You Use Mercury Thermometers? Eliminate Them.

Mercury thermometers should be replaced with non-mercury-containing thermometers. If and when a thermometer breaks and the mercury spills, it creates a toxic mercury exposure for a long time after the event. When disposing of the mercury-containing thermometers, make sure that they are disposed of in a safe manner. They are considered a hazardous substance. Call the person responsible for hazardous materials waste manager at your facility or in your city or county.

Do You Use Latex Gloves? Eliminate Them.

Because of the ubiquitous use of latex gloves in health care, the food preparation industry, and other places, there has been increased public exposure to latex and an increasing development of latex allergies. The mild symptoms include eye and nose irritation, but severe symptoms, including anaphylactic shock, have been experienced. Therefore the elimination of latex is recommended, replacing the gloves with nitrile or another non-latex-containing substance.

Does Your School Have a Pest Control Plan That Includes Regular Spraying of Pesticides in or Around the Nurse's Office? Initiate Healthy and Intelligent Pest Management.

If pesticides are regularly and widely applied in the school, this may be an opportunity to decrease unnecessary pesticide exposures, starting with the nurse's office. Speak with the people in charge of pest control (janitorial staff, contracted pest management company) and ask them about the pests of concern in your school and their pesticide application practices. Request that they not routinely spray in your area. (See chapter 17 for more information on pesticides.)

Are There Moisture Problems in Your Office? Make a Request to Have Them Addressed.

Check to see if there are leaks under the sink, leaky faucets, discolored ceiling tiles, or other signs of moisture problems and ask the facililtes manager/janitor to fix the problem. Moisture can promote mold and other microbial growth. Cockroaches and other pests require a source of water in order to exist.

Is Your Office Adequately Ventilated? Is There Room for Improvement?

Is there a fresh air vent in the health suite? Check to make sure that the air vents are not blocked or covered. Ask where the fresh air intake vents are. Are they near the area where buses are likely to idle? Are they on the ground, where herbicide or pesticide spraying may cause contamination of the fresh air as it enters the fresh air vents.

Do You Have Access to Natural Lighting?

If you do have access to natural lighting, it will enhance productivity, mood, and learning. If you do not have access, you can purchase full-spectrum lighting that can provide some of the same benefits as a natural light source.

STEPS THAT CAN BE TAKEN TO REMOVE ENVIRONMENTAL

HEALTH RISKS FROM INDOOR ENVIRONMENTS

1. Clean or replace contaminated heating, ventilation, and air-conditioning system components, including ducts and filters. By doing this, you will decrease asthma and allergy triggers. In addition, there will be decreased exposure to biological contaminants that may increase the risk for upper respiratory infections.
2. Remove water-damaged ceiling tiles, carpet, and other building materials. Control moisture. When shampooing carpets, avoid overwetting, allow sufficient time for thorough drying, and provide extra ventilation in areas with high humidity. This will decrease the exposure to molds, mildew, and other biological contaminants that can trigger asthma, allergies, and respiratory infections.
3. Prohibit smoking indoors.   This will reduce the risk of primary and secondary exposures and their resultant respiratory effects, ear infections, and other illnesses associated with environmental tobacco smoke exposure.
4. Use and store paints, adhesives, and solvents in well-ventilated areas. Purchase these items in small quantities to avoid storage exposure. Eliminate or limit the use of toxic and harmful chemicals by considering the selection of non-solvent-based materials and other less toxic products. Most paints, adhesives, and solvents release harmful chemicals (volatile organic contaminants) that may be neurotoxic, hepatotoxic, and carcinogenic.
5. Test for radon and remediate as appropriate. Chronic long-term exposure to radon places individuals at risk of cancer.
6. Encapsulate or remove asbestos (per AHERA). Exposure to asbestos places students and staff at risk of asbestos-related diseases such as cancer and asbestosis.
7. Maintain painted surfaces. Have buildings inspected for possible lead-based paint. (In the U.S., an estimated 52 million homes have some lead based paint.) Test soil for lead and, if necessary, limit indoor

exposure by using walk-off mats at doors and covering contaminated soil mulch or plantings. In older buildings, paint may be lead based. Ensuring intact lead-based paint decreases the risk of lead poisoning.

8. In school and office buildings, run HVAC systems whenever the school building is occupied. Begin operation at least one to two hours before the school is reopened to flush out accumulated pollutants. This will improve the air quality by maximizing the air exchange.

9. Control dust and dirt with damp mops or vacuum cleaners that have high efficiency particle air (HEPA) filters. Isolate building occupants from dust or fumes generated during renovation work. Use plastic sheeting, portable fans, and mechanical ventilation systems to prevent dust and fumes from reaching building occupants through hallways, doors, windows, and the HVAC system. This will reduce asthma and allergy triggers.

10. Control pest infestations through good housekeeping and repair, and limit the use of pesticides. Implement integrated pest management (IPM) by identifying pests; establishing regular inspections for pests; determining health and aesthetic tolerances to pest populations; preventing pest problems through sanitation, physical barriers, and environmental modifications; and selecting the least hazardous pesticides for targeted area only when nonchemical measures have failed. This will decrease asthma triggers and reduce the necessity for pest management.

TIPS TO IMPROVE AIR QUALITY THROUGH NON-TOXIC CLEANING

1. Read the label. Look for household cleaning products that contain non-petroleum-based surfactants, that are chlorine and phosphate free, and that are biodegradable. These products clean as effectively as their petrochemical counterparts, but do not pollute your home/school in the process. Avoid topical biocidal solutions. Avoid products containing urea-formaldehyde. Purchase in small quantities items that can leak pollutants into the air, such as paints, adhesives, solvents, and pesticides in order to avoid storage exposure. Use and store in well-ventilated areas. Use low-emission cleaning products and avoid purchasing products with strong odors.

2. When choosing maintenance products such as interior paint, use water-based latex paints that contain no solvents. Avoid solvents for thinning and cleanup; have low or zero volatile organic compounds that contain

no heavy metals or other ingredients that are harmful to human health or the environment.

3. Buy only non-chlorine-bleached paper products. Traditional paper products like bath tissue and paper towels are commonly bleached with chlorine. The process of chlorine bleaching releases dioxin into the atmosphere. Recent research has revealed conclusive links between dioxin and cancer, reproductive disorders among adults, deformities and developmental problems in children and immune system breakdowns. Look for paper products labeled "non-chlorine bleached" and buy recycled paper products.

4. Do not buy products containing chlorine. Found in a host of scouring powders, laundry bleach, dishwasher detergent, and basin, tub and tile cleansers, these chemicals are a potential cause of health problems.

5. Especially read the label for toilet bowl cleaner, oven cleaner, or furniture polish because they are very likely to contain potentially toxic chemicals, such as strong acids or alkalis, which are associated with damage to skin, eyes, and lungs. Such products, when in liquid form, may also contain petroleum distillates that can acutely affect lung tissue.

6. Use plain soap and water for cleaning agents whenever possible. Remove dust with vacuum cleaners and/or damp cloths. Do not use feather dusters or spray dust collectors. Cleaning solvents are an important source of volatile organic compounds. Select materials that can be cleaned with soap and water.

7. Avoid aerosols, including air fresheners, as they are common respiratory irritants. Air fresheners can be a problem for chemically sensitive people.

(Healthy Schools Network, Inc. Healthier Cleaning and Maintenance: Practices and Products for schools.)

FRAGRANCES

Fragrances are another contributor to the indoor chemical mix. Consumers' fascination with scent has increased with the manufacture of multitudes of scented personal products including cosmetics, lotions, soaps, oils, and perfumes. There are more than 1,000 body fragrances (Fisher, 1998). In addition, fragrances are now added to a range of cleaning products to tissues and from candles to diapers. The term "fragrance" on a label is often representative of a complex mixture of chemicals that commonly includes acetone, benzaldehyde, benzy alcohol, camphor, 1,8-cineole, ethanol, ethyl acetate, limonene, methylene chloride, and alpha-pinene, all of which are associate with a lengthy list of potential signs and symptoms. Choosing fragrance-free products can decrease the unnecessary load of potentially hazardous chemicals in indoor air. There is a growing subpopulation with multiple chemical sensitivity who may experience symptoms when exposed to chemical fragrances.

Multiple Chemical Sensitivity (MCS) is described as a syndrome "characterized by multisystem response to low-level chemical exposures commonly encountered in the ambient environment, that often follows exposures incurred in association with indoor air quality" (Oliver, 1998, p. 401). Symptoms are similar to those seen in SBS, but are of a more chronic nature, and in children they can include hyperactivity and attention deficit. The causal factors are thought to be chemical air pollutants.

In 1993, the Environmental Protection Agency established an Environmentally Preferable Purchasing program to assist federal agencies in considering environment (along with price and performance) when making their purchasing decisions. This program has been establishing guidelines for cleaning products, computer reuse, nontoxic paints, adhesives, and many other products. Some states have established programs to set guidelines and companies that have invested in environmental product development have seen their profits rise handsomely in response to these initiatives (Environmental Health Perspectives, 1999). Nurses can encourage their school districts to develop purchasing protocols for healthier products by following the guidance set by the EPA's program.

For additional information, refer to the general resources section (Appendix) for a list of products, vendors, organizations, agencies, how-to guides, and information on purchasing environmentally preferable products in your school.

ENVIRONMENTAL HEALTH AND SAFETY COMMITTEES

Nurses who work in school settings and nurses who are parents of children in school settings can play a significant role in affecting the environmental quality of the schools. Because there is no single person who can make a school environmentally healthy and safe, a good place to start is with a committee whose members may each play a role in improving the school's environment. In many workplaces, health and safety committees provide the structure in which to address the conditions that may pose risks. Because schools are workplaces for adults and learning places for children, creating an environmental health and safety committee can provide a forum in which a multidisciplinary team can learn about health and safety issues, develop and exercise assessment capabilities, prioritize concerns and issues, develop an intervention plan, and provide a feedback loop regarding the success of the remediation and other intervention activities. A health and safety committee can also propose policies. Some of the people who should be considered for a school health and safety committee are teachers, principals, parents, custodial staff, facilities managers, a school board representative, and even a student.

There are some quick fixes that can be accomplished for some problems. But many environmental health risks have existed in schools for years; identifying and reducing such risks may also take years. Some risks are quite complex and will require changes in purchasing practices, rehab and renovation specifications, and upgrades of ventilation systems. The best way to address any of the problems will be from an informed position and with the support of others in your educational setting. Health and safety committees can provide a win–win platform for creating environmentally healthy schools that will be safe workplaces and healthy learning places.

The nature of most environmental problems demands a multidisciplinary approach. In the school setting, nurses are singularly focused on the health and safety of the children and staff. Given this focus, they are uniquely positioned to help convene a committee to assess and address occupational and environmental health and safety risks that may exist in schools.

The first task in establishing a committee is determining who has responsibility for and authority over health and safety issues. This may be more than one person and may include the principal, facilities manager, and/or superintendent. Next, determine who has a vested interest in health and safety among the teachers and other school staff and parents. If the teachers and staff (including the school nurses) are represented by a union or professional association, they may have health and safety language articulated in their collective bargaining contract. If such contract language exists, it may provide a framework for the development of a health and safety committee. The Parent–Teachers Association should be formally represented on the committee in order to facilitate communication. Setting the tone of the committee will be very important, establishing trust and a sense of common ground will promote the committee's success.

At the first meeting, the committee as a whole should establish the operating principles: who will lead the meeting (one person, rotating people); how often will they meet (e.g., same time each month); who will record minutes and how will they be distributed (mail, email); how often will the committee do "walk-through" assessments; if a problem is identified, who will be responsible for addressing the problem; how will the committee's activities and findings be communicated to the affected community (parents, teachers, and staff). The committee may want to invite experts from the community to come in and talk with them about such health and safety issues as indoor air quality, pest management, and preventive building maintenance.

The committee may find a checklist helpful when they do their first walk-through of the school. There are several available. Included in the resource section is a checklist that was established by a parent group in Howard County, Maryland, with input from the school's facilities manager. Once the initial walk-through has been completed, a list of all of the concerns and observations should be developed. The committee can then rank the problems in priority order. Sometimes simple fixes should be on the top of the list so that they can be addressed immediately. The committee should then develop a plan of action for addressing the most pressing problems, recognizing once again that not all problems will be easily and quickly remediated. The next time the committee meets, the list should be reviewed to determine and discuss progress.

There are wonderful additional resources that can provide significantly more depth and directions on particular issues. For example, the Health and Safety Department of the American Federation of Teachers has created excellent materials on all aspects of health and safety concerns in schools, as well as information about setting up a health and safety committee. The Healthy Schools Coalition also has superb materials, including a very good website.

The "built environment" is the focus of increasing health-related concerns. Nurses in various settings can help educate and guide building occupants about the health risks associated with poor indoor air quality and the steps that can be taken to reduce the risks. Although some of the issues may be new, nurses are prepared with the requisite skills to provide education, do assessments, and develop intervention strategies and risk communication programs. With these skills, nurses can provide needed leadership to improve the environment in schools.

REFERENCES AND BIBLIOGRAPHY

Brooks, D., et al. (1995). *Indoor Air Quality: A Guide for Educators.* School Facilities Planning Division, California Department of Education. Sacramento, CA.

Children's Environmental Health Network. (2000). *Training manual on pediatric environmental health: Putting it into practice.* Children's Environmental Health Network. Available at: www.cehn.org

Daisey, J. M., & Angell, W. J. (1998). *A Survey and Critical Review of the Literature on Indoor Air Quality, Ventilation and Health Symptoms in Schools.* Indoor Environment Program, Energy & Environment Program, Energy & Environment Division, Lawrence Berkeley National Laboratory, Berkeley CA.

Environmental Health Perspectives. (1999). Environews forum. *Environmental Health Perspectives, 107,* 188–190.

Environmental Protection Agency website: www.epa.gov/children

Fisher, B. E. (1998). Scents and sensitivity. *Environmental Health Perspectives, 106*(12), 594–599.

Healthy Schools Network, Inc. (2000). *Guide to school renovation and construction: What you need to know to protect child and adult environmental health.* Albany, NY. HSN is the organization that published the guide. No author was attributed.

The Healthy School Environmental Action Guide. 1999.

Indoor Air Quality. The Little Institute for School Facilities Research.

Institute of Medicine. (2000). *Clearing the Air: Asthma and Indoor Air Exposures*, National Academy Press (Available through; National Academy Press,2101 Constitution Ave., N.W., Box 285, Washington, DC 20055, or call 1-800-624-6242 or visit National Academy Press' on-line bookstore at www.nap.edu).

McNeel, S. V., & Kreutzer, R. A. (1996). Fungi & Indoor Air Quality. *Health & Environment Digest, 10*(2), 9–12.

Salerno, M., Huss, K., & Huss, R. (1992). *Allergen Avoidance in the Treatment of Dust-mite Allergy and Asthma.* Nurse Practitioner, October.

Schettler, T., Stein, J., Reich, F., & Valenti, M. (2000). *In harm's way: Toxic threats to child development.* Greater Boston Physicians for Social Responsibility. Boston, MA.

U.S. Environmental Protection Agency. (1991) *Building Air Quality; A Guide for Building Owners and Facility Managers*, EPA Indoor Air Division

Woolums, J. (2000). *Managing Indoor Air Quality in Schools.* National Clearinghouse for Educational Facilties, May.

CHAPTER 22

Cross-Cultural Issues on the Mexican–U.S. Border

Maria Alvarez Amaya

Nursing practice settings often provide unparalleled opportunities for addressing environmental health hazards and health effects. The nursing capacity to integrate cultural concepts enhances environmental risk assessment and risk management. Yet, the importance of cultural competence in environmental health nursing is often undervalued. Cultural competence is paramount to understanding the dynamic interrelationships among environmental exposures, health beliefs, behavior, and health.

In the twenty-first century, geographic boundaries no longer define the cultural group contained within. According to Sohier (1995) Third World (new wave) immigration has created a situation in which nurses commonly do not speak the languages of their clients or understand their communication within a cultural context. Most nurses are members of nonminority U.S. cultures, yet the cultural mix in any given community affected by environmental health problems will be diverse.

Cultural groups share common values and beliefs about family, community, and environment that influence their perceptions of environmental health problems. These values and beliefs are often intergenerationally, and people tend to hold tenaciously to their views. Nursing interventions must be culturally relevant to maximize the attainment of desired outcomes.

Newly arrived groups tend to cluster in ethnic communities both by choice and necessity. Poverty, low educational attainment, and language barriers contribute to social isolation. Nurses typically encounter clients and families meeting basic survival needs, such as shelter, food, and basic health care. Confronted by environmental health issues, they may be unable or unwilling to perceive the threat in the same way as the nurse. This can be a source of frustration and a barrier to achieving desired outcomes.

Many immigrants come from countries with moral or philosophical beliefs about the environment that do not match the mainstream U.S. perception and mores, and that reflect differences between developed and developing regions. The mainstream (nonminority) U.S. culture with its affluent and highly educated populace contrasts sharply with the culture of poorly educated indigent immigrants. The less acculturated minorities are often most affected by environmental health problems while the more acculturated minorities hold beliefs and attitudes about the environment more like these of the mainstream group. Thus, values may be modified or changed by the process of acculturation. Nurses need to understand the acculturation process as it relates to changes in cultural values.

Cultural assessment data provide an invaluable tool for tailoring environmental health nursing interventions. It encompasses careful assessment of socioeconomic and religious factors, in addition to level of acculturation. Lassiter and Mitchem-Davis (1999) emphasize the importance of collecting data relating to regional social and cultural influences to facilitate health promotion initiatives for environmental health.

HISPANIC/LATINO CULTURE

The label "Hispanic" was given by the U.S. Bureau of Census to a diverse group of people who reside in the U.S. and who were born in or trace the background of their families to one of the Spanish-speaking Latin American nations or to Spain (Marin and Marin, 1991). Subgroups included are Mexican (65%), Puerto Rican (10%), Cuban (4%), Central and South American (14%) and other Hispanic (Spanish/Mexican/Native American) (7%) (U.S. Bureau of Census, 1999). Nearly half of all Hispanics living in the U.S. in 1999 were foreign-born (45%).

Regardless of subgroup, members share some common basic values that identify them as a cultural group. Marin and Marin (1991, pp. 11–17) summarized the cultural characteristics of Hispanics. The degree to which these characteristics may be expressed is determined by the level of acculturation.

1. Collectivism (allocentrism) is a prevailing regard for the well-being of the larger group. If personal objectives, attitudes, and values do not resemble those of the larger group, the expectation is that they should be relegated to secondary status. Hispanic groups tend to value smooth interpersonal relationships. Interpersonal conflict may be avoided by

several strategies, including acquiescence and agreeability. This characteristic contrasts sharply with individualistic, competitive, achievement-oriented cultures of nonminority U.S. groups.

2. *Familísmo* is a strong identification with and attachment to the nuclear and extended family. Individuals manifest a sense of obligation to the family as well as reliance on the family group for sustenance and approval.

3. *Respeto* means being respectful of others, particularly in interpersonal encounters. Every individual should feel that his or her personal power, whatever it may be, is acknowledged. This allows an elder who does not speak English and is undocumented to hold on to authority in a family unit that includes English-speaking legal residents and citizens. The practice of asking a younger English-speaking relative to translate for an elder is not recommended because it diminishes respect.

4. *Personalísmo* refers to the closeness permissible between two or more individuals during an interpersonal encounter. The amount of physical space considered appropriate between two interacting individuals is shorter than in non-Hispanic whites. The longer personal distance acceptable in the mainstream nonminority culture may seem cold and impersonal.

Emphasis should be given to how environmental health issues affect family structure and unity within the community. In many Hispanic families, the husband is the decision maker, but the extended family may also play a major role in decision making. Therefore, perception of gender roles should be part of the inventory.

ENVIRONMENTAL HEALTH AND CULTURE ON THE TEXAS-MEXICO BORDER

Centuries of interaction along the U.S.-Mexico border have resulted in a hybrid culture that is uniquely different than that found in the interior regions of either country. The Rio Grande (known as the Rio Bravo in Mexico) forms the 1,254-mile long international line dividing Texas and Mexico. Environmental health problems seen in this region may resemble those seen in developing countries. For example, the worst radioactive contamination in North American history occurred in Ciudad Juarez in 1983, just across the border from El Paso. Measured in terms of the total number of people exposed, the Juarez incident fell somewhere between the partial meltdown at Pennsylvania's Three Mile Island reactor in 1979 and the 1986 accident at Chernobyl (Sharp, 1998). Thousands were exposed to low-level radiation over an extended period when a hospital handyman hauled away a Picker 3000 radiotherapy machine.

Environmental health problems frequently occur in a milieu of political turmoil despite various national, state, and local agreements. Cultural issues are often at the forefront of misunderstandings and allegations. For example, information about environmental health risks often originates from the U.S. side of the border with proposed solutions often one-sided. Because environmental health problems do not respect international borders, nurses addressing environmental health concerns on the border often must work in binational, multicultural settings.

The following is a brief synopsis of current and emerging environmental health problems on the Texas-Mexico border. Nursing practice on the U.S.-Mexico border invariably brings one into contact with all or some of these problems at some point.

1. The agricultural areas along the Texas-Mexico border have significant problems with the use of pesticides, many of which are banned in the United States but are still used in Mexico.
2. Childhood lead exposure is an endemic problem on the Texas-Mexico border. A significant proportion of children along the Texas-Mexico border live in poverty and substandard conditions that predispose to lead exposure. These children are also exposed to lead from consumer products contaminated by lead-based ink used in the packaging labels on some foods and candy. Lead-based ink may also be found in children's erasers. Other consumer products, such as ceramic cookware, also pose a problem. Other consumer products have been identified as environmental hazards.
3. Herbal and mineral folk remedies may pose environmental health risks. For example, Greta is a powdered folk medicine used to treat colic and upset stomach that may contain as much as 80% lead oxide, a highly soluble form of lead. This is one of several cultural preferences that influence environmental health risks on the border.
4. Hazardous waste transport presents a risk that has precipitated a great deal of binational planning. *Maquiladora* (twin plant) agreements require that hazardous waste produced in Mexico by American-owned business be transported back to the U.S. for disposal. Each day finds trucks at the border crossings transferring hazardous materials from a Mexican truck to a U.S. truck, in full view of and proximity to the lines of cars waiting to cross the border. In particular, hydrofluoric acid transport is

an environmental disaster waiting to happen.

5. Significant environmental problems have occurred with illegal dumping in the vast desert regions of the border. Major problems emanate from improper disposal of batteries, oil, and construction materials. Illegal industrial hazardous waste dumping is not a rare occurrence.

6. Air pollution is caused by industrial sources in both Texas and Mexico. In addition, automobiles (particularly cars that use leaded gasoline), dust from unpaved roads, brickmakers burning tires for fuel, and coal-fired electricity plants contribute to high levels of particulate matter in the air.

7. The Rio Grande has been designated one of the most polluted rivers in the U.S. High levels of fecal coliform bacteria, pesticides, and salinity have been documented. One major source of pollution is untreated sewage waste from Mexico.

8. *Colonias* (unplanned developments) are manifestations of housing needs of a rapidly growing population in extreme poverty. Over 1,500 of them pepper the U.S. side of the border, and at least that many exist on the Mexico side. Myriad actual and potential environmental health problems exist in these neighborhoods (Sharp, 1998).

INTERVENTION: PREVENTING CHILDHOOD LEAD EXPOSURE ON THE U.S.-MEXICO BORDER

A growing body of scientific evidence supports the danger to children's health posed by low-level chronic exposure to lead. It is estimated that lowering the "safe" limit of lead exposure from 10 ug/dL to 5 ug/dL will result in prevalence rates of elevated lead levels in the millions. In addition to exposure pathways related to substandard housing and undernourishment, children on the U.S.-Mexico border have the added burden imposed by child-targeted consumer products tainted with lead.

While the use of lead-based ink on consumer products is a technical issue, it is also a politically sensitive issue. Health agencies in Mexico have tremendous difficulty addressing the public health threat in a climate of potential political backlash. Binational collaborative partnerships that include academia, government agencies, health care groups, and community-based organizations seek short- and long-term solutions to this problem.

There are approximately 1.6 million consumers on both sides of the El Paso and Ciudad Juarez international border. Cultural preferences and limited incomes contribute to a reliance on Mexican products. In cases where consumer products are unsafe, neither U.S. nor Mexican federal regulatory agencies can effectively monitor the problem. As transborder commerce increases, environmental health and safety issues will escalate.

The opportunities for nursing involvement in the process abound. Culturally relevant risk communication in Hispanic communities should focus on the family unit. and use popular cultural media forms, such as drama, in both visual and written form tailored for the region. Bilingual, linguistic appropriateness materials are essential.

This author has found that dramatic representations help promote lasting behavioral change by enhancing self-efficacy, and that self-efficacy is mediated by cultural norms. Perception of self-efficacy, according to Bandura's Social Learning Theory, is partly influenced by a history of personal success in performing a related activity. Positive role modeling provides vicarious experiences of success and reduces aversion.

The author produced a bilingual video and photo-novel in collaboration with volunteers, faculty and students from both sides of the border. Input was obtained from community members and government organizations using focus groups. A dramatic story line was developed to dramatize childhood lead exposure and prevention strategies in the home setting. The content addressed regionally specific as well as general exposure pathways. The recommended activities did not impose additional cost and were easy to accomplish. The characters used to model desired behavior, give verbally persuasive messages, and provide positive feedback were culturally and sociodemographically similar. The characters experience life on the border as it is lived by the majority. The drama also aroused emotions that reinforced cultural values for children, family, and community. Finally, it reinforces the notion that environmental problems know no borders, and that addressing them requires individual as well as collective efforts.

AFRICAN-AMERICAN CULTURE

African-Americans form a large, distinct, yet indigenous cultural group. Sudarkasa (1988) describes the cultural characteristics of African-American families.

1. Respect and reverence are core cultural values that originated in Africa. Respect involves having the esteem of others, particularly of parents, relatives, and community leaders. Reverence is the veneration of God, ancestors, and nature. In the U.S., this is exemplified by reliance on the church (and religion) as both a support mechanism and a conduit for

activism. The Environmental Justice Movement, born in African-American communities in the 1970s, was organized at the grass-roots level primarily through churches.

2. Responsibility among African-Americans extends beyond self-responsibility to include the extended family, the community, and even those who are less fortunate. Again, this value is reflected in environmental activism seen in many African-American communities.

3. Reciprocity involves giving back to the family and community in return for what has been given. This value embraces the principle of mutual assistance.

4. Restraint in decision making, reason in settling conflict, and reconciliation characterize interpersonal relations, particularly conflict resolution. These values reflect positive attitudes toward problem solving (Sudarkasa, 1988).

INTERVENTION: EDUCATING NURSES ON THE MISSISSIPPI DELTA FOR ENVIRONMENTAL HEALTH

The Mississippi delta region has reaped the benefits of economic development spurred by the great regional waterway, but has also been plagued by the environmental health problems created by polluting industries. These industries include oil refinery plants, chemical plants, and other petrochemical-allied facilities. "Cancer alley" is a region near the southern end of the Mississippi delta, so known because of the high prevalence of environmentally related health problems. Over the years, polluting industries were located near predominantly African-American neighborhoods. Thus, this group has been disproportionately at risk for environmental exposures.

Environmental justice issues such as low-paying jobs, poverty, and lack of political power keep millions of African Americans living and working in proximity to hazardous waste sites, such as the Devil's Swamp, one of the largest such dump sites near East Baton Rouge.

Louisiana sits squarely in the "cancer alley" region. This state has been characterized as one of the major industrial toxic waste dump sites in the nation, with about 700 hazardous waste sites. It ranks near the top in toxic emissions (Adeola, 1994).

Howard University, in collaboration with the Minority Health Professions Foundation and the Agency for Toxic Substances and Disease Registry, addressed the problem of inadequate educational preparation for nurses to address environmental health issues on the Mississippi delta. A modular curriculum was developed for integrating regionally specific environmental health concepts into nursing curricula (Howard University, 1999). Although it is specific for the Mississippi delta region, it is rapidly gaining nationwide attention. One module addresses the role of culture (Lassiter & Mitchem-Davis, 1999).

The project emphasizes the importance of cultural assessment in the environmental health nursing role. The purpose of cultural assessment is to develop a database from which to tailor locally relevant nursing care for clients and communities experiencing environmental health problems. Cultural assessment data are necessary to develop strategies for community empowerment.

SUMMARY AND CONCLUSIONS

Although Native American, Asian, and Pacific Islander cultures are not covered here, the purpose and basic principles of cultural assessment in environmental health nursing have been presented. Consideration of culture in environmental health nursing may be the single most important determinant of outcome, yet, cultural assessment is rarely given its due importance. The Mississippi Delta Project is notable in this regard for emphasizing the importance of cultural competence in environmental health.

Environmental health problems are regionally mediated. Focus is largely given to the natural and man-made environmental hazards that exist in a region. But in structuring solutions to these problems, it is equally important to consider the people that are affected. What economic and social factors mediate their risk of exposure? What cultural variables mollify or worsen the environment in which they live? Cultural nursing assessment provides answers to these crucial questions that allow the development of effective strategies to improve environmental health.

REFERENCES

Adeola, F. O. (1994). Environmental hazards, health, and racial inequity in hazardous waste site distribution. *Environment and Behavior, 26*(1), 99–126.

Howard University. (1999). *Environmental health & nursing: The Mississippi delta Project, a modular curriculum.* Atlanta: Minority Health Professions Foundation and Howard University.

Institute of Medicine. (1995). *Nursing, health, & the environment.* Washington, DC: National Academy Press.

Lassiter, P. G., & Mitchem-Davis, A. (1999). The role of culture, poverty, race, and economic development on environmental health. In Howard University, *Environmental health & nursing: The Mississippi Delta Project,* (pp. II/1–II/17). Atlanta: Minority Health Professions Foundation and Howard University.

Marin, G., & Marin, B. (1991). *Research with Hispanic populations.* Newbury Park, CA: Sage.

Sharp, J. (1998). *Bordering the future: Challenge and opportunity in the Texas border region.* Austin: Texas Comptroller of Public Accounts (Publication #96-599).

Sohier, R. (1995). Nursing care for the people of a small planet: Culture and the Neuman systems model. In B. Neuman (Ed.), *The Neuman Systems Model* (3rd ed., pp. 101–117). Stamford, CT: Appleton & Lange.

Sudarkasa, N. (1988). African and Afro-American family structure. In J. B. Cole (Ed.), *Anthropology for the nineties.* New York: Collier Macmillan.

U.S. Bureau of Census. (1999). Department of Statistical Information, Washington, DC. Available at http://www.census.gov/population/socdemo/hispanic/

PART IV

Integrating Environmental Health into Nursing Practice

CHAPTER 23

Occupational and Environmental Health History-Taking

Jane Lipscomb and Karen Sova

The Satterfields' strange run of nagging health problems began in late September, right after the weather turned cold in Baltimore. It would be more than 2 months before any of their health care providers asked the correct questions to get at the source of their problem. Mrs. Satterfield and her 8-year-old daughter came down with headaches, stuffiness, and coughs. She also had a growing sense of fogginess, while her daughter was dizzy and had fainted several times. Mrs. Satterfield's allergist renewed her prescriptions while her internist couldn't see her but told her to go to the emergency room if she felt seriously ill. The family pediatrician thought it was migraines and advised the child to slow down and skip physical education class. Mr. Satterfield had sinus pain and a run-down feeling. Their 11-year-old son began to have headaches and dizzy spells. Upon learning of the children's absence from school, Jan Brant, a nurse at the school, began to question what was making the whole family ill when no one had any sort of fever that might signal a shared infection. She suspected that it had to be the house and questioned a natural gas or carbon monoxide (CO) leak. She advised Mrs. Satterfield to call Baltimore Gas and Electric Company and have the house tested. Within 30 minutes of her call to the electric company a technician was at the home and found CO levels of 300 ppm. This is ten times the level at which CO detectors may alarm and more than eight times above the permisable level for occupational exposure. The source of the CO was the gas-fired furnace in the basement of their home. Prior to this life-threatening incident the Satterfield home contained no CO monitors (Roylance, 2000).

This case should demonstrate the critical need for astute clinical observation and thorough history taking to uncover occupational/environmen-
tal links with what otherwise may appear as common health complaints
or disease. It also demonstrates the fact that nurses are well positioned
to identify environmental illnesses within the context of their everyday
practice.

The purpose of this chapter is threefold: (1) to familiarize nurses and
other health care providers with the basic principles underlying occupational and environmental diseases, (2) to describe the purpose and benefits of taking an environmental history, and (3) to provide tools for collecting
basic environmental exposure data through history taking and referral to
specialists.

PRINCIPLES UNDERLYING HISTORY TAKING

Identification of an environmentally related disease depends on good (if
not great) history taking. A physical exam and laboratory testing can provide supporting and confirming data, but without a thorough history of
current and past occupational and environmental exposures, the appropriate laboratory testing and additional exam(s) needed may not be performed.
In addition, inappropriate laboratory tests might be performed and may
serve to further confuse the clinical picture. There are five major principles underlying occupational- and environmental-related disease. They
should be kept in mind when interviewing a client presenting with symptoms of an undetermined cause that could be occupational or environmental
in origin (Rosenstock and Cullen, 1994).

1. *Environmentally related diseases are often indistinguishable from diseases caused by nonenvironmental risk factors.* This fact alone makes
   history taking and drawing associations between environmental exposures and symptoms extremely challenging. In the case study presented
   above, several nonenvironmental causes were competing explanations
   for the presenting symptoms. Without a thorough occupational and/or
   residential history, carbon monoxide poisoning would never be identified and the family member would be returned to the environment that
   posed the risk. The client may even return to the hazardous environment with a false reassurance that a nonenvironmental agent is responsible. In the case of work-related illness, workers may even relax their
   own work practices in response to such a diagnosis. Unfortunately,
   unique or highly specific occupational and environmental illnesses are

the exception rather than the rule. This is especially true of environmentally related disease associated with lower-level community-based exposures. Therefore, clinicians need to consider an environmental cause as part of their differential diagnosis for more than just classic or sentinel occupational illnesses. At a minimum, environmental causes should be considered when evaluating individuals with skin disease, asthma, neuropathies, cancer, diminished hearing, and musculoskeletal disorders (Becker, 1992).

2. *Most diseases, including those caused or exacerbated by environmental exposures, have multifactorial causes.* In other words, the vast majority of diseases are caused by a combination of environmental and genetic factors. Even when an environmental exposure is implicated in disease causation, other factors usually play a role. In the case of environmentally caused lung diseases, it is incorrect to attribute them to air pollution or smoking alone. Efforts to blame one source of exposure (or individual behavior) rather than taking a comprehensive approach to primary prevention are counterproductive. It is critical to note however, that some sources of exposure are more easily and effectively controlled than others and therefore approaches to risk management may favor controlling environmental air pollutants, which are less voluntary in nature and can be controlled by engineering rather than by relying on changing an addictive personal behavior, such as cigarette smoking. It should also be recognized that in the case of work-related illnesses, workers' compensation applies to illnesses that are caused or exacerbated by the workplace; therefore there is no need to deny the fact that many workers with work-related pulmonary disease also have a history of cigarette smoking. Of course this does not relieve the client from the responsibility for making lifestyle changes or the health care provider from offering education and support for these changes. Similarly, it does not exonerate the workplace as a source of the hazard.

3. *For chronic diseases associated with environmental exposures, a biologically predictive latency interval usually exists and should be considered in history taking.* For example, asbestos exposure usually precedes the expression of lung cancer by at least 20 years. Therefore, asking clients about their current or even usual job or occupation will miss critical exposure data. In the event that the clinician suspects pulmonary fibrosis or lung cancer, a complete occupational history is needed, including a history of past employment, an assessment of hobbies such as auto repair, and a history of military service that may include asbestos exposure.

4. *A dose–response relationship exists for the majority of recognized environmental diseases.* For example, as the concentration and duration (or dose) of exposure to hazards such as coal dust or cotton dust increase, so does the incidence of pulmonary fibrosis in populations exposed to these dusts. An exception to this principle is the case of asbestos and mesothelioma (a unique cancer of the lining of the pleura of the lung and/or stomach), where a dose–response relationship is less clear. In fact, mesothelioma has been diagnosed in non-occupationally exposed individuals whose only exposure to asbestos occurred through the fibers carried home on the clothing of asbestos workers (U.S. Department of Health and Human Services, 1995). In addition, occupationally related asthma may present after a single exposure or following years of exposure.

5. *Large individual variability exists in human responses to environmental exposures.* We are only beginning to understand the nature and range of this variability. This factor poses extreme challenges to clinicians and researchers in environmental health who are accustomed to thinking in terms of a 40-year-old white male rather than, for example, an often underserved person of color and/or of poverty who is disproportionately affected by environmental hazards. It is also becoming apparent that ever within a group of individuals with similar demographics there is variability in individual susceptibility to illness.

PURPOSE AND BENEFITS OF HISTORY TAKING

There are numerous compelling reasons to incorporate environmental history taking and awareness into one's clinical practice. The primary motivation for taking an environmental history, whether it involves one or ten minutes of additional questioning, is to make an accurate diagnosis. The primary and secondary prevention of subsequent disease is dependent on this diagnosis. It is important to recognize that not all client visits require the same level of history taking or scrutiny. Rather, what is needed is a general awareness of the potential adverse effect of the environment on human health and a heightened awareness in those cases where a client presents with complaints for which there may be a recognized environmental link.

The primary prevention of environmental disease is dependent on case identification through history taking. In most cases, there are numerous other members of the work force or larger community who are similarly exposed and for whom making a link with the environment may prevent disease. In the case briefly described above, knowledge of the risk of exposure to carbon monoxide from home heating units will alert the public to a previously unrecognized hazard and lead to enhanced preventive actions on the part of the community. It can also alert other health care providers to the hazard and motivate them to incorporate education about the risk of carbon monoxide poisoning in their clinical practice.

In addition, appropriate history taking can prevent the aggravation of many underlying conditions that may not be caused by an environmental exposure but made worse by it. Asthma is the perfect case in point. We now understand that outdoor air pollutants such as nitrous oxides, sulfur dioxides, carbon monoxide, hydrocarbons, ozone, and particulate matter exacerbates asthma. In fact, children with asthma have been found to be a sensitive subpopulation for acute responses to outdoor air pollution (Mortimer and Etzel, 1999). The identification of these environmental triggers for disease is critical to reducing morbidity and mortality from many common health conditions.

An environmental history can also assist in the identification of potential new workplace or community hazards. Knowledge of these toxic effects will dramatically aid primary prevention of disease globally. The toxicity of a single chemical or exposure may provide insights into the toxic potential of structurally similar chemicals. This has been true of solvents and pesticides that have been tested and found to have similar neurological effects as the originally identified and chemically similar agent.

A compelling reason to take an occupational and/or environmental history is to establish documentation and a basis for compensation for work-related conditions or for environmental illnesses for which compensation may be available. The first U.S. workers' compensation act was passed in 1911 to provide a no-fault system for compensating workers for medical expenses and lost time resulting from injuries or illnesses incurred in the course of work. As such, the system does not require the examining clinician to establish fault on the part of the employer or employee. However, it does expect the examining physician to say whether a worker's illness was caused by or aggravated by work (Boden, 2000). This is why it is critical for clinicians to ask about work in the event of a potential work-related illness. Contrary to popular belief, the workers' compensation system is not a pot of gold for malingering workers. It is an opportunity for workers to receive medical care and partial coverage (usually two thirds) of lost wages in the event they are injured while at work or on duty. Most eligible workers do not file compensation claims for work-related illnesses. A study of occupational disease in Washington and California revealed that of the 51 probable cases of occupational respiratory conditions, only one was reported as a workers' compensation claim. When workers with chronic occupational diseases are compensated, they wait more than a year, on average, to receive compensation payments (Boden, 2000). Workers' compensation does not provide any payment for pain and suffering or punitive damages. The workers' compensation system precludes workers from suing their employer for work-related injuries or illnesses, even in the case of egregious workplace safety violations on the part of the employer. However, proper identification and documentation of occupational exposure/disease, can assist the worker in achieving more equitable worker compensation claims based on appropriate disability ratings for future medical bills, future lost wages, and vocational rehabilitation. By contrast, victims of environmental illness are not prevented from filing lawsuits against potentially responsible parties, including payment for pain and suffering. Class action lawsuits against the tobacco industry and the lead manufacturing industry are current examples of lawsuits involving environmental exposures.

Finally, incorporating environmental history taking into health care professional training and practice will assist in the larger effort to increase awareness about the potential environmental causes of disease among providers. Unfortunately, much work is needed to accomplish this goal.

TOOLS FOR HISTORY TAKING

Asking a client's occupation is not the same as asking what the client does in the performance of that occupation. A client answering "registered nurse" to a question of occupation tells us nothing about the myriad occupational exposures to which this client can be exposed. We also know that demographic information and the initial client history frequently get buried so far down in a record they are never reviewed again. Unless an astute health care provider suspects a correlation between presenting symptoms and an occupational/environmental exposure, clients may never again be asked their occupation or what they do in the performance of that occupation.

How does one go about incorporating an environmental history into every client encounter in the current managed care environment? What follows are several key screening questions or areas of concern for all providers to consider and select among, depending on the chief complaint and developmental stage of the client. If you suspect, even remotely, an environmental etiology to a presenting complaint, the following questions should be asked:

1. Where do you spend most of your time (i.e., home, school, place of employment)?
2. What are your current, past, and longest held jobs?
3. What kind of hobbies, home work, and leisure activities are you involved in?
4. Do you have exposure to any specific hazards, such as dust, fumes, chemicals, or biologic agents?

If the client's answers to the above questions indicate a linkage between current symptoms and activities at home, school or work, these additional questions may be asked:

1. Are symptoms worse at work (or in other environments)?
2. Do they improve on weekends, vacations, or when away from the suspect environment?
3. Are co-workers or other family members affected?
4. Have you changed jobs, hobbies, or leisure activities due to symptoms?

If the above screening questions indicate a suspected occupational cause of the presenting illness, the following in-depth questions can be included (where appropriate) regarding the work history:

1. Describe in detail the work site and a typical day's work.
2. Was protective clothing or equipment available and worn?
3. Is the workplace ventilated?
4. Is any specialized periodic testing or safety training done on the job?
5. What do you think is causing the illness?
6. Have you or your employer filed a first report of work injury or worker's compensation claim?

The following in-depth occupational and environmental health form was developed by faculty at the University of Maryland to train nurses and other health professionals in history taking. You may want to use the work history part of this form to elicit responses to the six questions listed above (Figure 23.1).

If your client is a child or someone who spends the majority of time at home you would want to inquire as to the age, location, and condition of the home. The Environmental Health Checklist for Home Assessment was developed by the Children's Environmental Health Network (1999) to assist

Work History

1. List your current and past longest held jobs, including the military:

Company	Dates Employed	Job Title	Known Exposures
_____	_____	_____	_____
_____	_____	_____	_____
_____	_____	_____	_____
_____	_____	_____	_____
_____	_____	_____	_____

2. Do you work full-time?   No   YES   How many hours per week?

3. Do you work part-time?   No   YES   How many hours per week?

4. Please describe any health problems or injuries that you have experienced in connection with your present or past jobs:

5. Have you ever had to change jobs due to health problems or injuries? YES NO
   If so, describe:

   Did any of your coworkers experience similar problems?

6 In what type of business do you currently work?

7. Describe your work (what do you actually do):

8. Have you had any current or past exposure (through breathing or touching) to any of the following?

__ acids	__ carbon	__ dichlorobenzene	__ manganese	__ pesticides	__ TDI or MDI
__ alcohols	tetrachloride	__ ethylene dibromide	__ mercury	__ phenol	__ trichloro-
__ alkalies	__ chlorinated	__ ethylene dichloride	__ methylene	__ phosgene	ethylene
__ ammonia	napthalences	__ fiberglass	chloride	__ radiation	— trinitrotol-
__ arsenic	__ chloroform	__ halothane	__ nickel	__ rock dust	uene (TNT)
__ asbestos	__ chloroprene	__ heat (severe)	__ noise (loud)	__ silica powder	__ vibration
__ benzene	__ chromates	__ isocyanates	__ PBBs	— solvents	__ vinyl chloride
__ beryllium	__ coal dust	__ ketones	__ PCBs	— styrene	__ welding
__ cadmium	__ cold (severe)	__ lead	__ perchloroethylene	-- toluene	fumes
					__ x-rays
					__ talc

9. Did you receive any safety training about these agents? NO   YES

    Explain:

10. Are you involved in any work processes such as grinding, welding, soldering, or polishing that create dust, mists, or fumes?

    NO _____   YES _____ (If yes, describe):

11. Did you use any of the following personal protective equipment when exposed?

____boots   ____glasses/goggles   ____safety shoes   ____sleeves
____coveralls   ____gloves   ____shield   ____welding mask
____earplugs/muffs ____respirator

12. Is your work environment generally clean? If not, describe:

13. What ventilation systems are used in your workplace?

14. Do they seem to work? Are you aware of any chemical odors in your environment? (If so, explain.)

15. Where do you eat, smoke, and take your breaks when you are on the job?

16. Do you use a uniform or have clothing that you wear only to work?

17. How is your work clothing laundered? (at home, by employer, etc.)

18. How often do you wash your hands at work and how do you wash them? (running water, special soaps, etc.)

19. Do you shower before leaving the worksite?

20. Do you have any physical symptoms associated with work? If yes, describe:

21. Are other workers similarly affected?

FIGURE 23.1 Comprehensive occupational and environmental history

Nursing, Health, and the Environment (1995)

clinicians in history taking (Figure 23.2). Because of the prevalence of environmental lead exposure in older homes and public buildings, questions regarding possible lead exposure must be considered in all pediatric clinical encounters.

Prior to 1997, the Centers for Disease Control (CDC) recommended universal screening of all preschool children at 12 and 24 months of age and at 36–72 months of age if not previously screened (Balk, Walton-Brown, & Pope, 1999). In 1997, because the prevalence of childhood lead poisoning had been reduced significantly (primarily in response to the elimination of lead from gasoline in the 1970s), CDC replaced the guideline with one of local risk assessment of exposure to lead. State and local health departments were given the responsibility of determining the level of risk of exposure and issuing policy guidelines for providers. In the

FAMILY NAME: _____

ADDRESS: _____

HOUSING

Type of housing?   Ownership?

    How old? _____   __Rental

    Condition?_____   __Owner Occupied

    _____   __Public Housing

Renovation/repairs occurring?   __ Yes   __ No   Describe:_____

Existence of rodents/insects?   __ Yes   __ No   Describe:_____

Existence of molds/fungi?   __ Yes   __ No   Describe:_____

What is source of drinking water? Describe:_____

HEATING SOURCE

Heating sources?_____

Uses gas stoves/ovens for heating?   __ Yes   __ No Adequate ventilation? __ Yes

                                                                                __ No

Uses fireplaces/woodburning stoves?   __ Yes   __ No   What is burned? _____

Wood smell indoors?   __ Yes   __ No

Evidence of smoke/soot?   __ Yes   __ No

Uses kerosene heaters?   __ Yes   __ No

ENVIRONMENTAL TOBACCO SMOKE

Household members smoke?   __ Yes   __ No

Regular visitors smoke?   __ Yes   __ No

Smoking allowed in the car?   __ Yes   __ No

INDOOR AIR POPULATION—FORMALDEHYDE AND ASBESTOS

Sources of formaldehyde?   __ Yes   __ No Describe: _____

(particle board, urea in foam insulation, other)

Potential asbestos hazards?   __ Yes   __ No Describe: _____

(friable pipe/boiler insulation, old vinyl linoleum, wall board repair, home renovation/repairs)

AIR POLLUTION—TOXIC ORGANIC HYDROCARBONS

Uses cleaners/polishes/air fresheners/disinfectants?   __ Yes   __ No

Uses glues/solvent/varnishes/building materials?__ Yes   __ No

Where are these materials stored? _____

PEST/MOLD/FUNGI CONTROL

Home garden?   __ Yes __ No Use of pesticides outdoors?

                                                              __ Yes   __ No

Evidence of rodents/insects?   __ Yes __ No Use of pesticides in home?

                                                              __ Yes   __ No

Use of pesticides on children?   __ Yes __ No What type?_____

Is re-entry after pesticide use according to instructions?   __ Yes   __ No

Evidence of molds/fungi?   __ Yes __ No

PETS   Are there pets in the home? __ Yes   __ No   Are the pets ill?
Describe: _____

LEAD

Paint in poor repair?	__ Yes	__ No
Uses leaded pottery/dishes?	__ Yes	__ No
Crafts/other activities with lead?	__ Yes	__ No
Drinking H_2O tested for lead?	__ Yes	__ No
House members lead-exposed at work?	__ Yes	__ No

PLAYGOUND HAZARDS
Where do children play? _____
Any hazardous play equipment or toys? _____

HOME/PARAOCCUPATIONAL ACTIVITIES
House members work with heavy metals/solvents/dust?   __ Yes   __ No
What materials are used? _____

MEDICATIONS
House members use home remedies?   __ Yes   __ No   Which ones? _____
Where are medications stored? _____

HOUSEHOLD MEMBERS' OCCUPATIONS & ACTIVITIES
House members' occupation and potential   House members' activities and hobbies:
exposures:

_____   _____
_____   _____
_____   _____
_____   _____

SURROUNDING NEIGHBORHOOD
Is home or school close to highways? __ Yes __ No Near to industries? __ Yes __ No
Are any of the neighboring business
  Dry-cleaning?   __ Yes __ No   Radiator/auto repair?   __ Yes   __ No
  Photoprocessing? __ Yes __ No

WHERE DO CHILDREN SPEND MOST OF THEIR TIME?

_____
_____

NOTES

_____
_____

ASSESSMENT COMPLETED BY: _____
DATE:: _____

FIGURE 23.2 Environmental hazards checklist for home assessments (CEHN, 1999)

absence of formal local guidance, "universal screening should be carried out" (CDC, 1997). "The Minimum Personal Risk Questionnaire" below may be used as a first-pass screening method, followed by blood lead testing if the answers indicate high risk. Overall, the sensitivity of the questionnaire designed to identify lead-poisoned children is 60–70% (CDC).

1. Does the child reside in or regularly visit a house that was built before 1950? (Include setttings such as a day care center and a babysitter's or relative, home.)
2. Does the child reside in or regularly visit a house built before 1978 undergoing recent (past 6 months) or current renovation?
3. Does the child have a sibling or playmate who has been diagnosed with lead poisoning?

In addition to occupational sources of dusts, fumes, chemicals, biologic agents, and childhood lead exposure, several other specific nonoccupational hazards or sources of exposure should be considered, including the client's source of drinking water (i.e., well or municipal reservoir). The National Research Council (NRC) reports that the drinking of water provides about half of all toxic exposures people commonly incur (Rosenstock and Cullen, 1994). Another exposure, environmental tobacco smoke (ETS), is a pulmonary irritant and the cause of approximately 3,000 cases of lung cancer in the U.S. among nonsmokers annually (Bofetta, Agudo, Ahern, Benhamou, Darby et al., 1998). ETS increases the prevalence of respiratory illnesses among children and adults. Environments in which exposure to ETS may occur include the home, work, and day care (especially in home day care). In addition, the heating source for the home should be considered in the case of respiratory complaints. Exposure to wood smoke or fireplace may precipitate or worsen respiratory symptoms (Honicky, Osborne, & Akpom, 1985). Respiratory irritants such as nitrogen dioxide, respirable particulates, and polycyclic aromatic hydrocarbons (PAHs) can be emitted in high concentrations from fireplaces and wood stoves that are not regularly cleaned or are improperly vented. Carbon monoxide, another combustion product, can cause fatigue at low concentrations and headache, dizziness, weakness, confusion, nausea, or even death at higher concentrations. Pesticide use in home or garden should be part of any environmental assessment (see chapter 17).

Certain signs, symptoms, and the associated diseases should be considered as potential sentinel occupational health events and worked up accordingly (see chapter 20). Certain types of cancer have been associated with specific occupational exposures including cancers of the lung, liver, bladder, brain, and blood-forming organs. As mentioned earlier, respiratory and neurologic complaints should be considered for environmental causes. Both obstructive and restrictive lung disease are associated with workplace dust and fibers. Solvents, heavy metals, and pesticides are associated with neurologic effects.

Numerous sources of exposure information are available to assist both generalists and specialists in their clinical assessment. An invaluable source of toxicologic and human data is the National Library of Medicine's web-based Toxicology and Environmental Health Information Program (http://www.nlm.nih.gov/). The program's resources include thirteen searchable databases, chemical and drug information/structures, fact sheets, database documentation, bibliographies, an interactive toxicology tutorial, and links to other related internet sites. The databases are easy to search using clinical search terms. The reference section of this book contains numerous other sources of information to assist nurses and other health care professionals in understanding potential environmental links to disease.

You should be familiar with and identify occupational/environmental health specialists and clinics in your area or region of practice. Referral to or consultation with an occupational/environmental specialists may be needed, depending on the primary care provider's comfort level with diagnosis and management of occupational/environmental disease and/or injury. Less complex exposures or injuries can be managed in a primary care practice; others might be managed in consultation with or referral to a specialist. As with all referrals, sending the client to the specialist with as much information about presenting symptoms and diagnostic tests as possible is essential to successful treatment. Basic testing to rule in or rule out nonoccupational/environmental disease should be done whenever possible. Consulting with the specialist prior to diagnostic testing may help eliminate future testing "assaults" by grouping tests needed for occupational diagnosis with initial testing.

A worksite evaluation is a critical step that can be done by or coordinated with an occupational health specialist. A walk through evaluation of the physical workplace can lead to the identification of workplace hazards, work practices, and the general condition of a workplace.

One excellent source of referral is the Association of Occupational and Environmental Clinics (AOEC). This clinic network consists of more than 60 clinics and more than 250 individuals across the U.S. committed to improving the practice of occupational and environmental medicine through information sharing and collaborative research. AOEC currently has clinics in 27 states, the District of Columbia, and 3 three Canadian provinces. They have individual members in more than 40 states. In a recent survey of AOEC members, 88% reported sharing their environmental health expertise with other health care professionals (www.aoec.org and personal communication with AOEC). Most, if not all clinics, have multidisciplinary practice.

Many workers believe that the organizations, institutions, and employers they work for and with provide safe and healthy environments at the workplace. We would all like to believe that our communities pose no threat to our health and that our homes are safe havens. In order to ensure these healthy environments, the analysis of every client encounter should include the awareness of occupational and environmental exposures. Key questions about present and past jobs, hobbies, home work, leisure activities, and the community are essential to primary and secondary prevention of occupational and environmental disease.

REFERENCES AND BIBLIOGRAPHY

Balk, S., Walton-Brown, S., & Pope, A. (1999). Environmental history taking. In *Training manual on pediatric and environmental health: Putting it into practice* (pp. 77–87). Children's Environmental Health Network/Public Health Institute.

Becker, C. E. (1992). Key elements of the occupational history for the general physician. *Western Journal of Medicine, 137*(6), 581–582.

Boden, L. I. (2000). Workers' compensation. In B. S. Levy, & D. H. Wegman (Eds.), *Occupational health: Recognizing and preventing work-related disease and injury* (pp. 237–256). Philadelphia: Lippincott, Williams & Wilkins.

Bofetta, et al. (1998). Multicenter case-control study of exposure to environmental tobacco smoke and lung cancer in Europe. *Journal of the National Cancer Institute, 90*, 1440–1450.

Centers for Disease Control and Prevention. (1997). *Screening for lead poisoning in young children*. Atlanta, GA: Author.

Children Environmental Health Network (1991). Environmental Health Checklist for Home Assessment. Emeryville, CA.

Honicky, R. E., Osborne, J. S., & Akpom, C. A. (1985). Symptoms of respiratory illness in young children and the use of wood burning stoves for indoor heating. *Pediatrics, 75*, 587–93.

Institute of Medicine (1995). *Nursing, Health and the Environment*. Washington, DC: National Academy Press.

Mortimer, X., & Etzel, R. (1999). Air pollution. *Training manual on pediatric and environmental health: Putting it into practice* (pp. 133–152). Children's Environmental Health Network/Public Health Institute.

Rosenstock, L., & Cullen, M. (1994). *Textbook of clinical occupational and environmental health*. Philadelphia: W.B. Saunders.

Roylance, F. D. (2000, December 23). School nurse hailed for lifesaving tip: Family's illness attributed to CO leak from furnace. *The Baltimore Sun*.

U.S. Department of Health and Human Services. (1995). *Report to Congress on worker's contamination study conducted under the worker's family protection act (29 U.S.C. 671a)* (DHHS [NIOSH] Publication No. 95-123). Cincinnati, Ohio: Author.

CHAPTER 24

Understanding Environmental Health Policy

Barbara Sattler

Who is in charge of our environmental health? This is not an easy question to answer. Our environmental health status is a function of the environmental exposures in our work, living, learning, and community environments from chemical, biological, and radioactive exposures and influenced by our general health status and phase of human development. So who provides environmental protection in our workplaces, communities, schools, and homes?

- *Workplace* health and safety is the purview of the Occupational Safety and Health Association (OSHA), which is a federal regulatory agency. Half of the states are under the jurisdiction of the federal OSHA and half of the states are deputized by federal OSHA to promulgate and enforce standards within their states (as long as the state regulations are at least as effective as the federal standards). See chapter 20 on occupational health policy for more detailed coverage of this subject.
- *Home environments* are protected by a variety of agencies. For example, the Consumer Product Safety Commission is responsible for ensuring healthy and safe consumer products. State, local, and federal agencies provide guidance and regulations regarding lead-based paint exposures. However, there are many exposures in our homes that do not have associated regulations and for which the homeowner or property owner is solely responsible. Drinking water from a private well is a perfect example. Although wells must be tested when they are initially dug, there are no other requirements for testing the water thereafter. This task is left entirely to the homeowner.

- *Schools* are another place in which the responsibility is shared by several agencies at local, state, and federal levels. Employee safety and health is the purview of OSHA, so the teachers and school staff are covered by exposure regulations, but there is not an equivalent agency that creates standards to protect the children. School environmental health policies may be decided on state or local levels or may be nonexistent. For example, several states have passed legislation requiring the implementation of Integrated Pest Management strategies. Other states have no policies regarding pesticide use.
- Environmental protection within our *communities* is the most complicated. Food quality is the responsibility of the Department of Agriculture and the Federal Food and Drug Administration. Radiation exposures are the responsibility of the federal Nuclear Regulatory Agency, and transportation of hazardous substances through our neighborhoods and on our highways is the responsibility of the Department of Transportation. With the evolving concern about biological warfare agents the responsibility is shared by several agencies including the Department of Health and Human Services, the Department of Justice, and a variety of local public health and law enforcement agencies.

This overview should give the reader some idea of how quickly the map of environmental health policy becomes complicated. Nonetheless, the primary regulatory agency responsible for our air, soil, water, and drinking water quality is the federal Environmental Protection Agency. The EPA is responsible for protecting the environment and often uses human health risks to guide its policies and regulations but sometimes uses other ecological parameters. The Department of Health and Human Services (DHHS) is responsible for our nation's health but has little relationship with the EPA. A new study completed by the Pew Foundation has found that the lack of a strong interrelated working plan between the EPA and DHHS among other factors has resulted in poor tracking of health effects that may be associated with environmental exposures. (Pew Environmental Health Commission, 2000).

An essential competency for environmental health assessments is knowledge of the health and environmental statutes, regulations, and practices regarding what data are collected and how they are accessed. Yet, very little is collected that specifically connects environmental exposures to disease outcomes. Making these connections has been left to researchers and has been investigated primarily on a case-by-case basis. For instance, in states where there are cancer, birth defects, or other disease outcome registries, data can be explored for the relationship to environmental exposures only where environmental exposure data exists.

Pollution monitoring is generally done by governmental agencies or by polluting industries and reported to the government. Some exposure data can be gleaned from permits issued by state departments of environmental protection that designate legal discharge of hazardous pollutants into the air and water. Several environmental statutes have been promulgated to specifically give the public the right to know about the hazardous chemicals in our environment. (See chapter 8 for more detailed information about access to information.)

The EPA and each state's equivalent entity are the primary agencies responsible for environmental protection. The EPA was established in 1970 in order to permit coordinated and effective governmental action on behalf of the environment. It endeavors to abate and control pollution systematically by integration of a variety of research, monitoring, standard setting, and enforcement activities and coordinates and supports research and antipollution activities by state and local governments, private and public groups, individuals, and educational institutions. Each state has a designated agency that is responsible for the regulatory oversight on all environmental regulations and standards. The EPA web site (http://www.epa.gov) is an excellent source for general information and, in some cases, geographically specific information. Additionally, all of the environmental acts, regulations, and standards can be accessed on the EPA's website.

Within the Centers for Disease Control is the National Center for Environmental Health (NCEH) and within the DHHS is the Agency for Toxic Substances and Disease Registry (ATSDR). Both of these relatively small, nonregulatory governmental agencies are responsible for environmental health issues. The ATSDR was established under Superfund legislation and is responsible for environmental health-related issues associated with hazardous waste sites including those that have been designated as Superfund sites. Their website is also quite useful to health professionals (http://www.atsdr.gov).

Superfund designation derives from the 1980 Federal Comprehensive Environmental Response, Compensation, and Liability Act created to identify and clean up industrial hazardous waste sites that pose a threat to human health. There are approximately 1,200 hazardous waste sites that are now on the National Priority List, indicating an active threat to human health, and approximately half of the sites have contaminated the ground water. Potential sources for human exposures from hazardous waste sites include contaminated air, ground water, drinking water, surface water, and soil. Additionally, there may be the physical risk of fire or explosion.

Environmental statutes and regulations may be promulgated and implemented on a federal, state, and sometimes even local level. Most environmental statutes are media specific meaning that regulations are created based on the polluted medium such as air, water, soil, and food. As with workplace health statutes, states must adhere to the federal environmental statutes. States may promulgate more stringent but not less stringent statutes and regulations.

The development and promulgation of environmental statutes and regulations is a study in civics. During the development stages, there are a number of opportunities for citizen input. During both legislative and regulatory policy development, there are opportunities for testimony from individuals, advocacy organizations, and professional associations. Yet, health care professionals have been conspicuously absent in all stages of the development of policies that purport to protect our environmental health.

The EPA and state agencies often have citizen advisory bodies. Attending the advisory body meetings is another opportunity to learn about the programs, plans, and deliberations about environmental health policies. This is another venue in which health care professionals are more often absent than present, but our presence could be quite positive. Having health care professionals advising our environmental protection agencies and policy makers might serve two functions: first, it could provide a more significant health perspective to discussions (which often take place without health experts) and second, it could help health professionals to better understand the environmental health policy context and decision-making process.

MAJOR ENVIRONMENTAL LAWS

The following are among the environmental laws enacted by Congress through which the EPA carries out its efforts.

THE NATIONAL ENVIRONMENTAL POLICY ACT (NEPA)

The National Environmental Policy Act established the EPA (1970) and a national policy for the environment and provided for the establishment of a Council on Environmental Policy. All policies, regulations, and public laws must be interpreted and administered in accordance with the policies set forth in this act.

Federal Insecticide, Fungicide, and Rodenticide Act (FIFRA)

FIFRA provides federal control of pesticide distribution, sale, and use. The EPA was given the authority to study the consequences of pesticide usage and requires users such as farmers and utility companies to register when using pesticides. Later amendments to the law required applicators to take certification exams, registration of all pesticides used in the U.S., and proper labeling of pesticides so that, if in accordance with specifications, they will cause no harm to the environment.

Clean Water Act (CWA)

The Clean Water Act sets basic structure for regulating pollutants to U.S. waters. The law gave the EPA the authority to set effluent standards on an industry basis and continued the requirements to set water quality standards for all contaminants in surface water. The 1977 amendments focused on toxic pollutants. In 1987 the CWA was reauthorized, and again focused on toxic pollutants, authorized citizen suit provisions, and funded sewage treatment plants.

Clean Air Act

The Clean Air Act regulates air emissions from area, stationary, and mobile sources. The EPA was authorized to establish National Ambient Air Quality Standards (NAAQS) to protect public health and the environment. The goal was to set and achieve the NAAQS by 1975. The law was amended in 1977 when many areas of the country failed to meet the standards. The 1990 amendments to the Clean Air Act intended to meet unaddressed or insufficiently addressed problems such as acid rain, ground level ozone, stratospheric ozone depletion, and air toxics. Also in the 1990 reauthorization, a mandate for Chemical Risk Management Plans was included. This mandate requires industry to identify worst case scenarios regarding the hazardous chemicals that they transport, use, or dispose of.

Safe Drinking Water Act (SDWA)

The Safe Water Drinking Act was established to protect the quality of drinking water in the U.S. The Act authorized the EPA to establish safe standards of purity and required all owners or operators of public water systems to comply with primary health-related standards. Under the reauthorization of the SDWA in 1996, a new right-to-know was created.

RESOURCE CONSERVATION AND RECOVERY ACT (RCRA)

The Resource Conservation and Recovery Act gave the EPA the authority to control the generation, transportation, treatment, storage, and disposal of hazardous waste. The RCRA also set forth a framework to manage non-hazardous waste. The 1984 Federal Hazardous and Solid Waste Amendments to this Act required phasing out land disposal of hazardous waste. The 1986 amendments enabled the EPA to address problems from underground tanks storing petroleum and other hazardous substances.

TOXIC SUBSTANCES CONTROL ACT (TSCA)

The Toxic Substances Control Act gives the EPA the ability to track the 75,000 industrial chemicals currently produced or imported into the United States. The EPA can require reporting or testing of chemicals that may pose environmental health risks and can ban the manufacture and import of those chemicals that pose an unreasonable risk.

COMPREHENSIVE ENVIRONMENTAL RESPONSE, COMPENSATION, AND LIABILITY ACT (CERCLA OR SUPERFUND)

This law created a tax on the chemical and petroleum industries and provided broad federal authority to respond directly to releases or threatened releases from waste sites of hazardous substances that may endanger public health or the environment.

SUPERFUND AMENDMENTS AND REAUTHORIZATION ACT (SARA)

The SARA amended the CERCLA with several changes and additions. These changes included increased size of the trust fund, encouragement of greater citizen participation in decision making on how sites should be cleaned up, increased state involvement in every phase of the Superfund program, increased focus on human health problems related to hazardous waste sites, new enforcement authorities and settlement tools, stressing the importance of permanent remedies and innovative treatment technologies in cleanup of hazardous waste sites, and Superfund actions to consider standards in other federal and state regulations. Under Superfund legislation the federal Agency for Toxic Substances and Disease Registry was established.

EMERGENCY PLANNING AND COMMUNITY RIGHT-TO-KNOW ACT (EPCRA)

The Emergency Planning and Community Right-to-Know Act, also known as Title III of SARA, was enacted to help local communities protect public health safety and the environment from chemical hazards. Each state was required to appoint a State Emergency Response Commission that was required to divide states into Emergency Planning Districts and establish a Local Emergency Planning Committee (LEPC) for each district.

NATIONAL ENVIRONMENTAL EDUCATION ACT (NEEA)

The National Environmental Education Act created a new and better coordinated environmental education emphasis at the EPA. This legislation also created the National Environmental Education and Training Foundation, which provides funding for environmental education programs.

POLLUTION PREVENTION ACT (PPA)

The Pollution Prevention Act focused industry, government, and public attention on reduction of the amount of pollution through cost-effective changes in production, operation, and raw materials use. Pollution prevention also includes other practices that increase efficient use of energy, water and other water resources such as recycling, source reduction, and sustainable agriculture.

FOOD QUALITY PROTECTION ACT (FQPA)

The Food Quality Protection Act amended the Federal Insecticide, Fungicide and Rodenticide Act and the Federal Food, Drug, and Cosmetic Act. The Act changed the way the EPA regulates pesticides and pesticide residues on foods. The requirements included a new safety standard of reasonable certainty of no harm to be applied to all pesticides used on foods. It also called for the explicit consideration of pesticide effects on children's health.

REGIONAL, STATE, AND LOCAL ENVIRONMENTAL PROTECTIONS

In addition to the main headquarters of EPA, there are ten regional EPA offices around the country. Each of these offices provides technical support and programming under the EPA statutory mandates. They also interface with the state agencies responsible for environmental protection. In some states, there is a designated environmental protection agency, while in other states, there is a combined health and environmental protection agency. In still others environmental protection is subsumed within the state health department.

The level of involvement by local health departments in environmental health is quite variable. Some health departments may only have a few services, such as food inspections and vector control, while other departments may have a wide range of services and programs like lead poisoning prevention, school environmental health, and training and education programs. Health professionals should familiarize themselves with the environmental health capabilities and services of their local health departments, as well as their state agencies.

In making an environmental health assessment, it is equally important to know who you can call when you suspect an environmentally related health problem as it is to identify the potential threat. As professionals newly venturing into the environmental health arena, nurses will be learning about the experts and services in state and local health departments and among federal agencies, as well as the gaps in expertise and services. It will be incumbent on us to help develop plans to fill the gaps, be they in exposure monitoring, health surveillance, data gathering, technical assistance, or the delivery of services. Additionally, it will be important to facilitate more effective interface among the health delivery sector, the public health sector, and the environmental protection sector. Health professionals can offer a distinct and important perspective on this interface, but in order to offer our perspective, we must be at the tables.

There are a number of ways to get involved in environmental health policies such as through our professional associations, through advocacy organizations such as the Health Care Without Harm Campaign, the Children's Environmental Health Network or the Sierra Club, through community-based associations, and even as individuals. Once health professionals begin their involvement in this policy area, they find that their input is very well received and that they really can make a difference in supporting good environmental health policies.

REFERENCE

Pew Environmental Health Commission (2000). America's Environmental Health Gap: Why the country needs a nationwide health tracking network. Reporting by Environmental Health Tracking Project. Johns Hopkins University School of Hygiene and Public Health, Baltimore, Maryland.

CHAPTER 25

Environmental Health Education

Barbara Sattler

Environmental education has been integrated into many aspects of K–12 education. The predominant attention is paid to the ecologic aspects of the environment based in biology and geology. Children learn about the life cycles of ponds and endangered species. They rarely learn about the human health threats associated with the environment. Undergraduates experience much of the same. Environmental courses in college focus on ecology, anthropogenic pollution, and environmental policies but seldom review the human health effects related to environmental degradation or protection. And when health professionals are in their basic training, they typically learn neither ecology nor environmental health. Because of this deficit, nurses and other health professionals, including physicians, are left with a critical gap in their knowledge about environmental health effects.

Because the teaching of environmental health is absent in our K–12, college, and professional school education, much of our "education" about environmental health has been derived from the popular media. The fact is that the popular media have actually been doing a fairly good job for the general population. When focus groups were held in Baltimore with inner city high school students about environmental health threats, the students were able to identify an almost identical list of health threats associated with environmental exposures as a group of medical residents, undergraduate nursing students, and nursing school faculty. This points to the success of the popular media in raising our awareness about many environmental health risks. All four groups of people identified lead-based paint, pests and pesticides, outdoor and indoor air pollution, water contaminants, old industrial sites, and other sources. Although this is a start, we have much work ahead of us.

COMMUNITY ENVIRONMENTAL HEALTH EDUCATION

The media have provided substantial general information about environmental health risks but have been significantly less attentive when providing solutions, including environmentally healthier purchases, practices, activities, and policies. Because our media-delivered education does not stress solutions, it is important when working with community members, or even individual patients, to include information about environmental health risks and the steps that can be taken to reduce exposures. It is extremely important to present incremental steps to solving problems. If the only solutions offered are grand and only attainable after years of struggle and policy changes, then the community may be paralyzed by the daunting tasks ahead. Organizations like the Sierra Club, Clean Water Action, and the Public Interest Research Groups (PIRGs) have a history of grassroots mobilization that starts with education and moves quickly to action.

YOUTH

Environmental health education can be delivered in myriad ways in the community. After the focus group mentioned above was completed with Baltimore youth, the young people decided they would like to learn more about the environment and health. A graduate student helped to convene the youth group every Saturday, during which time they learned about environmental health in an enjoyable and engaging way. Hank, a lanky 6'4" basketball player, had heard that there was an acceptable level of mouse parts that was allowed in sausage and hot dog products. When he made this statement, it launched the group to learn about food safety. This culminated in a field visit to the Parks Sausage factory where they watched the sausage-making process. This provided a great opportunity to ask questions about food quality control, to observe occupational conditions, and to eat free chitlings at the end of the tour!

As the Baltimore youth group progressed, they named themselves the Environmental Justice Youth Council (EJYC) and they planned a city-wide conference entitled *Endangered Species: Our Urban Youth*. They found co-sponsorship for their conference with the local Urban League where the conference was hosted, the Chesapeake Bay Foundation, the Maryland Department of the Environment, the Environmental Health Education Center at the University of Maryland, and others. The conference they organized was very interactive and creative. Each of the cosponsors provided a workshop, but the best session was the one for which the EJYC was completely responsible. Community service hours were offered to anyone who attended the conference for the whole day, creating incentives for students to attend an all-day Saturday event.

The EJYC wanted to do a session on lead poisoning that was reflective of their experiences, many of the youth had siblings or cousins who were lead poisoned. (In one of the communities from which they came, more than 10% of the children were lead poisoned.) They decided to write a play. Writing the play helped them to describe their own conditions, learn more about lead poisoning, and have fun. In the play, the physician character had to teach a mother about the signs and symptoms of lead poisoning, so the EJYC members had to look this information up. Another character was a lawyer who advised the mother about her rights as a renter. To get their facts straight for their script, they interviewed a law professor. When they performed the play, they received a standing ovation from a room packed with other teenagers from Baltimore. Immediately following the play, the real law professor came on stage to answer questions from the enthusiastic audience.

As children learn about environmental hazards and threats to the earth's ecosystems, they often react with fear and despair (Alimahomed and Keeler, 1995). However, children become less fearful and more hopeful by taking action to address environmental hazards, preserve resources, and protect the health of global and local ecosystems. They gain confidence in their ability to create a healthier environment through managing and minimizing environmental health hazards and through control of their future environment.

Young people are like sponges when it comes to environmental health issues. We just have to allow them to be a little self-directed, especially the adolescents. The National Institutes of Environmental Health Sciences generously supported the EJYC for five years. NIEHS also provided a number of national grants for the development of K–12 environmental health curricula that can be accessed by searching "K–12 education" on the NIEHS web site (www.niehs.nih.gov).

COMMUNITY-BASED ENVIRONMENTAL HEALTH EDUCATION

Environmental health education may go hand-in-hand with a risk communication program because the impetus for either is usually the real or perceived health threat associated with an environmental pollutant. Environmental health education can follow most of the health education and health behavior models, but often the solutions are beyond the purview of individual behavior such that solutions may require community-wide, political, and/or economic approaches. Regardless of the final resolution of an environmental health problem, there are certain basics that are critical to consider when offering or participating in environmental health education.

1. The community should help drive the educational activities.
2. The community should participate in identifying its educational needs.
3. Materials and presentations should be mindful of cultural, language, educational, and literacy issues within the community.

The deficit in our formal education demands that we help community members learn basic environmental health concepts, such as how chemicals get into our bodies and the nature of dose-response, how exposure–health effect relationships are derived, what we know and what we don't know about chemicals and chemical mixtures, and the basics of environmental regulations. In a working-class community in South Baltimore, where a medical waste incinerator was being expanded, the community was very concerned about the trafficking of medical waste through their neighborhood and the health effects associated with the emissions from the incinerator smoke stack. They asked nursing faculty who had worked with them on other issues to help them address their concerns.

A meeting of the community members was organized during which they identified their information needs. By the end of this meeting, information needs and a list of possible experts who could help the community understand the problems were identified. A teach-in was organized in which a combination of informed community members and outside experts gave short talks and then led a discussion on the history of the medical waste facilities; waste management, disposal, and the different environmental aspects of medical waste incineration; and the associated health effects. The outside experts included a university toxicologist, a legal specialist, a waste specialist, a representative from the Health Care Without Harm Campaign (who was a nurse), and a member of Physicians for Social Responsibility. The teach-in was facilitated by the nurse faculty. Because the community helped to frame their educational needs and choose the educators, there was a feeling of empowerment and a comfort level that perhaps would not have existed if they were not the driving force in their own education. The Center for Health and Environmental Justice, a non-profit organization that advocates for communities who are struggling with environmental health issues, provides technical assistance and a wealth of information for community environmental health education. Their materials are written for lay audiences and are extremely helpful (see www. chej.org).

Increasingly we are seeing opportunities for communities to partner with universities to address environmental health issues. Once again, the NIEHS has been a leader in fostering community–university partnerships. They continue to fund community-driven research in which universities work with community members to identify the research questions and methodologies. The EPA is also requiring that community outreach activities be part of their research center awards.

It has been equally important to bring community members into the classrooms of nursing schools so that students can understand the breadth of understanding that invested community members can have about their environmental exposures and the possible health outcomes.

CLINICAL SETTINGS AND ENVIRONMENTAL HEALTH EDUCATION

Too often we lose the opportunity to prevent environmentally related illnesses when we miss the teachable moments in health care delivery settings. For example, pregnant women and new parents are amazingly open to suggestions for how to create the best conditions for their newborns. There are a number of environmental health risks that can be reduced with relatively simple interventions: CO detectors; lead-paint testing and lead-safe nursery renovations; elimination of hazardous pesticides; removal of wall-to-wall carpeting (if possible replace with throw rugs that can be cleaned regularly); observation of fish advisories with regard to fish consumption, especially during pregnancy; review of drinking water status for unhealthy contaminants (check private well or check Consumer Confidence Report, if water is supplied); and, of course, not smoking.

Throughout this book, guidance and resources are provided for a variety of environmental health risks. It will now be up to the individual nurses who are reading it to determine what information should be integrated into their clinical settings. The roadmaps are still pretty uncharted in this area and we welcome and encourage nurses in different subspecialties to consider how to include environmental health considerations in their nursing practice and then to write about it or present it to their professional peers. This is how the field will advance.

NURSING AND ENVIRONMENTAL HEALTH EDUCATION

National Activities

After the publication of the Institute of Medicine Report, *Nursing, Health and the Environment, in 1995*, there was negligible initial response from the federal agencies (HHS, EPA, NIEHS) to support the development of a national strategy to implement the report's recommendations. As a result, individual nurses and others from around the country took the initiative to develop their own activities and to encourage federal agency support. The National Environmental Education and Training Foundation convened a multidisciplinary conference to develop a plan for the integration of environmental health into the health professions. In part as a result of this conference, a comprehensive training and education initiative was developed with the EPA and the Department of Health and Human Services on the diagnosis, treatment, referral, and prevention of pesticide poisoning. This effort has included the publication of the "Recognition and Management of Pesticide Poisoning" (full text can be found at www.epa/pesticides/safety/healthcare/), which serves as a model for the integration of other environmental health issues into health professional education and practice.

The University of Maryland School of Nursing worked with the National Environmental Education and Training Foundation and the Kellogg Foundation to create a faculty development project for nursing faculty on environmental health. Initially, this three-year project has trained over 200 faculty in the southern states, as well as provided several workshops at national nursing subspecialty conferences, such as the American College of Nurse Midwives, the American Public Health Association, and the National Association of School Nurses. The entire faculty workshop can be viewed on the web site that was created for nurses who are interested in environmental health (www.enviRN.umaryland.edu). In addition to viewing the workshop, the web site provides a one-stop shop for nurses about environmental health.

With support from the Agency for Toxic Substances and Disease Registry (ATSDR), several initiatives have been supported. Regional training programs have been convened for practicing nurses and nursing faculty on environmental health associated with Superfund issues. The ATSDR has also produced a two-hour video broadcast for nurses about basic environmental health and nursing concepts. Additionally, it funded Howard University School of Nursing for the Mississippi Delta Project, a curriculum development and training program for nursing school faculty and practicing nurses in and around the Mississippi delta.

The Environmental Protection Agency is now supporting several nursing and environmental health initiatives as well. The National Association of School Nurses is being supported to train school nurses on the reduction of asthma triggers in schools. A new training curriculum has been created that uses many concepts from the EPA's "Tools for Schools Kit." The American Nurses Association (ANA) is funded by the EPA's Office of Child Health Protection to create a series of paper-based and web-based continuing education programs on children's environmental health issues. (See: www.nursingworld.org for the on-line version) As part of the grant to the ANA, several workshops at national conferences will also be convened.

In additional to the recent federal agency and university educational activities, several national, nonprofit organizations have also contributed to the environmental health education of nurses. The Children's Environmental Health Network has created a terrific training manual (www.cehn.org/cehn/trainingmanual/manual-front.html), trained nurses and physicians at national workshops, and convened a number of national conferences. The Network also helped to organize several special issues of *Environmental Health Perspectives* (the official journal of the National Institutes of Environmental Health Science) on children's environmental health that are excellent educational resources for selected science and policy issues.

The national activities of the Health Care Without Harm Campaign have provided a number of educational opportunities for nurses and other health care providers. They have created a number of educational materials (www.noharm.org) and convene national and international conferences. Their materials are excellent resources for the integration of environmental health issues into nursing education because of their immediate relevance to nursing students, both undergraduates and graduates.

EXAMPLES OF SCHOOLS OF NURSING ACTIVITIES

In the short period of time that the University of Maryland has been integrating environmental health into the undergraduate and graduate nursing curriculum, there have been excellent responses from the faculty and students. The following are some examples of how the university has begun the integration. They are intended to provide some food for thought to educators who are reading this book.

In the required undergraduate community health course, a mock hearing has been used as a way of introducing environmental health issues to the students. An introductory lecture is offered on common environmental health risks in homes, schools, workplaces, and the community. The community risks include air and water contamination and other ambient environmental exposures. During their clinical placements students are encouraged to consider the potential for environmental health risks.

The mock hearing is the capstone event for the class. The class is divided into 10 groups of approximately 10 students each. Each semester a new environmental health topic is introduced and the students are assigned roles to play in a mock public hearing on the subject. For instance, during the semester that lead poisoning was the topic, some students played landlords, parents with lead-poisoned children, state regulators, and advocacy organizations. This activity helped the students learn about environmental health problems but also about the incredible complexity of environmental health issues.

Another semester the hearing was focused on creating environmentally healthy hospital settings. The following is a list of the topics about which students had to present. They had to develop policies, propose the cost of implementing the policies, identify the elements of the implementation, and identify the possible barriers to implementation.

1. Create a policy to reduce *latex* exposure in health care (check ANA web site).
2. Create a policy to eliminate *mercury* thermometers and reduce or eliminate other mercury-containing hospital equipment (see www.noharm.org and Health Care Without Harm publications, as well as EPA materials).
3. Create a policy to eliminate *DEHP (Di(Z-ethylhexyl)Pthalate)* use in IV tubing and its impact on health (see www.noharm.org and the National Toxics Program's new position on DEHP).
4. Create a policy to eliminate *PVC plastic* in hospitals (see www.noharm.org and make sure that students review the health effects associated with dioxin [the combustion product created when PVC plastic is incinerated]).
5. Explore waste management policies in the health care settings in which the students work. How can *medical waste* be managed in the hospital in an environmentally sound way? Have the students find out where all the waste goes from their own hospitals—paper, plastic, infectious waste, hazardous chemical waste, kitchen waste, computers (and other electronic equipment), batteries, construction waste. Batteries are particularly interesting because almost all of them are made from toxic metals that create health threats if they are released to the environ-

ment. There are a half dozen ways in which infectious waste can be processed, all of which have pros and cons regarding health risks that they pose. Have students compare and contrast methods focusing on the occupational and environmental health and safety issues as well as costs. Create a policy to manage

6. *sharps-related injuries and illnesses.* Review current policies in the hospital and the new OSHA directives (see the ANA website).

7. Evaluate the extent to which *back injuries* account for lost work days in the health industry (looking at local hospitals and nursing homes) and review the new OSHA Ergonomic Standard. Have the students consider an ideal ergonomic policy for a hospital setting.

8. Review *bloodborne pathogen* policies at local health care facilities. How well are undergraduate nurses prepared regarding their understanding of "universal precautions"? Have them survey other nursing students or medical students (third and fourth year) to see how much training they have had and what they know about the policies. For example, precisely what do you do if you get a "stick" and what are the responsibilities of the hospital?

9. Examine *hepatitis A, B, C* policies in the local hospital setting. What are the worker exposure issues and worker protection policies? What are the postexposure policies? (OSHA, the ANA, and the American Liver Foundation have materials on this).

10. Review the *sterilants and disinfectants* that are used in hospitals, clinics, and nursing homes and their associated health risks. Ethylene oxide (used in autoclaves) and gluteraldehyde are two very toxic chemicals that are commonly used in health care settings. What are the ideal policies to prevent hazardous human exposures? (Check OSHA, ANA, and the National Library of Medicine's Toxnet databases for toxicity info.)

At the graduate level, a new environmental health nursing course has been added to the Masters Degree Program in Community Health Nursing at the University of Maryland. This is a survey course that provides the community health nurse with a framework for assessing and addressing environmental health. One of the most telling exercises that the students do is to identify an article in *Environmental Health Perspectives* that they consider relevant to nursing practice and then to search the nursing literature for any articles on the subject. They very rarely find anything in the nursing literature and quickly realize the necessary work to be done in this new and emerging subject area of environmental health for nurses.

The graduate students in their spring policy course are required to actively follow a bill through the state legislature. There are always environmental bills with health implications and the students have become enthusiastic advocates for the bills they have chosen. A most recent group of students chose to follow a bill that requires the state to collect data on the veterinary use of antibiotics in livestock feed. (Antibiotics are creating the conditions for the development of antibiotic resistant organisms both in the livestock, which becomes our food, and in the environment, including the soil and water.) This is another activity that helps the students learn environmental health science as they learn about the political and economic complexities of environmental health protection. During this process the students may have an opportunity to provide environmental health education to legislators, the press, and the community.

The University of Maryland School of Nursing now has an Environmental Health Track in their Community Health Masters Degree, as well as a new Post Masters Certificate in Environmental Health Nursing. (See: www.enviRN.umaryland.edu)

CONCLUSION

Nurses, whether practicing in a clinical setting, community setting, or educational settings have a wonderful opportunity to be creative and to develop environmental health education activities. With the advent of the Worldwide web, we all have access to extraordinary resources, including resources on environmental health. The nursing profession provides a perfect vehicle for environmental health education to be delivered to individual patients and to whole communities.

REFERENCES

Alimahomed, S., & Keeler, B. (1995). The role in creating a healthy future for the earth: An examination of the link between collective action for the environment and the emotional health of children. *Environmental Health Perspectives, 103*(Suppl. 6), 63–66.

EPA (1995). Indoor Air Quality. Tools for Schools; Action kit: Document # EPA 402-k-95-001 2nd Ed.

CHAPTER 26

Advocating for Environmental Justice: Protecting Vulnerable Communities from Pollution

Dorothy Powell and Diann Slade

Fair treatment means that no group of people should bear a disproportionate share of negative environmental conse- quences resulting from industrial, municipal, and commercial operations or the execution of federal, state, local, and tribal programs and policies.

Environmental Protection Agency, 1997

Environmental justice was a term coined in the early 1990s to denote the application of fair strategies and processes in the resolution of inequality related to environmental contamination. The fact that such a term exists suggests several things: (1) that we as a nation have done things to our environment that place people at risk; (2) that remedies have been enacted to rectify environmental contamination and the associ- ated threats to health and well-being; and (3) that all people have not been treated the same when it comes to enacting these remedies. Minorities and low income communities face a much higher level of environmental expo- sure and risk than majority populations, especially in the areas of haz- ardous waste disposal, transport, and containment. As a result, these communities bear a disproportionate share of the nation's air, water, and waste contamination problems (Gaylord, 1993). For instance, the largest hazardous waste facility in the United States is located in Emelle, AL, a poor, predominately African-American community. It receives toxic materials from forty-five states and several foreign countries. Similarly, along the 2,000 mile U.S.-Mexico border are canals black with dangerous chemicals, where waste management is almost nonexistent, and where tires, plastics, and unknown chemical waste are burned in dumps and backyards (Motavalli, 2000).

The purpose of this chapter is to elevate consciousness among nurses about environmental justice and the opportunities and imperatives for advocacy with communities that disproportionately carry the burden of discrimination from unfair environmental decisions. This chapter establishes a context of environmental contamination in this country, followed by a description of how contamination, historically and currently, is unequally addressed. Further, it describes the movement that propelled injustices to the forefront of national policy. Findings from key federal and nonfederal studies that document environmental injustices and their impact on the health of individuals and communities are explained. Federal and state responses to actual and potential injustices, through the creation of federal agencies and the passage of federal and state laws, are chronicled. Last, the chapter discusses various advocacy strategies that nurses, nursing groups, and coalitions might adopt in addressing environmental injustice with communities.

SETTING THE CONTEXT OF ENVIRONMENTAL CONTAMINATION

Every industrialized country on the face of the globe has the continuing challenge of how to dispose of trash and waste products. Historically, the remedy was to burn it, bury it, or dump it, with little consideration for the potential implications for future generations. The "chemical revolution" of the 1940s and 1950s ushered in the production of potentially toxic and radioactive substances, including munitions associated with World War II. These substances posed potential threats to health and well-being for decades and centuries to come. Workers in the defense industry and communities neighboring manufacturing facilities were exposed to highly radioactive substances, their byproducts, and the waste discharged into the air, soil, and water systems bordering plants and reservations where the chemicals were produced (Freeze, 2000).

The chemical revolution led to the manufacture of miracle drugs, more effective solvents, adhesives, dyes, paints, and wood preservatives (Freeze, 2000), now known to have highly toxic effects. The use of fertilizers, such as DDT, and pesticides to enhance plant growth had, paradoxically, the unfortunate effect of polluting the environment and placing farm workers who labored in the fields at risk.

Industrialization led to an era of mass production, packaging, and the creation of disposable containers made of glass, paper products, and, ultimately, plastics. Automobile tires, for instance, became a major source of noxious fumes and toxins when disposed of by burning. Ours became a throwaway society that created trash in exponential quantities. The open burning of trash piles and later incinerators, waste dumps, and landfills grew in relation to the growing consumption of disposable products by the American people. During the 1950s and 1960s, there were few, if any, controls or standards for emission into the environment. The burning of hazardous and nonhazardous waste created unknown risks to the people who lived within reach of fumes and particulates as they dissipated in the atmosphere.

INEQUALITY IN ENVIRONMENTAL CONTAMINATION AND REMEDIATION

More than 1327 Superfund sites were identified by 1992 (www.boma. org\suprissa.htm) with a disproportionate number located in poor or minority communities (Government Accounting Office, 1995; United Church of Christ Commission on Racial Justice, 1987). Despite federal efforts to clean up evidence of prior contamination, to impose strict standards on emissions from industrial sites, and to enact safeguards to protect the public in the siting of industrial and waste treatment facilities, the net effect has not been and continues not to be equitable across all racial and socioeconomic classes. Poor and minority communities experience a disproportionately heavier burden from environmental contamination than more affluent and nonminority communities (Bullard, 1990, 1993, 1994; Department of Justice, 2000; Gaylord, 1993; Levine, Epelbaum, Nelson-Knuckles, et al., 1997; USEPA 1992, 1997; Wigley and Shrader-Frechette, 2000). Race is the most significant factor associated with the location of hazardous waste sites. Low income and minority groups are also more likely than affluent and nonminority groups to live near landfills, incinerators, and hazardous waste treatment facilities (United Church of Christ, 1987) and eat contaminated fish (Calderon, et al., 1993; USEPA, 1992) Three out of four southern waste dumps are located in African-American communities (Government Accounting Office, 1983; Heitgerd, Burg, and Strickland, 1995). Other data show that a significantly higher percentage of minority populations live in communities with commercial hazardous waste facilities and near NPL sites than nonminority populations (Powell, 1999). Three of the largest hazardous waste landfills, containing more than 40% of the total national permitted commercial capacity, remain in two African-American communities, supporting the notion that "waste tends to flow toward communities with weak response capacity" (Heiman, 2000). Many Superfund sites are located in or close by residential areas populated by ethnic minorities and people in the lowest economic stratum (Hirschhorn, 2000). Kelly (2000) reported that even when income is controlled, race continues to be a significant factor in the siting of waste facilities, particularly hazardous and nuclear facilities. Additionally, middle-class communities of color tend to have more waste facilities than poor white communities.

This phenomenon has been described as *environmental discrimination* or *environmental racism* (Bullard, 1990, 1993; Russell, 1989) and substantiates that past environmental practices, policies, and decisions were not fair. Weintraub (2000) notes that environmental racism is "the intentional siting of hazardous waste sites, landfills, incinerators, and polluting industries in communities inhabited mainly by African American, Hispanics, Native Americans, Asians, migrant farm workers, and the working poor."

While discrimination is often a challenge to prove, it is clear that low income and disadvantaged communities and populations are exposed and susceptible to hazardous substances to a greater degree than the population as a whole (Sexton, 1993,1997; Zimmerman, 1993, 1997). Susceptibility may be a function of minority communities being perceived as powerless. Communities known as passive, lacking political power, not well informed, unorganized, and with "an eager and docile work force" (Bullard, 1990; Weintraub, 2000) are the most likely targets for environmental contamination and abuse, and the least likely to receive remediation once dangers to the community are noted (Lavella and Coyle, 1992). Consistent with these findings, Heiman (2000) suggests that politics, demographic shifts, corruption, economics, permitting of fraud, discrimination, and weak community response capacity are at the root of decisions to site hazardous facilities in poor and minority areas.

Examples of environmental racism provide the most convincing evidence of unfair, intentional, and discriminatory decision making and/or neglect in the siting of toxic and other waste facilities. Such examples are reflective of the fate of Chester, Pennsylvania, and Alsen and Covent, Louisiana. Chester, a former industrial urban center, changed from 20% to 65% minority between 1950 and 1980 as the city decayed following the decline in the steel industries. It left in its wake the rise of new industries specializing in waste management. Chester has the fourth largest garbage-burning incinerator in the nation located directly across the street from residential housing; the largest infectious and chemotherapeutic medical waste autoclave in the nation; and a sewage treatment facility (DELCORA) handling 90% of the sewage from Delaware County and from refineries including Sunoco, British Petroleum, and Scott Paper. Chester also has the largest infant mortality and low birth weight rates in the state, a lung cancer rate 60% higher than other areas in Delaware County, and an unacceptably high blood lead level among 60% of the city's children (Ewell, 2000). Alsen and Covent are low-income communities of 1,500 that are 98.9% African-American with 65% unemployment. They house the fourth largest hazardous waste landfill in the U.S., 10 chemical plants, a plastics plant, lead smelters, landfills, tank car washers, petroleum coke yards, and two Superfund sites. In Covent, where plants were cited as violating federal environmental laws 100 times between 1980 and 1985, the average resident is exposed to 4,517 lb of toxic chemical releases per year compared to an average American level of 10 lb (Motavalli, 2000).

ENVIRONMENTAL JUSTICE

In an effort to address evidence of racism in environmental decision making and the disproportionate burden of contamination in communities of color, *environmental justice* became a part of the federal jargon in the early 1990s. During this period, the EPA Office on Environmental Equity was established, followed by the Office of Environmental Justice in 1992. In 1994, the National Environmental Justice Advisory Council (NEJAC) was founded to provide independent advice, consultation, and recommendations to the administrator of the EPA on environmental issues. In 1991, the first National People of Color Environmental Leadership Summit was held and affirmed through principles and strategies that environmental justice must ensure that all people should have an opportunity to live in a healthy environment and are entitled to breathe clean air, drink clean water, and consume uncontaminated foods (First National People of Color Environmental Leadership Summit, 1991).

THE ENVIRONMENTAL JUSTICE MOVEMENT

This federal response to evidence of environmental injustices and the potential for injustice, however, did not emerge voluntarily but was preceded by a grass-roots movement nestled within the civil rights movement of the late 1960s. A series of significant protests and displays of civil disobedience was staged to demonstrate public outrage at the consequences or intended consequences of environmental decisions or prevailing practices that placed people of color at significant risk. In 1967, students at predominately black Texas Southern University in Houston demonstrated following the drowning of an 8-year-old girl in a garbage dump where she played at a site unprotected and undeterred by a fence or warning signs. A year later in 1968, Martin Luther King, Jr. led a campaign for better working conditions for largely African-American garbage workers in Memphis, Tennessee. The handling of undifferentiated waste placed these workers at heightened risk for exposure to toxic substances.

The most widely recognized protest against a deliberate action of injustice occurred in 1982 in Warren County, North Carolina. Bullard (1990) recounts in detail how more than 32,000 cubic yards of soil contaminated with highly toxic PCBs (polychlorinated biphenyls) were dumped by a private trucking company along the roadway in 14 North Carolina counties in 1978. This act was later found to be illegal, the perpetrators jailed, and an EPA-mandated cleanup begun some four years later. The governor of North Carolina chose to bury the contaminated oils in the Afton community of Warren County, which was 84% African-American and one of the poorest counties in the state. Despite strong evidence that the site for the intended landfill was scientifically unsuitable and that the toxic chemicals would certainly over time leach into well water, the process of transferring nearly 6,000 truckloads of the chemical began in 1982. More than 400 protestors who lay across the highway to block the trucks were arrested. Despite broad national attention to this unfair and unfounded site for disposal of a highly toxic chemical, the demonstrators failed to block the creation of this egregious landfill (Bullard, 1990). The tremendous media attention surrounding the North Carolina incident no doubt gave impetus to ensuing federal responses.

Powell (1999) chronicles the salient milestones propelling environmental justice to a prominent position on the federal agenda. In 1983, a year after the PCB incident in North Carolina, the Government Accounting Office issued a landmark report documenting that three out of four of the largest operating hazardous waste sites in the U.S. were located in southern African-American communities (EPA, 1992). In 1985, the first African-American environmental organization, The Center for Environment, Commerce and Energy, was founded. In the same year, the National Council of Churches'

Eco-Justice working group began addressing environmental issues.

FEDERAL ENVIRONMENTAL JUSTICE LEGISLATION

Federal legislation in response to a growing awareness of the inequities of environmental contamination in communities of color and poor communities was passed, beginning with the landmark Superfund legislation of 1986. In 1993, the Environmental Justice Act, the Environmental Equal Rights Act, the Environmental Health Equity Act, and the Waste Export and Import Prohibition Act were enacted.

The Environmental Justice Act of 1993 directs the EPA to publish a list, in rank order, of the total weight of toxic chemicals released in each county or other geographic unit in the most recent five-year period for which there are available data. The act requires that potential health effects be identified and that remedies be legislated. (See [www.nativenet.uthscsa.edu/archive/nl/9311/0125.html].)

The Environmental Equal Rights Act of 1993 (H.R. 1924) gives "citizens of a state the right to petition to prevent the siting and construction of proposed polluting facilities scheduled to be placed in 'environmentally disadvantaged' communities" (Jewish Council for Public Affairs, 1994–1995). For the purpose of this act, environmentally disadvantaged communities are defined as communities that already have a similar facility, located within two miles of a proposed facility, and have a specific demographic mix of minority and low-income residents.

The Environmental Health Equity Act of 1994 (H.R. 1925) mandates data collection by the EPA on race, income, gender, ethnic origin and education level in communities adjacent to toxic sites (JCPA, 1994–1995).

The Hazardous and Additional Waste Export and Import Act of 1991 prohibits the export of waste to countries opposed to waste and countries that will manage waste in an environmentally unsound manner. The Act enjoins the export and import of hazardous and some nonhazardous waste, such as municipal solid waste, municipal incinerator ash, and infectious waste. However, the act permits some exceptions to the provisions when bilateral agreements exist between the United States and the receiving or sending country on waste management and with the consent for shipment by any transit countries. Other exemptions are included on recycling certain radioactive and spent nuclear materials not defined under other legislation (rs9.loc.gov/cgi-bin/query/z?r102:E20MY1-187).

Executive Order 12898, signed by President Clinton in 1994, mandates that federal agencies make environmental justice part of their mission by identifying and addressing disproportionately high and adverse human health or environmental health effects of their programs, policies, and activities with minority populations. Also, the Order requires that meaningful opportunities be provided for the involvement of communities in the development of, compliance with, and enforcement of federal laws, regulations and policies pertaining to human health and the environment regardless of race, color, national origin, or income (Report to the President on Executive Order 12898; USEPA, 1995, pp. 6–9).

The level of a community's participation in environmental legislation depends on its awareness, sophistication, sense of power, economic base, organizational skills, and access to knowledge. The community's affiliations and networks are, critical indicators of its performance when threatened by an environmental issue and are useful predictors success of its response to immediate and long-term implications of environmental decision making (Bullard, 1990). The resources of poor and minority communities are often undermatched when faced with contrary intentions of big business and developers.

Poor and minority communities are less likely than more affluent communities to know and understand environmental laws and regulations, to have access to environmental data, and to use such data in seeking remedies where there is an excess of environmental toxins. These communities are less likely to be aware of the hazard associated with specific environmental toxins and the long-term impact on health of generations to come. Such communities are also less likely to respond to environmental concerns arising out of industrial abuse or proposed citing of plants with the potential to pollute. Fear of reprisal, the need for employment, and economic stability are often priorities over the threat to health. Cultural habits and the vestiges of a subservient mentality (Lassiter, 1999) contribute to a sense of powerlessness and inactivity in the face of real environmental concerns.

ADVOCACY STRATEGIES

Nurses can assist in leveling the playing field through their role as advocates. Nurses have a historical presence in the types of communities where instances of environmental injustice are most likely to occur. Through roles as public and community health nurses, long-existing and trusted relationships have developed and constitute the basis by which nurses can help empower communities to better represent themselves in matters of actual and potential environmental contamination. Nurses are trusted and well respected as sources of information and inspirers of positive health behaviors (Lipscomb, 1994; Salazar and Primomo, 1994; Tiedje and Wood, 1995). Thus, all nurses, but most especially those working in community-based settings need to be well equipped with advocacy strategies, an understanding of and sensitivity to environmental issues, and effective assessment skills.

There are two major types of advocacy; case advocacy and class advocacy. The former involves actions taken on behalf of individual patients and is generally associated with the role that nurses play by acting on behalf of patients or representing them when they are unable to do so for themselves (Powell, 1999). Class advocacy is aimed at changing conditions that are detrimental to populations. It involves such strategies as lobbying, use of media, mediation, expert testimony, and community organizing.

The effective use of any of these advocacy skills is predicated on several basic nursing practices.

- Acute *observational skills* are essential. Seeing instances of environmental injustice and not really seeing them is a common practice among people who grow up in communities where the presence of inequities is perceived as "just the way it is." Historical demarcations that separated communities along racial lines continue to be part of the U.S. culture, despite decades of efforts for full integration and laws that make racial separation in housing and access to housing illegal. In the South, poor and African-American communities were commonly referred to as those communities "on the wrong side of the tracks," making reference to where the train tracks divided privileged from underprivileged neighborhoods. The underprivileged neighborhoods were the sites most likely to house the trash disposal facilities, the waste treatment plants, and the smoke stack industries, while the privileged communities were characterized by green lawns and stately residences. Observing these differences without recognizing the prevailing value systems that contributed to these demarcations begins to explain, in part, the context of environmental discrimination. Nurses' observational skills, which involve, need to be sufficiently acute to perceive the differences that exist and to recognize potential threats to health.
- *A questioning mind* is critical to identifying threats to communities and assessing the level of community awareness about potential instances of environmental contamination, sources of contamination, and patterns of health concerns. It is not uncommon that community residents are unaware of potential threats to their health related to the emission of

certain chemicals into their environment. There is often an unquestioning level of trust among communities; a belief that local and federal standards that regulate environmental emissions are properly and consistently followed. Where health advisories may be posted, there may be a lack of full community compliance due to knowledge deficits. For instance, community members may continue to fish in bodies of water polluted with PCBs, believing that cleaning fish or adding such condiments as vinegar or wine will negate the effect of the chemical (Slade, 2001) Nurses need to have an investigative mind and use a scientific approach when determining if potential problems exist in communities. Nurses need to be competent in conducting environmental assessments and taking exposure histories. Knowing how to access data from public documents and through various Internet environmental resources is important to substantiating evidence of chemical releases or the potential of such releases within communities. Skills in questioning and collaborating with other health and environmental personnel are likewise important in substantiating evidence of environmental threats. Also, knowledge of environmental laws and regulations is fundamental to making judgments relative to the degree of protection that should exist for communities.

- *Political astuteness* is an essential competency for nurses engaged in advocacy. This means knowing how the legislative system works and the points of influence. It also means being able to sway decision making through formal and informal processes. Formal influence include voting, providing testimony, and writing position papers. Informal influence occurs through social relationships and networks, the power that comes from building indebtedness (such as through volunteering and supporting political campaigns), affect over blocks of votes, and similar quid pro quo circumstances. Communities that are often victimized by environmental injustices are perceived as powerless because they lack substantial monetary resources, have high unemployment rates, are uninformed or underinformed about the issues and their rights, and tend not to vote (Bullard, 1990). Nurses can help communities to become more powerful and influential by providing information, facilitating coalition building, and helping organize and recognize rights and potential.

- *Cultural sensitivity and cultural competency* are important perspectives that nurses engaged in community-based work and advocacy must possess. To be helpful to communities, nursing activities need to be within the context of the communities' orientation and consistent with their values and priorities. This level of awareness, competence, and comfort is learned either by deliberate actions or result from the nurse's own cultural orientation. Openness to seeking the communities' perspectives and respecting those perspectives is critical. Care to not let one's own sense of ethnocentricity interfere is an important balancing phenomenon. Awareness of one's own culture is an essential first step, followed by the need to know and understand the other's culture (Purnell and Paullanka, 1998). Respect for differences is critical when helping communities develop capacities to address their environmental concerns. Helping communities through information sharing, supporting them through decision making, and adapting services to be congruent with their orientation are important steps in empowering them to address the toxic challenges that may confront them. It is also important for the nurse in his or her potential role as an intermediary to be sensitive to the cultural difference that may exist between communities targeted for potentially harmful industrial/economic development and profit-driven entrepreneurs who may select for industrial siting what are believed to be powerless communities with low skills and high unemployment (Bullard, 1990).

Common advocacy strategies include the following.

- *Lobbying* is defined as acts aimed at influencing and promoting legislation and/or encouraging the enforcement of laws, rules, and regulations. This may take the form of letter writing, face-to-face meetings with legislators or their staff, formal and informal social interactions, and other such activities. Objective data and evidence born out of specific examples from the communities are compelling arguments when lobbying. Elected officials tend to respond to issues that particularly affect their power base. Politicians are often influenced by circumstances that favor their election and approval ratings.
- *Media* are possibly the most dominant sources of information and influence. Nurses are highly respected as sources of information. Nurses interested in working with communities in an advocacy capacity would be well served to take media training. Armed with knowledge of environmental issues, the public's trust, and competency with handling the media, nurses are an extremely important source of information and influence. Examples of actual cases or situations do much to influence politicians and other local, regional, and federal officials to act.

- *Mediation* is the act of arbitrating opposing opinions of persons or groups of persons for the purpose of facilitating resolution of their differences. This might take the form of problem solving with community members and the producers of toxic discharge. Some basic skills include facilitating group dialogue and the logical steps of decision making and conflict resolution. Objectivity, impartiality, and neutrality are critical characteristics of a mediator. It is the group, not the mediators that reaches solutions, although the mediator may suggest creative and reasonable ideas for consideration in facilitating the process.

- *Expert testimony* occurs when nurses give evidence out of their professional knowledge and scope of responsibilities about the impact or implications of some phenomenon, such as contamination, on human health. Maintaining records on observations, environmental exposure histories, and environmental assessments collected within the context of the nurse's scope of practice can provide data from which the nurse can profile the community and draw inferences about the health status of its members. Given their knowledge and experience, nurses can play a critical role in hearings and litigation where environmental injustices have been charged.

- *Community organizing* involves bringing together cross-sections of community residents and building coalitions for strategic problem solving. In coalition building, citizen groups, professional groups, and other key stakeholders and supporters partner around common interest and concerns. Citizen participation and partnerships are essential for community growth and development and response to real and potential threats. Communities with fewer resources and weaker linkages with dominant and more powerful communities are vulnerable for exploitations (Lassiter, 1999; von Bertalanffy, 1952; Warren, 1963). Strengthening the knowledge base and self-advocacy strategies, coalescing disparate formal and informal groups, and broadening the economic and political power bases enable communities to address and respond to actual and potential circumstances of environmental injustices. Nurses are in a position to facilitate strengthening communities and building coalitions based on existing relationships with community members and potential networks with resources and power. In order to assist communities in addressing injustice issues, nurses need basic principles and the knowledge and skills fundamental to working with communities, including community development and community empowerment.

- *Program development* involves organizing and instituting educational programs in response to identified community needs. Program development and implementation can be effective due to the knowledge base of nurses and their role as teachers. Responding to community needs by offering health awareness, health promotion, and health education is of considerable value in empowering communities to address issues of environmental injustice. Developing and providing an educational program for citizens to make them aware of potential toxic emissions from manufacturing plants situated in their community and the relationship of the toxins to health and disease is an example of an important class advocacy strategy.
- *Protest* has historically facilitated many major societal changes and, as such, is an effective class advocacy strategy. Indeed, environmental justice is rooted in the civil rights movement and peaceful protest. Successful protests are well planned, involve coalitions, attract media attention, and have an impact on the operations, productivity, or economics of the targeted organization. Civil demonstrations must be organized and executed in accordance with the local laws that govern the right of American citizens to protest. Because protest is an adversarial strategy that makes a statement about one position against another prevailing set of principles or practices, care must be taken to act in ways to ensure the safety of protestors and property. Nurses can play meaningful roles in protests from assistance in organizing to being expert speakers at rallies to providing supportive health care services.

Environmental inequities disproportionately threaten the health and well being of far too many poor and minority citizens, as well as communities deemed powerless, ill informed, and economically depressed. Environmental justice is a goal by which inequalities can be minimized and health disparities diminished. Well-informed nurses using the vast array of environmental resources and networks can assist vulnerable communities to address real and potential environmental threats. Nursing advocacy is a fundamental nursing role that takes on great significance when applied to communities facing environmental threats. The strategies and knowledge base described in this chapter are tangible tools and resources to empower nurses and vulnerable populations in their efforts to achieve the goal of environmental justice for all.

REFERENCES AND BIBLIOGRAPHY

AAEA (2001). Maryland loses Clean Air Enforcement Authority to Fed. Retrieved

December 16, 2001 from MSN On line Web: http://communities.msn. com/aaea/maryland.msnw.

Agency for Toxic Substances and Disease Registry: Child Health Initiative: Presidential Executive Order 13045. (1997) *Protection of Children from Environmental Health Risks and Safety Risks* [announcement; online]. Washington, DC, William J. Clinton, April 21, 1997. Available: http://www. atsdr.gov/child/press497.html [March 3, 2001].

American Lung Association. (2001). Minority Lung Disease Data 2000-Focus: Asthma. Retrieved December 18, 2001 from American On line Web: http://www.lungusa.org/pub/minority/asthma_00.html

American Public Health Association (1997). *Community-base environmental health: Assembling the evidence and coordinating the plan.* CE Institute No. 1, November 8, 1997, p. 81.

Bullard, R. D. (1990). *Dumping in Dixie: Race, class, and environmental quality.* Boulder, CO: Westview Press.

Bullard, R. D. (Ed.). (1993). *Confronting environmental racism: Voices from the Grassroots.* Boston: South End Press.

Bullard, R. D. (Ed.). (1994). *Unequal protection: Environmental justice and communities of color.* San Francisco: Sierra Club Books.

Centers for Disease Control and Prevention, Office of the Associate Director for Minority Health. (1995). *Minority health is the health of the nation.* Atlanta, GA: CDC.

Community Center Environmental Justice Passaic county Report Distribution of Risks (2001). Distribution of Risks by Race/Ethnicity and Income In New Jersey. [On-line]. Available: http://www.scorecard.org/community/ej-risk.tcl?ftps_state_ code=34&ftps_county_code=3.

Chiras, D. D. (1994). *Environmental science: Action for a sustainable future.* Redwood City, CA: Benjamin/Cummings Publishing.

Department of Justice. (2000). *Guidance concerning environmental justice.* Available: http://www.usdoj.gov./enrd/ejguide.html.

Environment Protection Agency (EPA). (1997). Envirofacts Warehouse Homepage. [on-line]. Available: http://www.epa.gov/enviro

Environment Protection Agency (EPA) (2001). National Priority Site Fact Sheet. [on-line]. Available: http://www.epa.gov/region02/superfnd/site_sum/0202931c. htm

Ewell, M. (2000). *Environmental racism in Chester.* Available: http://www.pen-wed.org/chester/ewell_article.html.

Ewell, M. (2002). *Guidance concerning environmental justice.* Available: http://www.penwed.org/chester/ewell_article.html.

Executive Order No. 12898, 59 C.F.R. 7629 (February 16, 1994). Washington, DC: *Federal Register.* Vol. 59. No. 32.

First National People of Color Environmental Leadership Summit. (1991, October 24–27). *Principles of environmental justice.* Washington, DC.

Freeze, R. A. (2000). *The environmental pendulum: A quest for the truth about toxic chemicals, human health, and environmental protection.* Berkeley: University of California Press.

Gaylord, C. (1993). Environmental equity and empowerment. In *Patriots: Black History Commemorative Edition.* Silver Spring, MD.

Goldman, B. A. & Fitton, L. (1993). *Toxic waste and race revisted: An update of the 1987 report of racial and socioeconomic characteristics of communities with hazardous waste sites.* Washington, DC: The Center for Policy Alternatives, National Center for the Advancement of Colored People, and United Church of Christ Commission on Racial Justice.

General Accounting Office (1983). *Siting of Hazardous Waste Landfills and Their Correlation With Racial and Economic Status of Surrounding Communities.* Washington, DC: GAO.

Government Accounting Office. (1995). *Hazardous and nonhazardous wastes: Demographics of people living near waste facilities.* Washington, DC: Author.

Heiman, M. K. (2000). *Race, waste, and class: New perspectives on environmental justice.* Environmental Studies, James Center, Dickerson College, Carlisle, PA: http://www.penweb.org/er/rwc.html.

Heitgerd, J., Burg, J., & Strickland, H. (1995). A geographic information systems approach to estimating and assessing national priority lists site demographics: Racial and Hispanic origin composition. *International Journal of Occupational Medicine and Toxicology, 95*(4), 343–363.

Hirschhorn, J. S. (2000). *Two Superfund environmental justice case studies.* Wheaton, MD: Hirschhorn & Associates. Available: http://www.igc.org/envjustice/hirschhorn.html.

Jacobson, J. L., Jacobson, S. W. & Humphrey, H. E. B. (1990) Effects of in utero exposure to polychlorinated biphenyls and related contaminants on cognitive functioning in young children. *Journal of Pediatrics.* Vol. 116 (1), pp. 38.

Kelly, M. (2000). *Thc history of Chester.* http://www.penweb.org/chester.html.

Lassiter, P. G. (1996). *Group approaches in community health.* In M. Stanhope & J. Lancaster, (Eds) Community health nursing: Promoting the health of aggregates, families and individuals. (4th ed.). (pp. 433–448). St. Louis, MO: Mosby.

Lassiter, P. G. (1999). Community perspectives as related to community organizations: Empowerment, partnering and education. In Howard University Division of Nursing, *Environmental health and nursing: The mississippi delta project, a modular curriculum.* Atlanta, GA: U.S. Department of Health and Human Services, ATSDR.

Lavelle, M., and Coyle, M,. (1992). *Unequal protection: The racial divide in environmental law.* The National Law Journal, September 21, 1992.

Levine, R., Epelbaum, M., Nelson-Knuckles, B., et al. (1997). *Preliminary mortality and morbidity profile of the Mississippi Delta Region.* Unpublished manuscript. Meharry Medical College, Division of Preventive Medicine, Nashville, TN.

Levine, R., Epelbaum, M., Nelson-Knuckles, B., Meltzer, A., Pellet, H. & Knuckles, M. E. (1997a). *Preliminary mortality and morbitiy profile of the Mississippi Delta Region.* Unpublished manuscript, Nashville, TN: Meharry Medical College, Division of Preventive Medicine.

Levine, R., Epelbaum, M., Nelson-Knuckles, B., Meltzer, A., Pellet, H. & Knuckles, M. E. (1997b). *A sociodemographic and health profile of the Misssissippi Delta Region.* Unpublished manuscript, Nashville, TN: Meharry Medical College Division of Preventive Medicine.

Motavalli, J. (2000). *Toxic targets: Polluters that dump on communities of color are finally being brought to justice.* Available: http://penweb.org/ej/Estory.html.

National Council for Jewish Affairs (2000). *Jewish security and the bill of rights.* Available: http://www.jewishpublicaffairs.org/publications/JPP_94-95_security_environment.html.

Needleman, H. L. (1997). Lead exposure and antisocial behavior: A neglected effect. In Conference Report, *Children's Environmental Health: Research, Practice, and Prevention Policy.* Children's Environmental Health Network/Public Policy Institute.

New Jersey Work Environment Council. (2001). Available: www.njwec.org /alert%20environmental%20racism.htm.

Pollution Locator Environmental Release Report (2001). *Environmental Release Report: Indian River Power Plant.* [On-line]. Available: http://www.scorecard.org/env-releases/facility.tcl? tri_id=19966NDNRVRTE33.

Pope, A. M., Synder, M. A., & Mood, L. A. (Eds) (1995). *Nursing, health, and environment: Strengthening the relationships to improve the public's health.* Washington, DC: National Academy Press.

Powell, D. L. (1999). Environmental justice, In Howard University Division of Nursing, *Environmental health and nursing, The Mississippi Delta Project, a modular curriculum.* Atlanta, GA: U.S. Department of Health and Human Services, ATSDR.

Powell, D., Stewart, V. (Eds). (2001). Pediatric clinics of North America. *Children's Environmental Health, 48*(5), 1291–1305.

Purnell, L., & Paullanka, B. (1998). *Transcultural health care: A culturally competent approach.* Philadelphia, PA: F. A. Davis.

Report to the president on executive order 12898. (1994, February 16). (Executive order no. 12898, 59 C.F.R. 7629).

Russell, D. (1989). Environmental racism: Minority communities and their battle against toxic. *Amicus Journal, 11*(2), 22–32.

Schettler, T., Stein, J., Reich, F., & Valenti, M. (2000). *In harm's way: Toxic threats to child development.* Cambridge, MA: Greater Boston. Physicians for Sound Responsibility.

Sexton, K. & Zimmerman, R. (2000). The emerging role of environmental justice in decision making. In Sexton, K. Marcus, A. A., Easter, W., et al. *Better*

Environmental decision: strategies for governments, Businesses and communities. 419–443.

Slade, D. (2001). *Fishing in the Anacostia River.* Unpublished manuscript, Howard University: Division of Nursing.

Sterling, D. A., Roengner, K. C., Lewis, R. D., Luke, D. A., Wilder, L. C., Burchette, S. M. (1999). Evaluation of four sampling methods for determining exposure of children to lead-contaminated household dust. *Environmental Research.* 1999 Aug: 81(2): 130–41.

United Church of Christ Commission on Racial Justice. (1987). Toxic waste and race in the United States: A national study of racial and socio-economic characteristics of communities with hazardous waste sites. New York: *American Journal of Public Health, 87*(5), 731.

United States Environmental Protection Agency. (1992). *Environmental equity: Reducing risk for all communities* (Vols. 1–2). Washington, DC: Office of Solid Waste and Emergency Response.

United States Environmental Protection Agency (EPA). (1994). *Serving a diverse society: EPA's role in environmental justice.* (EPA Publication No. 200-F-93-001). Washington, DC: US Environmental Protection Agency.

United States Environmental Protection Agency (EPA). (1995). *Environmental justice 1994 annual report: Focusing on environmental protection for all people.* (EPA Publication No. 200-R-95003). Washington, DC: US Environmental Protection Agency.

Von Bertalanffy, L. (1952). *Problems of life: An evaluation of modern biological and scientific thought.* New York: Harper.

Vyner, H. M. (1988). *Invisible trauma: The psychosocial effects of invisible environmental contaminants.* Massachusetts: Lexington Books.

Warren, R. L. (1963). *The community in America* (2nd ed.). Chicago: Rand McNally.

Weintraub, I. (2000). *Fighting environmental racism: A selected annotated bibliography.* Library of Science and Medicine, Rutgers University. Available: http://egj.lib.uniaho.edu/egj01/wein01.html

Wigley, D. C., & Shrader-Frechette, K. (2000). *Environmental racism and biased methods of risk assessment.* Available: http://www.fplc.edu/RISK/vol7/winter/wigley.html

Calderon (1993). Presently searching for complete citation.
Tiedje & Wood (1995). Presently searching for complete citation.
Salzar & Primomo (1994). Presently searching for complete citation.

Other Internet Resources

http://communities.msn.com/aaea
http://www.census.gov
http://www.epa.gov/region02/superfnd/site_sum/0202931c.html
www.nativenet.uthscsa.edu/archive/nl/9311/0125.html

www.scorecard.org/cummunity/ej_summary.tcl?fips_county_code=10005#dist
www.scorecard.org/env-release/facility.tcl?tri_id=19966DNRVRTE33
www.scorecard.org/env-release/state.tcl?fips_state_code

CHAPTER 27

Conclusion

Barbara Sattler

W e are living in a time of incredible possibilities. We are also living in a time of troubling contradictions. So many of our essential practices—energy production, food production, transportation, and even the provision of health services—are not sustainable, not compatible with a healthy environment and thereby healthy people. Nurses, as the foot soldiers and generals in the defense of our public's health, have the potential to lead our patients and communities, our policy-makers and elected officials to a new way of seeing the relation between our life's choices, both individual and societal, and their impact on health.

The authors hope that this book has helped the reader explore some of the environmental health risks posed in our workplaces, homes, schools, and communities. Gaining information about such risks is the first step towards integrating environmental health principles and actions into our nursing practices. Dr. Claudia Smith, in her community health text, *Contemporary Problems in Community Health Nursing*, has developed a set of suggested points of integration in a framework of primary, secondary, and tertiary prevention.

PREVENTION INTERVENTIONS FOR ENVIRONMENTAL SAFETY AND HEALTH

PRIMARY PREVENTION

- Advocate safer environmental design of products, automobiles, equipment, and buildings.
- Teach home safety related to falls and fire prevention, especially to families with children and elderly members.

- Counsel women of childbearing age regarding exposure to environmental hazards.
- Advocate vehicle protection systems, such as seat belts.
- Advocate use of protective devices, such as earplugs for noise.
- Immunize occupationally exposed workers for hepatitis.
- Develop worksite health and safety programs.
- Develop programs to prevent back injuries at work.
- Support the development of exposure standards for toxins.
- Support disclosure of radon and lead concentrations in homes at time of sale.
- Advocate for safe air and water.
- Teach avoidance of ultraviolet exposure and use of sunscreen.
- Advocate for waste reduction and effective waste management.
- Support programs for waste reduction and recycling.

SECONDARY PREVENTION

- Assess homes, schools, worksites, and communities for environmental hazards.
- Routinely obtain occupational health histories for individuals, counsel about hazard reduction, and refer for diagnosis and treatment.
- Screen children from 6 months to 5 years for blood lead levels.
- Monitor workers for levels of chemical exposure.
- Screen at-risk workers for lung disease, cancer, and hearing loss.
- Participate in data collection regarding the incidence and prevalence of injury and disability in homes, schools, and worksites.

TERTIARY PREVENTION

- Encourage limitation of activity when air pollution is high.
- Support cleanup of toxic waste sites and removal of other hazards.
- Provide appropriate nursing care at worksite or in the home for persons with chronic lung diseases and injury-related disabilities.
- Refer homeowners to approved lead abatement resources.

As more nurses, particularly those in nursing subspecialties, build their basic assessment and intervention skills in environmental health, our activities will become more sophisticated and targeted. For those nurses interested in joining the growing number of pioneers in environmental health, there are already a great many resources that will prove very useful. The

Appendix to this book offers a selection of organizational and web-based resources.

Several organizations, including nursing organizations, are taking active roles in encouraging expansion of nurses' roles in environmental health. The American Nurses Association has passed several environmental health-related resolutions, including a call for nurses to actively engage in pollution prevention. With Health Care Without Harm, the American College of Nurse Midwives has assisted in the creation of a booklet entitled "Green Birthdays," in which they describe the environmental health risks to pregnant women and newborns in hospitals and birthing facilities. It also guides midwives in the creation of environmentally healthier birthing places. See www.noharm.org for "Green Birthdays". In this way, nurses can provide the necessary leadership to encourage primary prevention of environmentally related illnesses.

There are some natural allies for nurses who are interested in working on the juncture between health and the environment. The environmental movement has spawned a number of excellent organizations, nationally and locally. At the national level, the ones that have some focus on health and environment issues are the Natural Resources Defense Council, the Environmental Defense (formerly the Environmental Defense Fund), Sierra Club, Environmental Working Group, and Clean Water Action. On the state and national levels, the Public Interest Research Groups (PIRGs) have often addressed issues associated with the environment and health. Other, more targetted groups have been described throughout the book.

In terms of occupational health, there are several nongovernmental organizations that provide technical assistance and advocacy. The National Institute of Occupational Safety and Health funds several universities throughout the country as Education Resource Centers. These Centers are often associated with occupational health nursing and occupational medicine training programs. In several states, Committees on Occupational Safety and Health (COSH) provide training and advocacy. The labor movement has wonderful health and safety resources at many of the union's national offices. And the American Association of Occupational Health Nurses is the professional home for nurses.

The Association of Occupational and Environmental Clinics is a national organization with both clinic and individual members. It has an excellent library of educational resources. Its web site describes these resources and its member clinics around the country are home to a wide variety of environmental health specialists.

In recent years, Physicians for Social Responsibility, an international Nobel Peace Prize-winning organization, has expanded its work to encompass environmental health. Its national office in Washington, DC, monitors activities on Capitol Hill that relate to environmental health and provides training and education programs on such issues as drinking water quality and antibiotic use in agriculture. Its web site provides several important full-text works such as *In Harm's Way*, a book on children's health effects associated with persistent pollutants in our environment. (www.igc.org/psr/ihw-report_dwnld.html)

Another ally for nurses interested in environmental health is the community of academics, government employees, and activists who are working on "sustainability," the art and science of living in a manner that is both friendly to the environment and healthy for all. Some of the campaigns that have evolved in the sustainability movement include: Smart Growth, "Reduce, Re-use, and Recycle" activities, Green Buildings, and the Health Care Without Harm campaign. Alliances with the sustainability community will help to build a practical and multi-disciplined approach to creating a positive environmentally-sustainable future.

Finally, many of the faith-based communities have addressed environmental stewardship in the context of religious imperatives. This is a powerful movement to tap for those who are interested in environmental health. The earth's health is seen as inextricably related to our spiritual health and our children's health, and we, as stewards of the earth, have a moral responsibility to care for ourselves, our children and the earth.

As nurses venture deeper into environmental health, they should be heartened by the fact that many of the paths they will go down are already populated with practitioners, educators, and activists from other disciplines who will be very happy to have nurses join their journey. In other instances, nurses may be forging new trails. Taking the lead is also familiar territory to nurses and our environmental health leaders are growing in numbers every year.

APPENDIX

Environmental Health Resources

GENERAL RESOURCES ON ENVIRONMENTAL HEALTH

The Agency for Toxic Substances and Disease Registry (ATSDR)
www.atsdr.cdc.gov

This is an agency of the U.S. Department of Health and Human Services whose mission is to prevent exposure, adverse human health effects, and diminished quality of life associated with exposure to pollutants in the environment. ATSDR's ToxFAQs is a series of summaries about hazardous substances that is being developed by the ATSDR Division of Toxicology and can be found at http://www.atsdr.cdc.gov/toxfaq.html. ATSDR's Hazardous Substance Release/Health Effects Database, HazDat, available at http://www.atsdr.cdc.gov/hazdat.html#A3.1, is a database developed to provide access to information on the release of hazardous substances from Superfund sites or from emergency events.

American Public Health Association (APHA)
http://www.apha.org

This is a multidisciplinary organization of health care professionals working in the public health arena. They can be reached at The American Public Health Association, 800 I. Street, NW, Washington, DC 20001-3710, Telephone: (202) 777-APHA (2742), Fax: (202) 777-2532.

Association of Occupational and Environmental Clinics (AOEC)
http://www.aoec.org

This is a nonprofit organization committed to improving the practice of occupational and environmental health through information sharing and collaborative research. Its web site has educational resources and links to local pediatric environmental health units. They can be reached at 1010 Vermont Ave., NW #513, Washington, DC 20005, Telephone (202) 347-4976, Fax: (202) 347-4950.

Centers for Disease Control (CDC)
http://www.cdc.gov

The CDC develops and applies disease prevention and control, environmental health, and health promotion and education activities in the United States.

National Center for Environmental Health (NCEH) is part of the CDC (http://www.cdc.gov/nceh/default.htm). The NCEH web site offers fact sheets, brochures, books, a searchable index of Morbidity and Mortality Weekly Reports (MMWR), and articles and publications by NCEH authors on different environmental health topics. Their mailing address is Centers for Disease Control and Prevention, National Center for Environmental Health, Mail Stop F-29, 4770 Buford Highway, N.E., Atlanta, GA 30341-3724.

Environmental Hazards Epidemiology Response Program: The Health Studies Branch (HSB) of CDC's National Center for Environmental Health is responsible for investigating the human health effects associated with exposure to environmental hazards and to natural and technological disasters. (http://www.cdc.gov/nceh/emergency/factsheets/envhaz1.htm)

Environmental Health Listserv is an easy way to communicate among Environmental Health Professionals. (http://www.cdc.gov/nceh/ehserv/ephs/factsheets/listserv.htm).

Center for Health, Environment and Justice (CHEJ)
http://www.chej.org

CHEJ promotes citizens' rights to environmental justice, the principle that people have the right to a clean and healthy environment regardless of their race or economic standing. This site provides assistance with organizing and an on-line bookstore with pertinent data and information about national campaigns. Phone: (703) 237-2249, Fax: (703) 237-8389, Email: info@chej.org, 150 South Washington Street, Suite 300, P.O. Box 6806, Falls Church, VA 22040.

Consumer Product Safety Commission (CPSC)
http://www.cpsc.gov

This is an independent federal regulatory agency that was created in 1972 to protect the public against unreasonable risks of injuries and deaths associated with consumer products. To report an unsafe consumer product or to inquire about a product, call the CPSC toll-free hotline at (800) 638-2772 or (800) 638-8270 for the hearing and speech impaired. To request a free copy of publication listings, write to U.S. Consumer Product Safety Commission, Washington, DC 20207.

Environmental Health Coalition (EHC)
http://www.environmentalhealth.org
EHC is one of the oldest grass-roots organizations in the United States, using social change strategies to achieve environmental justice. Their mailing address is EHC, 1717 Kettner Blvd., Suite 100, San Diego, CA 92101, Phone: (619) 235-0281.

Environmental Protection Agency (EPA)
http://www.epa.gov
This is the U.S. government agency that handles environmental problems and issues. It has an extensive site on a wide variety of environment-related topics.

The Toxics Release Inventory (TRI), published by the U.S. EPA, is a valuable source of information on toxic chemicals that are being used, manufactured, treated, transported, or released into the environment (http://www.epa.gov/tri/tri97/index.htm).

EPA's Integrated Risk Information System (IRIS) is an electronic database maintained by the EPA on human health effects that may result from exposure to various chemicals in the environment (http://www.epa.gov/ncea/iris.htm).

Food and Drug Administration (FDA)
http://www.fda.gov
The U.S. FDA's web site regulates the safety of food and drugs in the United States. Its web site has information on publications, manuals, references and industry guidance. They can also be reached at U. S. Food and Drug Administration 5600 Fishers Lane, Rockville MD 20857-0001, Phone: 1-888-INFO-FDA (1-888-463-6332).

Johns Hopkins University, Pew Environmental Health Commission
http://pewenvirohealth.jhsph.edu
The mission of this group is to strengthen the country's public health response to environmental health threats. Reports available include "Asthma Report," "Healthy From the Start: Why America Needs a Better System to Track and Understand Birth Defects and the Environment" and "Why the Country Needs a Nationwide Health Tracking Network."

MapCruzin
http://www.mapcruzin.com/index.html

This site provides census data and maps, sources of free data on the internet, environmental justice resources, conferences information, and more.

National Association of County & City Health Officials (NACCHO)
http://www.naccho.org

NACCHO is a nonprofit membership organization serving all of the nearly 3,000 local health departments nationwide, in cities, counties, townships, and districts. NACCHO provides education, information, research, and technical assistance to local health departments and facilitates partnerships among local, state, and federal agencies in order to promote and strengthen public health. Their web site has a many EH-related topics.

National Institute of Environmental Health Sciences (NIEHS)
http://www.niehs.nih.gov

NIEHS is one of the National Institutes of Health. It conducts basic research on environmental health. This web site contains fact sheets and pamphlets on environmental health topics. It also includes a link to copies of *Environmental Health Perspectives*, a journal that reports extensively on matters related to environmental health issues.

National Institute for Occupational Safety and Health (NIOSH)
www.cdc.gov/niosh/homepage.html

NIOSH is part of the CDC. It is the federal agency responsible for conducting research and making recommendations for the prevention of work-related disease and injury. Telephone: 1-800-35-NIOSH (1-800-356-4674).

Occupational Safety and Health Administration (OSHA)
http://www.osha.gov

OSHA's mission is to prevent work-related injuries, illnesses, and deaths. OSHA and its state partners have approximately 2,100 inspectors, plus complaint discrimination investigators, engineers, physicians, educators, standards writers, and other technical and support personnel spread over more than 200 offices throughout the country. This staff establishes protective standards, enforces those standards, and reaches out to employers and employees through technical assistance and consultation programs. Contact information: U.S. Department of Labor Occupational Safety & Health Administration, Office of Public Affairs—Room N3647, 200 Constitution Avenue, Washington, DC 20210, Telephone: (202) 693-1999.

Rachel's Environment & Health Weekly
http://www.monitor.net/rachel/rehw-home.html.
Providing news and resources for environmental justice, the site provides access to back issues and offers on-line subscription to the weekly. Their address is Environmental Research Foundation, P.O. Box 5036, Annapolis, MD 21403-7036.

HEALTH CARE AND THE ENVIRONMENT

American Nurses Association (ANA)
http://www.nursingworld.org
At ANA's Occupational Safety and Health homepage (http://www.nursingworld.org/dlwa/osh/) there is information on safety and health including position statements, collaborations with other organizations, brochures, and other literature. Topics include latex allergy, needlestick injury, ergonomics, and pollution prevention in health care. They can be reached at 600 Maryland Avenue, SW, Suite 100 West, Washington, DC 20024, Telephone: (202) 651-7000, 202/651-7001, Fax: (1-800) 274-4ANA (4262).

ANA House of Delegates Resolution: Reduction of Health Care Production of Toxic Pollution (http://www.nursingworld.org/dlwa/osh/hodpoll.htm).

Becoming a Mercury-Free Facility: A Priority to be Achieved by the Year 2000
American Society for Healthcare Environmental Services, 1997. Catalog #197103. Contact: American Hospital Association, Telephone: (800) AHA-2626.

Consortium for Environmental Education in Medicine (CEEM)
www.ceem.org
CEEM strives to bring environment and health perspectives into medical education. This web site has information on workshops and a variety of resources and tools that support the incorporation of environment and health perspectives into curricula and programs.

99 Chauncy Street, Sixth Floor, Boston, MA 02111-1703, Telephone: (617) 292-7771, Fax: (617) 292-0150, Email: ceem@secondnature.org.

EnviRN
http://www.envirn.umaryland.edu
EnviR.N. is dedicated to supporting nursing professionals seeking information on environmental health and nursing.

EPA Fact Sheet: Mercury in Medical Facilities
http://www.epa.gov/seahome/mercury/src/title.htm

FDA Medical Bulletin: Natural Rubber Latex Allergy
http://www.fda.gov/medbull/natural.html

Health Care Without Harm (HCWH)
http://www.noharm.org

HCWH is an international coalition of more than 270 organizations in 17 countries dedicated to eliminating environmental pollution from health care. Their web site has information regarding the environmental impact health care practices have on the environment and actions to address the problem. For more information about the Health Care Without Harm Boston Project, contact Bill Ravanesi at (617) 244-2891 or ravanesi@mediaone.net, or the national office at the Health Care Without Harm web site.

The National Environmental Education & Training Foundation (NEETF)
http://www.neetf.org

NEETF educates health care professionals about how the environment affects human health. It includes information about grants and the Nursing & Environmental Health Initiative. It can be reached at Foundation, 1707 H Street, NW, Suite 900, Washington, DC, 20006, Telephone: (202) 833-2933, Fax: (202) 261-6464.

National Library of Medicine (NLM)

NLM produces *MEDLINEplus* (http://www.nlm.nih.gov/medlineplus), which provides access to extensive information about specific diseases and conditions to both health professionals and consumers. There are web pages on environmental health and related topics such as air pollution, pesticides, and asthma.

Toxnet website from NLM (http://toxnet.nlm.nih.gov) is a cluster of databases on toxicology, hazardous chemicals, and related areas.

Nightingale Institute for Health and the Environment (NIHE)
http://www.nihe.org

NIHE assists health care professionals to recognize the link between human and environmental health and their role in creating change in the practices of health care systems so they have less environmental impact. They have a number of publications on topics such as dioxin, hospital waste reduction planning and implementation, and reducing mercury use in hospitals.

OSHA Technical Information Bulletin—*Potential for Allergy to Natural Rubber Latex Gloves and Other Natural Rubber Products.*
http://www.osha-slc.gov/html/hotfoias/tib/TIB19990412.html

Physicians for Social Responsibility (PSR)
http://www.psr.org
The Environment and Health section of this web site features fact sheets and news updates on persistent organic pollutants, drinking water, children's health and other environmental health-related topics. Physicians for Social Responsibility, 1101 14th Street N.W., Suite 700, Washington, DC 20005, Telephone: (202) 898-0150, Fax: (202) 898-0172, Email: psrnatl@psr.org

In Harm's Way: Toxic Threats to Child Development: A report by Greater Boston Physicians for Social Responsibility. Available on-line and downloadable in PDF format at the GBPSR web site (http://www.igc.org/psr).

Preventable Poisons: A Prescription for Reducing Medical Waste in Massachusetts, a report by Greater Boston Physicians for Social Responsibility and the Toxics Action Center) by Ted Schettler and Erick Weltman. (http://www.nihe.org/prevntpoisons.html).

Preventing Allergic Reactions to Natural Rubber Latex in the Workplace
http://www.cdc.gov/niosh/latexalt.html

Sustainable Hospitals
http://www.sustainablehospitals.org
This site has a number of reports on topics such as strategies for reduction of mercury, PVC, and latex use in hospitals, including specific product recommendations. The reports include *10 Actions to Promote Environmentally Preferable Purchasing (EPP) (Fact Sheet)* (http://www.sustainablehospitals.org/HTMLSrc/TenEPP.html).

FILMS

The Health Care Industry's Impact on the Environment: Strategies for Global Change (Originally aired as an interactive teleconference.)
Pub: University of Vermont, 1998.
First Do No Harm: Polyvinyl Chloride and Medicine's Responsibility
Our Waste, Our Responsibility, Moving Toward a Pollution Prevention Approach in the Healthcare Industry, Pub: University of Vermont.
No Time to Waste: Resource Conservation for Hospitals
by Ben Achtenberg and Ann Carol Grossman
Pub: Fanlight Productions
http://www.fanlight.com/catalog/films/156_nttw.htm

MAJOR ENVIRONMENTAL GROUPS

Audubon Society
Founded in 1905, this major conservatory organization focuses on birds and other wildlife.
http://www.audubon.org/

Environmental Defense
http://www.environmentaldefense.org
Environmental Defense is a national nonprofit organization that links science, economics and law to create innovative equitable solutions to environmental problems. This site has information on publications, action steps, and a link to Scorecard (http://www.scorecard.org), an information service on local environmental conditions listed by zip code. Environmental Defense Membership (1-800) 684-3322.

The Environmental Working Group
http://www.ewg.org
1718 Connecticut Ave., N.W., Suite 600, Washington, DC 20009
Telephone: (202) 667-6982, Fax: (202) 232-2592.
The Environmental Working Group (EWG) is a leading content provider for public interest groups and concerned citizens who are campaigning to protect the environment.

GreenAction
http://www.greenaction.org
An organization working for health and environmental justice.

Greenpeace
http://www.greenpeace.org
An international conservation society. It can also be contacted at 702 H Street N.W., Washington, DC 20001, Telephone: (1-800) 326-0959.

Natural Resources Defense Council (NRDC)
http://www.nrdc.org
NRDC uses law, science, and the support of more than 400,000 members nationwide to protect the planet's wildlife and wild places and to ensure a safe and healthy environment. Its web site has information on various environmental issues and provides links to related web sites. Natural Resources Defense Council, 40 West 20th Street, New York, NY 10011, Telephone: (212) 727-2700, Fax: (212) 727-1773.

The Nature Conservancy
http://nature.org
The Nature Conservancy practices conservation science to protect natural habitats. For more information it can be contacted at International Headquarters, The Nature Conservancy, 4245 North Fairfax Drive, Suite 100, Arlington, VA 22203-1606, Telephone: (1-800) 628-6860.

Sierra Club
http://www.sierraclub.org
The web site has information on a wide variety of environment-related topics. They can also be reached at Sierra Club, 85 Second St., Second Floor, San Francisco, CA 94105-3441. Telephone: (415) 977-5500.

World Wildlife Fund (WWF)
http://www.worldwildlife.org
WWF is dedicated to protecting the world's wildlife and wildlands.

SPECIALIZED RESOURCES

AIR QUALITY

California Indoor Air Quality Program Infosheets and Related Links
http://www.cal-iaq.org/iaqsheet.htm
This web site provides web addresses of other sites that deal with the topics of mold, ozone, air cleaners, healthy schools, asbestos, radon, VOCs, and sites that give guidance for hiring IAQ consultants.

EPA Office of Indoor Air Quality
http://www.epa.gov/iaq
Indoor Air Pollution: An Introduction for Health Professionals.
http://www.epa.gov/iaq/pubs/hpguide.html
Secondhand Smoke
http://www.epa.gov/iaq/ets

NACCHO (1996) Indoor Air Quality Desk Reference
This reference put out by NACCHO and the EPA enables local health departments to adequately respond to indoor air quality (IAQ) problems that arise in their communities. Copies may be obtained from NACCHO for $20 by writing or calling the National Association of County and City Health Officials, 440 First Street, N.W., Washington, DC 20001, Telephone: (202) 783-5550, Fax: (202) 783-1583. It can also be ordered from their web site bookstore (www.naccho.org/index.cfm).

ALLERGIES AND ASTHMA

American Lung Association (ALA)
http://www.lungusa.org
The ALA web site offers information about lung diseases including asthma, lung cancer, and COPD. You can call your local Lung Association at (1-800) LUNG-USA (1-800-586-4872).

Asthma and Allergy Foundation of America, (AAFA)
http://www.aafa.org
The AAFA site provides educational materials and programs for health care professionals to use with a variety of audiences. They can be contacted at (1-800) 7-ASTHMA (1-800-727-8462).

CDC Fact Sheets
Molds in the Environment
http:///www.cdc.gov/nceh/asthma/factsheets/molds/moldfacts.htm
Questions and Answers on Stachybotrys chartarum and other molds
http://www.cdc.gov/nceh/asthma/factsheets/molds/default.htm

EPA Fact Sheets
Mold
http://www.epa.gov/iaq/pubs/moldresources.html#
Cockroach and Pest Allergens
http://www.epa.gov/iaq/asthma/triggers/pests.html
Dust Mites
http://www.epa.gov/iaq/asthma/triggers/mites.html#Links
House Dust
http://www.epa.gov/iaq/asthma/triggers/dust.html

CHILDREN AND SCHOOLS

Children's Environmental Health Network (CEHN)
http://www.cehn.org
Provides information on the organization's activities to promote a healthy environment for the fetus and child with consideration of the special vulnerabilities of children to environmental health hazards, as well as many links to other organizations that support that mission. Their *Resource Guide on Children's Environmental Health*, available on-line, is a collection of profiles of many organizations and projects. Also available at the site is the *Training Manual on Pediatric Environmental Health: Putting it into Practice*, which contains guidelines and teaching tools that health care fac-

ulty can use to teach pediatric environmental health. Contact information for CEHN is 110 Maryland Avenue N.E., Suite 511, Washington, DC 20002, Telephone: (202) 543-4033.

Children's Health Environmental Coalition Network (CHEC)
http://www.checnet.org
CHEC is a charitable, nonprofit organization dedicated to educating the public, specifically parents and caregivers, about environmental toxins that affect children's health. The site provides information about toxins in the home. They have compiled a number of studies that make the link between childhood cancer environmental toxins.

EPA Office of Children's Health Protection
http://www.epa.gov/children

EPA IAQ Tools for Schools
http://www.epa.gov/iaq/schools/tools4s2.html.
Tools for Schools is a program to address environmental conditions in schools and includes. There are informative fact sheets on indoor air quality in schools and asthma triggers such as radon, dust mites, mold, and cockroach and pest allergens.

EPA Region 7:A Case Study of Environmental, Health and Safety Issues Involving the Burlington, Massachusetts Public School System.
http://www.epa.gov/region07/kids/dresser.htm
Tips, suggestions, and resources for investigating and resolving environmental health issues in schools. Prepared by Todd H. Dresser, Environmental Engineer, Burlington Board of Health, 29 Center St., Burlington, MA 01803. Telephone: (781) 270-1956.

Handbook of Pediatric Environmental Health (book)
American Academy of Pediatrics (AAP).
A guide to the identification, prevention, and treatment of pediatric environmental health problems. Available from the AAP bookstore at: http://www.aap.org/pubserv/.

Healthy Schools Network
http://www.healthyschools.org
Advocates for the protection of children's environmental health in schools. Web site offers fact sheets and information packets (usually $3 each)

designed by and for parents with professional and technical reviewers to help parents and others resolve school environmental problems, or to help schools adopt environmentally healthier practices.

The Indiana Department of Environmental Management (IDEM)
http://www.state.in.us/idem/kids

IDEM has several resources available on children's environmental health in schools. Resources include "A Self-Assessment for Child Care Facilities," designed by IDEM to help identify potential environmental, health and safety threats in childcare facilities (http://www.state.in.us/idem/kids/5star/selfassessment.pdf).

Also available is "Protecting Children From Environmental Threats: Guidance for Indiana's Child Care Facilities." This document gives explanations and demonstrations of the environmental, health, and safety rules with which child care facilities must comply. While it is specific to Indiana it also gives guidance on how to "go beyond the rules to be an environmental steward in your community." Also from IDEM: "Simple Steps to Help Make Our Environment a Safer Place."

The Integrated Pest Management in Schools List Server

This list is open for membership to any person interested in integrated pest management (IPM) in schools and who wishes to discuss the subject with others on the list. It will also be used to inform subscribers of additions and updates to the School IPM web site that the University of Florida Entomology and Nematology Department is developing with an EPA Region 4 grant. You subscribe or unsubscribe to this mailing list by sending email to mailto:listserv@lists.ufl.

Minnesota Department of Health
http://www.health.state.mn.us

This web site has a page on Children's Environmental Health (CEH) with information on lead poisoning and lead in school drinking water, pesticide use in schools with model pesticide notices for schools, and children's health risks from chemical exposures with fact sheets on chemicals and a great deal more information on CEH.

Minnesota School District 742 Case Study
http://www.facilitiesnet.com/fn/NS/NS3a0ea.html

This case study gives an outline of how one school district addressed its IAQ problem by forming a planning committee that agreed on a vision and six goals for an IAQ plan for their district.

National PTA's Environmental Action & Awareness Program
http://www.pta.org/programs
The Environmental Resource Library provides an assortment of resources focusing on a healthy environment at home, at school, and in the community.

New York Healthy Schools Network
http://www.cehn.org/cehn/resourceguide/nyhsn.html
The New York Healthy Schools Network is a statewide coalition of parent, environment, health, and education organizations working to assure every child and school employee an environmentally healthy school that is clean and in good repair, through shared advocacy, information, and referral.

Pest Control in the School: Adopting Integrated Pest Management.
This booklet can be obtained at no cost by contacting the following address and referencing the booklet code (EPA 735-F-93-012) from EPA Public Information Center, 401 M Street, S.W. Washington, DC 20460.

Washington State Dept. of Health (1995), School Indoor Air Quality Best Management Practices Manual
http://www.doh.wa.gov/ehp/ts/iaq.pdf
Sections in this 175-page manual include the following topics: "Why Manage School Indoor Air Quality?" "Factors Influencing Indoor Air Quality," "Basic Strategies for Good Indoor Air Quality," and several others.

FOOD SAFETY

Alliance for the Prudent Use of Antibiotics (APUA)
www.healthsci.tufts.edu/apua/apua/html
75 Kneeland Street, Boston, MA 02111-1901. A nonprofit organization "dedicated to preserving the power of antibiotics," through advocating their appropriate use.

The Fight Bac! Campaign
www.fightbac.org
This site was developed by the Partnership for Food Safety Education. Founded in 1997, PFSE is a private-public coalition developed to educate the public about safe food handling and avoiding foodborne illnesses.

Institute for Agriculture and Trade Policy
www.iatp.org
2105 1st Avenue South, Minneapolis, MN 55404, Telephone: (612) 870-3418. Founded in 1986, this nonprofit organization's mission is "to create

environmentally and economically sustainable communities and regions through sound agriculture and trade policy."

HOMES

EPA's Asbestos Home Page
http://www.epa.gov/oppt/asbestos

EPA's What you can do around the home.
http://www.epa.gov/children/ucando/ucd_home.htm
Information on composting, gardens, garage, IPM.

Farm*A*Syst/Home*A*Syst
http://www.uwex.edu/farmasyst
Farm*A*Syst is a partnership between government agencies and private business that enables you to prevent pollution on farms, ranches, and in homes, using confidential environmental assessments. Some of the issues that Farm*A*Syst can help you address include quality of well water, livestock waste storage, storage and handling of petroleum products, managing hazardous wastes, and nutrient management. They are also available at Farm*A*Syst, 303 Hiram Smith Hall, 1545 Observatory Drive, Madison, W.I., 53706-1289, Telephone: (608) 262-0024.

LEAD

CDC Lead Information
Screening Young Children for Lead Poisoning: Guidance for State and Local Public Health Officials, November 1997. To obtain a printed copy of this guidance document, call toll-free (1-888) 232-6789.
(http://www.cdc.gov/nceh/lead/guide/guide97.htm)
   CDC Childhood Lead Poisoning Prevention Program
   (http://www.cdc.gov/nceh/lead/lead.htm)
   What Every Parent Should Know About Lead Poisoning in Children
   (http://www.cdc.gov/nceh/lead/faq/cdc97a.htm)
   The Childhood Lead Poisoning Surveillance: State Reports and Publications Resource Guide
   http://www.cdc.gov/nceh/lead/surv/states/states.htm

The National Center for Lead-Safe Housing (NCLSH)
www.leadsafehousing.org/NCLSH
NCLSH was founded in 1992 to bring the housing, environmental, and public health communities together to combat childhood lead poisoning.

The site provides information on scientific research, technical assistance and training rules, regulations and policies, and immediate strategies to reduce childhood lead poisoning in high-risk communities. They can be reached at The National Center for Lead-Safe Housing, 10227 Wincopin Circle, Suite 205, Columbia, MD 21044, Telephone: (410) 992-0712, Fax: (410) 715-2310.

The National Lead Information Center (NLIC)
http://www.epa.gov/lead/nlic.htm
(1-800) 424-LEAD (5323). The National Lead Information Center (NLIC) provides the general public and professionals with information about lead hazards and their prevention.

Protect Your Family From Lead In Your Home
http://www.hud.gov/lea/leadhelp.html

State Reports and Publications Resource Guide
http://www.cste.org
This collection of state surveillance documents, prepared by the Council of State and Territorial Epidemiologists, serves as a reference for childhood lead poisoning prevention and surveillance programs in state health departments and facilitates sharing among states on the different ways surveillance data are being used.

STELLAR
http://www.cdc.gov/nceh/lead/surv/stellar/stellar.htm
STELLAR is a software application provided free of charge to state and local Childhood Lead Poisoning Prevention Programs (CLPPPs), allowing a practical means of tracking medical and environmental activities in lead poisoning cases.

MERCURY

Case Against Mercury: Rx for Pollution Prevention
This is a 10-page multicolor brochure that describes mercury's health effects and its sources in health care. It covers safe handling techniques for spills, housekeeping suggestions, and pollution prevention tips. Telephone: (202) 833-8317.

Vermont Agency of Natural Resources
http://www.anr.state.vt.us/dec/ead/mercury/SchoolCleanout/invabcs.htm
Mercury Education & Reduction Campaign, includes school cleanout information.
    See also the Health Care and the Environment Section.

PESTICIDES

Beyond Pesticides/National Coalition Against the Misuse of Pesticides (NCAMP)
http://www.beyondpesticides.org/index.html
NCAMP is a nonprofit organization that provides the public with useful information on pesticides and alternatives to their use. They can be reached at 701 E Street S.E. #200, Washington, DC 20003, Telephone: (202) 543-5450, Fax: (202) 543-4791, Email: info@beyondpesticides.org.

EPA Office of Pesticide Programs
http://www.epa.gov/pesticides
Telephone: (703) 305-7090.

Extension Toxicology Network (EXTOXNET)
http://ace.ace.orst.edu/info/extoxnet
Provides science-based information about pesticides to health care providers treating pesticide-related health concerns.

National Pesticide Telecommunications Network (NPTN)
http://ace.orst.edu/info/nptn/
Source of a wide variety of objective science-based pesticide information based at Oregon State. Subjects include pesticide products, recognition and management of pesticide poisoning, toxicology, and environmental chemistry. Telephone: (1-800) 858-7378, Email: nptn@ace.orst.edu.

New York Coalition for Alternatives to Pesticides
http://www.crisny.org/not-for-profit/nycap
Information about Integrated Pest Management (IPM), tips on helping schools eliminate pesticides.

Pesticide Action Network of North America (PANNA)
http://www.igc.org/panna/about/about.html
PANNA is a campaign to replace pesticides with ecologically sound alternatives.

Pesticide Watch
http://www.pesticidewatch.org
PW is a California-based organization. Its web site provides information about pesticides and the problems associated with pesticide use. Some useful tools regarding pesticide use in schools are included.

WATER

Bottled Water/Home Water Filter Information
http://www.druc.org
Provides information on bottled water.

Clean Water Action
http://www/cleanwateraction.org
Clean Water Action is a national citizen's organization working for clean, safe, and affordable water, prevention of health-threatening pollution, creation of environmentally safe jobs and businesses, and empowerment of people to make democracy work. Telephone: (1-202) 895-0420.

The Clean Water Action Plan
http://www.cleanwater.gov
The key actions described in this Action Plan focus on achieving cleaner water by strengthening public health protections, targeting watershed protection efforts at high priority areas, and providing communities with new resources to control polluted runoff and enhance natural resource stewardship.

EPA Information on Water
Safe Water Web site **(http:www.epa.gov/safewater)**
"Surf Your Watershed" Database (http://www.epa.gov/surf)
Information on private wells (http://www.epa.gov/safewater/pwells1.html).

Healthy Drinking Water
http://www.healthywater.com
Learn about your drinking water, bottled water, water filters, chlorination, fluoridation, reverse osmosis, distillers, and more. Understand the relationship of drinking water to heart disease and cancer.

Newsletter of the Healthy Water Association
http://www.execpc.com/~cc/hwanews.html
The purpose of the Healthy Water Association is to identify and promote those waters that are most healthful and beneficial to consumers.

Safe Drinking Water Hotline (1-800) 426-4791.

WASTE MANAGEMENT

Alameda County Waste Management Authority and Source Reduction and Recycling Board
http://www.stopwaste.org
This is an agency that promotes source reduction and recycling. It has tools applicable nationally.

California's Integrated Waste Management Board
http://www.ciwmb.ca.gov
This web page offers hyperlinks to the state's waste reduction programs that aim to divert 50% of waste from landfills.

The Recycled Paper Coalition
http://www.papercoalition.org
The Recycled Paper Coalition strives to conserve natural resources and reduce waste by purchasing environmentally preferred paper products and by using paper more efficiently.

Index

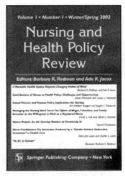

Springer Publishing Company

Hispanic Health Care International

Journal of The National Association of Hispanic Nurses

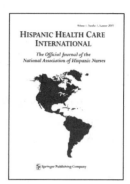

Nilda Peragallo, RN, DrPH, FAAN
and **Sara Torres,** RN, PhD, FAAN, Editors-in-Chief

Clare Hastings, PhD, RN, **Maria R. Warda,** PhD, RN,
Mary Lou De Leon Siantz, PhD, RN, FAAN
Ildaura Murillo-Rhode, PhD, Med, RN, CS, FAAN,
and **Joyce J. Fitzpatrick,** PhD, MBA, RN, FAAN, Associate Editors

This new peer-reviewed journal will serve as an interdisciplinary forum for the dissemination of information for clinical practice, education, research and policy on issues concerning Hispanic/Latino populations in the United States and Latin America. A unique feature will be the availability of all abstracts in both English and Spanish. The interdisciplinary editorial board is comprised of experts in a variety of clinical, policy and research areas. This is the official journal of the *National Association of Hispanic Nurses* which serves as an interdisciplinary state of the art resource for educators, researchers, administrators, policy makers and health care providers on Hispanic/Latino health care.

Partial Contents:

• Editorial, *I. Murillo-Rohde*

• Use of Visual Analog Scales With Spanish Speaking Individuals, *J.W. Lange*

• Latina's Perspective on HIV/AIDS: Cultural Issues to Consider in Prevention, *N. Peragallo, et al.*

• Sexual Behavior of Latino Pre-Adolescents and Adolescents: The Relationship of Acculturation and Generational History, *A.M. Villarruel, C. Lanfield, and C.P. Porter*

• Income Inequality and Population Health in Latin America and the Carribbean

Volume 1, 2002 • ISSN 1540-4153

---

536 Broadway, New York, NY 10012 • Telephone: 212-431-4370
Fax: 212-941-7842 • Order Toll-Free: 877-687-7476
Order On-line: www.springerpub.com